THE WORLD HEALTH ORGANIZATION BETWEEN NORTH AND SOUTH

The World Health Organization between North and South

Nitsan Chorev

CORNELL UNIVERSITY PRESS, ITHACA AND LONDON

First published 2012 by Cornell University Press
Printed in the United States of America

Library of Congress Cataloging-in-Publication Data

Chorev, Nitsan.
   The World Health Organization between north and south / Nitsan Chorev.
     p. cm.
   Includes bibliographical references and index.
   ISBN 978-0-8014-5065-5 (cloth : alk. paper)
   1. World Health Organization.   2. World health.   3. Public health—
International cooperation.   I. Title.
   RA8.A4C46 2012
   362.1—dc23   2011042191

Cloth printing   10   9   8   7   6   5   4   3   2   1

Contents

Preface

International organizations have been a prominent feature of the post–World War II order and have become even more central in the current global era. In the last half-century, the number of international organizations has proliferated, and their roles have expanded substantially as they have acquired broader powers and responsibilities. Using their normative and legal authority, international organizations have had a substantive impact on the dissemination of ideas and practices worldwide. International financial institutions have been particularly noted for their influence, but other intergovernmental organizations, including the World Health Organization (WHO), which is the subject of this book, have similarly shaped the views and decisions of governments.

The WHO is the United Nations (UN) agency responsible for global health policies and programs. Countries are interdependent in controlling diseases, as clearly illustrated by HIV/AIDS and the recent cases of SARS and avian flu, so WHO member states should be and have normally been deeply invested in the successful functioning of that organization. Developing countries in particular have welcomed international cooperation, because the delivery of public health services may require heavy reliance on advanced science and complex technology. The influence of the WHO on national health policies, especially in poor countries, has been apparent: WHO technical and operational assistance has affected which populations are provided with care, what types of treatments are recommended, and other similarly fundamental decisions that have had substantial impact on the health conditions of a large number of people in need.

Mainstream theories of international relations offer potentially conflicting views as to how these evidently consequential global health policies are formed. We know that member states have great, and greatly uneven, influence over the decision-making process in international negotiations. We also know, however, that international organizations are not simple arenas. International bureaucracies, such as the WHO secretariat, have their own interests and potential capacity to act on those interests. But how can international bureaucracies act on their independent interests if these clash with the preferences of their member states? How do international bureaucracies respond to external demands that may not be compatible with their own perceptions and goals? This inquiry motivates this book.

To answer this question I look at two particularly contentious periods in the history of the WHO and other UN agencies: the period from the early 1970s till the early 1980s in which the WHO bureaucracy had to respond to developing countries' call for a New International Economic Order; and the period from the late 1990s to the 2000s, in which the WHO bureaucracy, following a decade-long crisis, began to respond to the neoliberal expectations of developed countries. In both phases, the WHO staff and leadership have played a surprisingly influential role. Member states have certainly imposed their demands on the organization, but the WHO secretariat was able to reframe the content of these demands to fit its own institutional culture. The book identifies the adaptive strategies available to international bureaucracies that enable them to respond to external demands in a way that satisfies the member states making those demands while protecting the organization's material interests and core principles.

Studying the turbulent history of an international organization as complex as the WHO is a daunting task. If I have been able to meet the challenge of writing this book, it is due to the invaluable help of many individuals. I first thank the many WHO insiders and other participants in the global health field who took the time to patiently answer my detailed questions about their work. Their intimate knowledge of global health issues is manifested in the many quotations and references throughout the book. Their insightful comments were essential not only for my analysis of specific events but also for my ability to capture what I concluded was the nature of international health politics. For earlier parts of the history of the WHO I relied heavily on archival materials in numerous libraries and archives. Of the many helpful archivists and librarians, I thank in particular Marie Villemin, of the WHO library in Geneva, who helped me find, in a somewhat disordered archive, the many materials I was looking for. Research assistants were helpful in gathering and ordering the materials, including Roxanne Carter, A. Graham Cumberbatch, Lorraine Fryer, Daniel Kleinman, Osarenoma Okunbor, and Kimberly Stickels at Brown University, and Marissa Brescia and Sarath Ganji at the Woodrow Wilson International Center for Scholars. Most of the transcriptions of the interviews were done by the very competent Kathleen E. Wood. Special thanks also to two patient editors, Kelley Smith and Eoin Ryan. My research for this book received support from several institutions, including research and writing fellowships from the International Institute at the University of California-Los Angeles and from the Woodrow Wilson International Center for Scholars, and from my home institution, Brown University.

Once parts of the manuscript were done, I benefited greatly from the opportunity to present it in conferences, seminars, and meetings, including those held by the Department of Sociology at Boston University, the Department of Sociology at the University of Connecticut, the Center for European Studies at Harvard

University, the Department of Sociology at the University of California-Berkeley, the Graduate Center of the City University of New York, the Social Science Research Council, and the Department of Sociology and Anthropology at Central European University. The experience of collective thinking never ceases to amaze me. Both the narrative of this book and its sociological argument emerged much improved as an outcome of these events.

The greatest debt I owe to the many colleagues and dear friends for their constant support and critical guidance. Most of all, I thank Greta Krippner and Andrew Schrank, who read the entire manuscript and provided invaluable suggestions. Many others were incredibly helpful in forcing me to think more clearly about the project and giving me useful advice. In particular, I would like to thank Peter Andreas, Sarah Babb, Emily Barman, Tim Bartley, Patrick Heller, Jim Jasper, and Victoria Johnson. Many thanks also to Ebony Bridwell-Mitchell, Jose Itzigsohn, Cynthia Hooper, Margot Jackson, Gail Kligman, Ahmed Abdel Latif, Nancy Luke, David Miller, Leo Rotman, and Samer Shehata. I owe special thanks to Roger Haydon, at Cornell University Press, for his enthusiastic support and incredible responsiveness. I also very much appreciated the helpful comments of two reviewers. I could not have hoped for a more constructive, helpful, and enjoyable process.

I dedicate this book to my family. Their continued support means so much to me.

THE WORLD HEALTH ORGANIZATION BETWEEN NORTH AND SOUTH

THE WORLD HEALTH ORGANIZATION

In his address before state delegates at the World Health Assembly, on May 15, 1975, the director-general of the World Health Organization (WHO), Dr. Half-dan T. Mahler, spoke of the "changes that are rapidly taking place in the political and economic relationships between Member States." He boldly predicted that "1974 will be remembered by many of us, and possibly by future historians, as a turning point in our thinking about the future social and economic development of mankind."[1] In 1974, the United Nations (UN) General Assembly had passed a resolution calling for a New International Economic Order (NIEO), which was indeed a turning point in the relations between developing and developed countries. It was also a decisive moment for the WHO, which saw in the following years a radical transformation in its priorities, policies, and programs. In a later speech, Mahler insisted that in making these changes, the WHO was "merely respond[ing] to the imperatives of contemporary history."[2]

Mahler's statements echo a familiar sentiment in the scholarly literature—that international organizations are nothing more than carriers for the wishes of their member states. But Mahler's remarks were disingenuous, for he knew well that the WHO was not simply mirroring external imperatives. Rather, the

---

1. "WHO's Mission Revisited," Address by Dr. H. Mahler, Director-General of the WHO, in Presenting his Report for 1974 to the Twenty-Eighth World Health Assembly, 15 May 1975. WHO Library.
2. "The Political Struggle for Health," Address by Dr. H. Mahler, Director-General of the WHO at the Twenty-Ninth Session of the Regional Committee for the Western Pacific, Manila, 21 August 1978. WHO Library.

WHO leadership and staff were able to advocate a global health agenda that, while acceptable to developing countries, also reflected the WHO's own principles and interests. In this book I argue that international bureaucracies, including at the WHO, have the capacity to restructure global ideational regimes that member states impose on them, and that they restructure these regimes to fit their own institutional cultures.

Through coercion or learning, some elements of external regimes such as the NIEO are successfully transmitted, but others are transformed, with the result that the policies of international organizations are only selectively aligned with member states' demands. Policies and priorities at the WHO during the 1970s only partly corresponded to the call for a New International Economic Order. Similarly, in the 1990s, the WHO's policies did not fully reflect the dominant neoliberal logic. The experience of the WHO was hardly unique: policies and programs in other international organizations, such as the International Labor Organization and the UN Children's Fund, have also often significantly deviated from the principles defining the dominant logic in accordance with the organizations' own agenda. My purpose is to identify and explain the capacity of such international bureaucracies to protect their interests in the face of external demands.

The WHO in Comparative-Historical Perspective

The WHO was established in 1948 as a specialized agency of the United Nations responsible for directing and coordinating authority for international public health. As the designated agency on worldwide health matters, the WHO was tasked with setting norms and standards, articulating policy options, providing technical support to countries, monitoring and assessing health trends, and shaping the global health research agenda.[3] The overall objective of the organization, as defined in the founding constitution, was particularly ambitious: "The attainment by all peoples of the highest possible level of health" (WHO 1958: annex 1). This wording established two commitments at the heart of the organization's mission: the notion that universal access to health services is its principal objective, but that it is simultaneously concerned with the quality of those health services. The constitution, which was adopted by the fifty-one member states participating in the International Health Conference in July 1946 (WHO 1958: 38–45), also offered a progressive definition of health as "a state of complete

---

3. See http://www.who.int/about/en.

physical, mental, and social well-being and not merely the absence of disease or infirmity," which committed the WHO to the viewing of health beyond its biomedical focus. The constitution declared that "the enjoyment of the highest attainable standard of health is one of the fundamental rights of every human being without distinction of race, religion, political belief, economic or social condition" and further committed the WHO and its member states to the pursuit of equality by declaring that "unequal development in different countries in the promotion of health . . . is a common danger." The last preamble of the constitution announced, "Governments have a responsibility for the health of their peoples, which can be fulfilled only by the provision of adequate health and social measures" (WHO 1958: annex 1).

Given the desperate health conditions of the poor and other vulnerable populations across the globe, the objective of universal access of quality health care has been, and remains, a daunting task.[4] In 1946, when the WHO constitution was signed, and still today, challenging physical environments, inadequate social and economic conditions, and limited health care infrastructure have provided fertile ground for poor health. In 1950, life expectancy in low-income countries was forty years, and twenty-eight of every hundred children in those countries died before the age of five.[5] Infectious diseases were prevalent. Malaria, for example, affected some 300 million persons yearly and caused about 3 million annual deaths, and smallpox affected almost 200,000 people per year. Over the last half-century some conditions have improved in the poorest countries, but avoidable diseases and excess mortality have persisted. By 1990, life expectancy in developing countries had increased to sixty-three years, and child mortality improved but remained high, with ten deaths for every hundred children. Treatable infectious diseases have remained a major cause of death. According to the most recent estimates, in 2008, malaria caused about 250 million clinical episodes and about 850,000 deaths. Over 9 million people become sick with tuberculosis (TB) each year, and there are almost 2 million TB-related deaths worldwide. The devastating HIV/AIDS epidemic over the past twenty-five years has further complicated efforts at improving global health and eradicating health disparities. In 2009, around 33 million people were living with HIV and 2.6 million people

---

4. For the historical and current data cited in this and the following paragraph, see WHO 1958, WHO 1968, World Bank 1993, WHO 2008, CSDH 2008, UNAIDS 2010.

5. Throughout this book I use the WHO and World Bank categorizations to describe the countries under consideration. Economies are classified as low-, middle- or high-income according to gross national income per capita, calculated using the World Bank Atlas method. Following World Bank practices, I refer to low- and middle-income countries as developing countries and high-income economies as developed countries. I also use the terms *poor/rich, South/North,* and *Third World* when appropriate.

were newly infected; 1.8 million AIDS-related deaths occurred that year. It is estimated that 25 million people have died of AIDS-related deaths so far. Lack of available resources—the annual expenditure on health in developing countries in 1990 was $41 per capita, compared to $1,860 per capita in Western economies—means that the toll of ill health has fallen mostly on the Global South.

In the face of such suffering on the one hand and limited state capacity on the other, how was the World Health Organization to fulfill its mandate? As in other international organizations, the inevitable tension between technical possibilities and political and economic constraints was reflected in the institutional arrangements in place.[6] Like its mission and objectives, the organizational structure and working procedures of the WHO were also defined by the member states participating in the International Health Conference. The result was a three-layered organizational structure made of the World Health Assembly, the Executive Board, and a secretariat headed by a director-general.[7]

The World Health Assembly (WHA) is where member states enjoy direct representation, and it is therefore the more overtly political layer. Delegates to the assembly are representatives of their designated states, usually elected from the national health administrations and competent in the field of health. However, governments with large delegations often send, in addition, delegates familiar with issues of foreign affairs. The assembly meets annually, usually at the WHO's headquarters in Geneva, Switzerland. At the meetings, the assembly decides on the organization's policies, approves a general program of work, reviews and approves the budget, and gives directives to the Executive Board and to the director-general (WHO 1958: 84). Decisions are made through votes. Like the UN General Assembly and most specialized agencies (but unlike the Security Council, the World Bank, and the International Monetary Fund [IMF]), the assembly follows the principle of one-country/one-vote.

The Executive Board (EB), which meets twice a year, considers the program and budget estimates prepared by the director-general and submits them to the assembly with its comments and recommendations. The board also submits proposals and prepares general programs of work for approval by the assembly (WHO 1958: 92–95). Board members are elected by the assembly for three-year terms. Originally, the board was to consist of between twelve to eighteen persons (WHO 1958: 41), but that number has increased to improve representation of

---

6. On the role of institutional arrangements in determining policy outcomes, see Steinmo, Thelen, and Longstreth 1992, Chorev 2007.

7. The discussion here focuses on the organizational structure of the WHO headquarters in Geneva, Switzerland. The WHO member states are also divided into six geographical regions, each having a regional office.

new members and today the board is composed of thirty-four individuals. The rules of rotation do not allow member states to be elected consecutively, so that even the largest contributors to the organization can be part of the board only every other term. Unlike delegates to the assembly, members of the Executive Board are expected to act as experts on behalf of the whole conference and not as representatives of their respective governments (WHO 1958: 41).

Finally, the WHO has a secretariat, the bureaucratic body of the organization, which comprises the technical and administrative personnel of the organization and is responsible for carrying out the WHO's programs and campaigns. Since the 1950s, the WHO staff has grown from around a thousand to more than eight thousand personnel in professional and general service positions. Professional positions are most often held by medical doctors, public health specialists, scientists, epidemiologists, and more recently, by experts in the fields of health statistics and economics. Member states have no authority over the appointment of staff. The function of the staff is to implement the organization's activities, conduct studies and author reports commissioned by the assembly, and otherwise assure the functioning of the organization. The director-general, who heads the secretariat, is nominated by the Executive Board and elected by the World Health Assembly to a five-year term and can be reelected. Among the many significant responsibilities of the director-general, one of the most important is the authority to suggest the annual budget, which identifies the organization's priorities and commits member states to provide the funds to pursue them (WHO 1958: 106, Lee 2009).

The prominent role of the World Health Assembly, and therefore of member states, in the process of decision making has secured the dominance of geopolitical logic in the global health agenda. Especially in the first few decades of the WHO's history, the Cold War division between East and West directly shaped international health priorities (Litsios 1997, Manela 2010). Following decolonization, the World Health Organization, along with the rest of the UN system, was greatly affected by the demands of the newly independent countries of the Global South for a New International Economic Order. In the mid-1980s, in turn, the NIEO logic was replaced with a U.S.-led neoliberal agenda, best expressed in what has become known as the "Washington Consensus" (Williamson 1990). For UN specialized agencies, including the WHO, each period was characterized by the emergence of a distinct global ideational regime and by exogenous pressures to follow that regime. An overview of the policies formulated by the WHO staff and leadership and adopted by the executive and the assembly illustrates, however, that these policies did not faithfully echo the call for a New International Order in the 1970s nor the neoliberal principles of the 1990s.

The WHO Responds to the New International Economic Order

In the 1960s, with the undoing of colonialism, the large number of newly in-dependent nations that were now recognized by the United Nations radically changed the conversations, debates, and declarations in the entire UN system, where developing countries had become the majority. Encouraged by the ability of oil-producing countries to raise the price of oil, which suggested to other poor countries that the power of their majority vote could be backed by the dependence of industrial countries on their raw materials, they called for economic and political change. Following a successful political mobilization of the Group of 77 (G-77), a coalition of Third World countries unified in their determination for an improved position in the capitalist world system, in 1974 the UN General Assembly adopted a number of resolutions that articulated the call by developing countries for a New International Economic Order. The NIEO contained a number of principles regarding the obligations of developed countries and the rights of developing countries that would reduce the inequities among states by allowing poor countries to achieve economic and social development, mostly through industrialization and improved terms of trade for primary commodities. Thus the G-77 advocated the principle of states' economic sovereignty over their natural resources and economic activities in their territories, including the right to restrict the activities of multinational corporations. The G-77 also called for a stronger regulatory capacity of those international organizations that followed a one-country/one-vote rule and a limiting of the influence of the international financial institutions that rich countries dominated through weighted votes. Developed states were asked to help shift industrial production to the South, transfer Western technology, and provide aid and debt relief. In an attempt to reduce both exploitation and dependence, the NIEO also contained a commitment to collective self-reliance.

In response to the call for a New International Economic Order, the WHO—which in the 1950s and 1960s focused on biomedical determinants and technological solutions—adopted a new agenda, with an unprecedented commitment to address the political, social and economic causes of poor health. This shift came with a novel focus on the question of equity—a concern with the systematic disparities in health between more and less advantaged social groups. Most centrally, the WHO leadership and staff mobilized member states around the unprecedented goal of "Health for All by the Year 2000" and advocated the novel approach that a focus on primary health care was the most adequate means to achieve that goal. The primary health care approach rejected the costly high-technology, urban-based, and curative care that led to skewed resource allocation in the national health systems in many developing countries. Instead, it prioritized universal access to essential health services. These essential services were to be provided at the community level, by nonprofessional workers trained for that activity. The rejection of costly or otherwise inappropriate technologies applied also to drugs, and the WHO staff prepared a model list of "essential" drugs, which aimed to help governments to rationalize their imports of expensive medicines. Directly challenging multinational corporations, the WHO criticized the unethical marketing of infant formula and of inappropriate drugs.

These new programs corresponded, but not quite fully, with the principles underlying the call for a New International Economic Order. The main objective of the NIEO was the attainment of economic development in poor countries, mostly through industrialization and improved terms of trade. Social development, namely, improvements in living conditions and quality of life, was a secondary concern. At the World Health Organization, this order was reversed: the WHO's main concern was the contribution of health to social development. Provocatively, the pursuit of social development was claimed to be attainable even under conditions of scarce resources—that is, independently of the need for economic development. The WHO's concern with equity also deviated from the original principle. The G-77, identifying long-lasting relations of exploitation between industrial capitalist countries and the Third World, called for a more equitable distribution of world resources. Developing countries did not intend UN agencies to influence how additional resources gained by poor countries would be internally distributed. The WHO programs concerned with addressing the issue of equity, however, focused not on equity among states but on equity within states. Health for All by the Year 2000 offered the promise of greater equity in access to health care, and the primary health care approach, including the call for "appropriate" technologies, required the spending of scarce resources on poor populations, thereby identifying practical steps toward equitable distribution at the national level. The WHO also deviated from the call in the UN General Assembly and other venues for increased financial aid. Instead, the primary health care approach was framed around the notion of self-reliance, which required health services to be at a cost that the country could afford to maintain. Finally, while many of the WHO's core initiatives, including the rejection of inappropriate technology, the list of essential drugs, and statements against unethical marketing, reflected support for economic sovereignty and followed developing countries' desire to confront multinational corporations, the WHO secretariat opposed a code of conduct regulating the marketing of pharmaceutical products.

The WHO Responds to Neoliberalism

The G-77 mobilization, which American critics called "Third World Radicalism," was doomed to failure as soon as the economic leverage that developing countries believed they had held all but disappeared with the debt crisis, which started in Mexico in 1982 and affected the entire Global South. The New International Economic Order was soon dead. It was replaced with articulations of the interests of the North, which were effectively encapsulated in the so-called Washington Consensus that was comprised of a number of basic market-liberalizing prescriptions (Williamson 1990). This new, U.S.-led logic, which was based on neoliberal economic premises, positioned markets, rather than governments, at the center of international development. The objective was still economic growth, but the means to achieve growth were markedly different and included encouraging free and open international markets (trade liberalization), reducing barriers to the flow of private capital investment (financial liberalization), encouraging policies that limit the role of government in the economy, including in public sectors such as health and education (budget cuts, deregulation, privatization). The concept of individual responsibility, or helping countries and people who are ready to help themselves, was an important part of this approach. It was assumed that social development would automatically follow once economic growth was achieved. The U.S. government expected UN specialized agencies to follow this neoliberal logic when recommending policies and implementing programs in poor countries, often by means that involved market-driven solutions and private-sector participation. In line with antigovernment principles, the U.S. government also demanded that UN agencies reform themselves. Budgets had to stop growing and managerial reforms were expected.

The collapse of the New International Economic Order and the rise of neoliberalism resulted in a period of severe crisis at the WHO. Starting in the late 1980s, the organization suffered from serious financial difficulties and from threats to its authority as the World Bank and other international organizations became involved in global health matters. A lack of effective leadership exacerbated the crisis. However, after a decade-long period of some paralysis, in the late 1990s the WHO secretariat finally emerged out of the crisis by embracing a radically new agenda. A new WHO leadership responded to the external pressures by promoting health programs and policies aimed at contributing to economic growth rather than to social development. In addition, commitment to primary health care was replaced with disease-specific interventions, and the WHO secretariat accepted cost-effective calculations as means to prioritize among alternative interventions. The WHO leadership also supported policies that offered market-driven solutions, such as charging for bed nets or subsidizing the pharmaceutical sector. Organizationally, many WHO programs were now designed as "partnerships" that incorporated new actors, including private foundations and multinational companies. Another indication of the willingness to rely on the private sector was renewed support for technological solutions, including a focus on the distribution of existing drugs and vaccines and the development of new ones, both with the active participation of pharmaceutical companies.

The new commitment to economic growth and cost effectiveness led to programs that corresponded largely but not quite completely with the economic logic of neoliberal thought. For example, the WHO leadership called for greater investment in health rather than for the budget cuts in the public health sector that neoliberal reasoning would prescribe. While adhering to a cost-effective logic, the WHO secretariat also maintained its focus on infectious diseases affecting the poor, including malaria, tuberculosis, and HIV/AIDS, and advocated for a "new universalism"—the delivery of high-quality essential care to all. Following neoliberal prescriptions, the WHO actively sought to improve its relations with the private sector, but the WHO staff also mobilized its member states to sign a treaty aimed against the tobacco sector and, in attempts to improve access to AIDS drugs, objected to intellectual property rules that were supported by the pharmaceutical sector.

In short, an examination of the WHO policies in the 1970s–1980s and the 1990s–2000s reveals a substantial shift in focus from social development to economic growth and from equity to cost effectiveness, which reflects a *selective* correspondence with the shift in the dominant logic at the international level.[8] While the dominant logic in each era clearly influenced the content of health policies and programs adopted by the WHO, there were also significant gaps between both logics and the WHO's respective response.

The origins of the selective correspondence between WHO policies and the dominant logic challenges the common perception of international organizations as arenas where policies and programs are determined by the power disparities of member states. At the WHO, policies and programs did not reflect the capacity of some members to use their economic, procedural, and/or normative leverage to convince or force other members to support their position. Rather, the deviation from the New International Order in the 1970s–1980s and from the neoliberal logic in the 1990s–2000s was the doing of the WHO leadership and

---

8. These are only generalized tendencies. The WHO, like any other complex organization, is not entirely coherent, and it combines multiple tendencies and orientations. While equity was the primary objective in the 1970s–1980s and effectiveness was the dominant concern in the 1990s–2000s, both of these missions were permanent considerations at the WHO. For particularly helpful accounts of the history of the WHO that make a similar point, see Thomas and Weber 2004, Brown, Cueto, and Fee 2006, Italian Global Health Watch 2008, Lee 2009.

staff. The WHO functioned not as a "site" but as an "agent," with the organization's bureaucracy actively participating in the making of policies. As an agent, in turn, the secretariat did not act as a neutral mediator between competing member states but used its position to promote independent goals and preferences.

The analysis of the WHO secretariat reveals, as constructivist and principal-agent theories of international organizations have also claimed, that international bureaucracies are partially autonomous actors who have material interests in ensuring sufficient resources and effective authority, as well as ideational positions regarding the meaning of their mandate and how to pursue it (Barnett and Finnemore 2004, Hawkins et al. 2006). The experience of the WHO secretariat also shows that the ability of international bureaucracies to act according to their preferences is potentially limited. The limits arise from international organizations' dependence on members' funds (resource dependence), votes (procedural dependence), and legitimacy (normative dependence): member states can shape the position of an international organization by threatening to withhold their contributions, to vote against proposals, or to undermine the organization's standing. International bureaucracies cannot ignore or defy exogenous demands and expectations without risking punitive measures. Hence international organizations are purposive actors who function within limits of external constraints.

This conceptualization raises the question that is at the core of the investigation here: How can an international bureaucracy advance its independent goals given its dependence on member states? In other words, how can an international organization successfully deviate from exogenous pressures? I argue that when the goals of an international bureaucracy are not compatible with the exogenous demands, it can employ various strategies to protect its preferences, and I identify the strategies available to an international organization's staff and leadership in their attempt to protect those goals.

Building on Christine Oliver's typology of organizational responses, which range "from passive conformity to active resistance" (Oliver 1991: 146), I make a distinction not only between conformity and resistance, as Oliver and others do, but also between "passive" and "active" responses. A response is passive when the organization takes the pressures "as a given constraint to be obeyed or defied." A response is active, or what I call strategic, when the organization attempts to redefine the meaning of the exogenous pressures before adhering to or resisting them (Oliver 1991: 159). When confronted with incongruous demands, the WHO secretariat often avoided passive compliance, that is, adherence to the original demands, where the preferences of the organization would have been sacrificed. The WHO secretariat also avoided passive resistance, that is, explicit defiance of the original demands, where the chances of success were low and the risk of being penalized was high. Rather, the WHO leadership and staff relied on strategic responses. In instances of strategic compliance, the WHO secretariat altered the meaning of the exogenous demands so that they were compatible with the organization's agenda before it adhered to those demands. For example, in the 1970s–1980s, the WHO leadership was able to present the primary health care approach as compatible with the New International Economic Order by drawing on principles of equity and justice but referring to intrastate equity rather than the NIEO's original concerns with interstate equity. In the 1990s–2000s, the WHO leadership was able to present investment in health as compatible with the neoliberal agenda by drawing on the neoliberal concern with economic growth while insisting that investment in health could contribute to such growth. In instances of strategic resistance, the WHO secretariat altered the meaning of the dominant logic, not in order to comply but so that refusal to comply with the exogenous demands would be considered consistent with that logic. For example, in the 1970s–1980s, the WHO leadership was able to oppose an international agreement on the marketing of pharmaceutical products by arguing that such an agreement would contradict the NIEO principle of sovereignty. In the 1990s–2000s, the WHO leadership was able to promote an international agreement on tobacco use by suggesting that, given the tobacco industry's undisputed unethical behavior, this was a legitimate exception to the organization's otherwise probusiness attitude.

International bureaucracies, then, are able to promote policies that reflect their preferences without alienating their member states by means of what I call strategic adaptation: instead of fully adhering to the external demands, international bureaucracies may first try to alter the meaning of the demands so they more closely correspond with their preferences before complying with them; in other cases, instead of simply defying the external demands, international bureaucracies may alter the meaning of the demands so that their decisions will not be considered to be in defiance of these expectations. Not all international bureaucracies employ strategic responses, and not all strategic responses succeed. When strategic responses are successful, however, they may create significant gaps between the dominant logic and the policies and programs that are put in place in the name of that logic. It is through strategic adaptation, then, that international organizations do not simply embrace the dominant logic, but transform it.

In short, international organizations are not neutral arenas where member states negotiate agreements that reflect their relative bargaining leverage. The bureaucracies put in place do not merely facilitate such negotiations but develop an inherent interest in the outcome. Under certain conditions, these bureaucracies have the ability to have an impact on the negotiations and to shape the policies and programs that define a given world order—such as those that establish international commitments on public health, but also women's rights, nuclear proliferation, world heritage, international debt, wars and genocides, and protection of refugees. Constructivist and principal-agent theories of international relations have contributed greatly to our understanding of international organizations as agents. Thus far, however, those theories have paid little attention to the question of how dependent organizations can protect their agendas, deflect criticism, and avoid compliance with the demands of powerful states. By identifying international bureaucracies not only as purposive actors, but as *strategic* ones as well, the purpose of this book is to contribute to this emerging conversation.

Why the WHO?

The immediate post–World War II period, with the establishment of the United Nations and the promise of a revived international arena, brought with it a wave of studies on international organizations. In February 1947, the first issue of a new journal, *International Organization,* was published. The introductory note announced that "international organization . . . is becoming an increasingly important part of the study and understanding of international relations" (Bundy 1947). But this interest in international organizations as organizations has since waned. The state-centered approach to international politics, which has dominated international relations theories, produced no theoretical interest in the internal functioning of international organizations, as they were often considered causally epiphenomenal (Kratochwil and Ruggie 1986, Rochester 1986, Barnett 1997). Recently, however, this tendency seems to have been reversed, with an increased interest in political science and sociology especially in the Bretton Woods institutions, namely, the World Bank, the IMF, and the General Agreement on Tariffs and Trade and its successor the World Trade Organization (WTO).[9] The focus on these three institutions is likely due to the fact that these were the international organizations that spearheaded the neoliberal transformation at the international and domestic levels. While not as commanding as the international financial institutions, other UN agencies, which have been generally overlooked in this recent wave of interest, also matter greatly, especially to developing countries. Through financial support, technical assistance, the advocacy of policies, and the initiation of programs, UN agencies influence many domestic policies, including in fundamental areas such as human rights, labor, education, health, and the environment (Meyer et al. 1997, Hafner-Burton and Tsutsui 2005,

---

9. On the World Bank, see Weaver 2008, Chwieroth 2008b, Babb 2009, Lavelle 2011; on the IMF, see Babb 2007, Abdelal 2007, Chwieroth 2008a; on the WTO, see Chorev 2007, Chorev and Babb 2009, Conti 2010.

Schofer and Meyer 2005, Torfason and Ingram 2010). Moreover, examination of other UN agencies can shed light on issues that the study of the World Bank, IMF and WTO may not. Most important, significant differences in institutional arrangements, including voting procedures and sources of funds, suggest that what we know about the responses of the World Bank and the IMF to external forces may not apply or may apply differently in other multilateral agencies.

Among UN agencies, the WHO is of particular interest. Because the WHO is the specialized agency responsible for global health policies and programs, and given the interdependence of countries in controlling diseases, all WHO member states have been generally supportive of the organization. As a result, it is one of the largest agencies, in its budget, scope of mandate, and actual programs. The influence of the WHO on national health policies, especially in poor countries, has been apparent, with WHO technical and operational assistance having substantial impact on which populations receive care, what types of treatments are recommended, and so on. The WHO's activities and impact, in turn, have been of interest to many actors, including donor countries, recipient countries, pharmaceutical and other multinational corporations, and consumer and health activists. As a result, the WHO has historically been particularly exposed to exogenous demands and expectations.

My research covers the period from the 1970s to the 2000s and encompasses the WHO's response to the NIEO in the 1970s and early 1980s and, following a period of relative inaction, to neoliberalism in the late 1990s and early 2000s.[10] The comparison between the two periods reveals the WHO's strategic responses in the face of very different environments—in the 1970s–1980s demands came from the Global South, whereas in the 1990s–2000s they came from the North. The two cases also reveal the conditions under which strategic adaptation is likely.

My historical narrative and theoretical interpretations rely on archival research and interviews, as well as invaluable secondary materials. I collected primary data from the library at the WHO headquarters in Geneva, Switzerland, and the library of the Pan-American Health Organization (PAHO), the regional office of the WHO in Washington, DC. These libraries hold collections of minutes of the World Health Assemblies (WHA) and the two WHA committees, and of the Executive Board meetings.[11] These minutes provide an invaluable source for identifying the

---

10. Chapter 3 provides a brief account of WHO policies between the 1940s and the 1960s; in the conclusion I analyze some of the more recent developments.

11. Many issues at the assembly are first discussed in one of two committees. Committee A is predominantly responsible for program and budget matters, and Committee B is predominantly responsible for administrative, financial, and legal matters. Minutes of the assembly and the two committees are provided verbatim (translated to the WHO formal languages). The Executive Board meetings are reported in the second person.

positions of the representatives of member states and of the WHO leadership and staff. The archives of the WHO also hold many publications, studies, reports, and correspondence with member states and other interested parties. I also conducted research in a number of archives and presidential libraries in the United States (the U.S. National Archives in Washington, DC; the Nixon Presidential Materials Project in Washington, DC; the Gerald R. Ford Presidential Library in Michigan; the Jimmy Carter Presidential Library in Georgia; and the Ronald Reagan Presidential Library in California); in England (the National Archives, Surrey); in Canada (the Library and Archives, Ottawa); and in Israel (the National Archives, Jerusalem). These archives and libraries hold useful correspondence between government officials and the respective state representatives attending WHO meetings.[12] They also hold evaluative reports of the United Nations in general and the WHO in particular. Among many other official documents, I studied congressional hearings in the United States, where Congress negotiated, often quite contentiously, appropriations for the WHO. In addition to archival research, I conducted fifty-three formal interviews with relevant informants[13] and conducted a large number of informal conversations at the WHO headquarters in Geneva, including while observing the annual World Health Assembly, in May 2008.

An Outline of the Book

The book offers a detailed empirical investigation of the World Health Organization's response to external pressures in two contentious periods: that of the call for a New International Economic Order in the 1970s and early 1980s, and when a neoliberal logic was particularly prevalent, in the 1990s and 2000s. For each period, I identify the exogenous demands and then analyze the adaptive strategies used by the WHO secretariat in protecting the organization's goals. Chapter 2 provides the theoretical foundations for my empirical claims. Drawing on insights from organizational sociology, I offer in this chapter an approach to international organizations that identifies and explains the capacity

---

12. In addition to corresponding with the respective health ministries, it is a common practice for delegations to report to, and receive instructions from, foreign offices or departments of foreign affairs.

13. The interviews were conducted between March 2008 and May 2009, with WHO staff, governmental officials in the United States and South Africa, and officials of the World Bank, the Global Fund to Fight AIDS, Tuberculosis and Malaria, the Joint United Nations Programme on HIV/AIDS, and public-private health partnerships, including Medicines for Malaria Venture, International AIDS Vaccine Initiative, and Drugs for Neglected Diseases initiative. I also interviewed local and transnational health activists in Geneva, Washington, DC, and South Africa (Médecins Sans Frontières, Consumer Project on Technology, and Treatment Action Campaign), representatives of pharmaceutical and other companies, and the International Federation of Pharmaceutical Manufacturers and Associations.

of international bureaucracies to achieve their organization's independent goals in spite of their dependence on member states. I describe the inevitable tension between the dependence of international bureaucracies on member states and their tendency to develop independent material and ideational goals. I also identify the types of strategic responses available to international bureaucracies to satisfy exogenous pressures while protecting some of their goals. Last, I discuss the implications of this study on our understanding of organizational change and analyze the conditions under which an international organization is likely to engage in strategic adaptation. In chapters 3 and 4, I provide a careful historical account of the WHO's strategic response to the call for a New International Economic Order. In chapter 3, I show how by reinterpreting the meaning of the principles of economic and social development, equity, and self-reliance, the WHO secretariat was able to present its central agenda—Health for All by the Year 2000 through promotion of primary health care—as loyally following the logic of the New International Economic Order, while carefully safeguarding the organization's commitment to its constitution and to new perceptions in public health knowledge. In chapter 4, I analyze the adaptive strategies leading to the WHO's policies and programs that threatened the commercial interests of multinational companies. I describe the three WHO initiatives that were in line with NIEO principles and that pharmaceutical companies vigorously opposed: a model list of essential drugs, which was intended to help developing countries to purchase drugs rationally; programs supporting the local manufacturing of drugs; and international codes of conduct for regulating the marketing practices of the infant formula sector and the pharmaceutical sector. I describe how, in a conscious attempt to avoid harm to its reputation, the WHO leadership was able to narrow the scope of the essential list's applicability, withdraw its support for local manufacturing, and strategically resist developing countries' demands for a pharmaceutical code of conduct. In chapter 5, I describe the rise of a neoliberal logic in the mid-1980s, and the deep financial, authority, and legitimacy crises that the WHO experienced due to this shift in the exogenous environment. In chapters 6 and 7, I examine how the WHO, under new leadership, was able to overcome the most pressing financial difficulties and regain some of its authority over global health programs by strategically adapting to neoliberal principles. In chapter 6, I look at how, by recruiting economists to show that health could contribute to economic growth, the WHO bureaucracy was able to present investment in health as a productive, rather than wasteful, spending of public funds; and how the WHO bureaucracy relied on cost-effective reasoning to introduce the concept of "new universalism," which supported the provision of cost-effective services to everyone, as an alternative to market-oriented approaches that relied on people's ability to pay. In chapter 7, which focuses on the WHO's relations with business, I analyze the strategic resistance of the WHO in two instances: a WHO campaign against the tobacco industry that led to the first binding treaty signed by WHO member states, and a WHO opposition to an international agreement protecting intellectual property rights, which threatened the capacity of member states to manufacture or purchase generic versions of patented AIDS drugs. In the conclusion, I draw on the findings described in the rest of the book to offer a systematic comparison between the "international organization" of the 1970s–1980s and the "global governance" of the 1990s–2000s and to evaluate the structural transformations of the global health regime over time. I then conclude with an analysis of the WHO bureaucracy's recent response to the still-in-formation post–neoliberal global order.

THE STRATEGIC RESPONSE OF INTERNATIONAL ORGANIZATIONS

How can we explain the selective correspondence between external pressures—the call for a New International Economic Order in the 1970s–1980s and neo-liberal thought in the 1990s–2000s—and WHO policies and programs in the respective periods? I address this question by analyzing the strategic response of international bureaucracies to exogenous demands. To that end, the first part of the chapter describes my approach to international organizations. Like constructivist and principal-agent theories, this approach conceptualizes international bureaucracies as purposive actors who function within limits of external constraints. By emphasizing the likely tensions between international bureaucracies and member states, however, this approach invites us to address a question that is frequently ignored: Given the dependence of international organizations on member states, what allows international bureaucracies to protect their goals and interests when those clash with exogenous demands? The analysis offered relies not on the power or authority of international organizations (Barnett and Finnemore 2004) but on their strategies.

I draw on organizational sociology in the second part to identify the strategies available to international bureaucracies to protect their goals in the face of incongruous demands. In some cases, an international bureaucracy will employ a "passive" response, either simply following the dominant logic, hence sacrificing its own goals, or else trying to resist the dominant logic, at the risk of being penalized by the member states on which it is dependent; each option is passive in that the dominant logic remains untouched. Often, however, an international organization will employ a strategic ("active") response, which involves altering the meaning of the external demands. By adopting policies that follow the logic of the altered expectations, the international bureaucracy is able to comply with external demands in a way that is compatible with the interests of the organization, hence minimizing the cost of compliance, or to refuse compliance in a way that is not considered resistance, thereby minimizing the risk of sanctions. As this book shows, the WHO secretariat employed such strategic responses to circumvent the call for a New International Economic Order and then the principles of neoliberal thought.

International Organizations as Partially Autonomous Agents

Common perceptions of international organizations, including neorealism (Mearsheimer 1994, Gruber 2000) and neoliberal institutionalism (Keohane 1984, Keohane and Martin 1995) in the field of international relations, and world society (Meyer et al. 1997, Krücken and Drori 2009) in the sociological literature, view international organizations as sites where member states are the only carriers of interests and the only ones capable of acting. Neorealists generally view international institutions as "arenas for acting out power relationships" and grant them no causal power of their own (Evans and Wilson 1992: 330). Neoliberal institutionalists do allow for states' participation in international organizations to have causal relevance. Institutional arrangements "change the incentives for states to cheat; they . . . reduce transaction costs, link issues, and provide focal points for cooperation" and in this way transform states' preferences, their behavior, and ultimately, policy outcomes (Keohane and Martin 1995: 49). Although neoliberal institutionalists see institutional frameworks as imposing constraints on states, they agree with neorealists that international organizations have no capacity to act, and they accept the neorealist assumption that policy outcomes reflect the power relations and interests of states (see Barnett and Finnemore 2004). The world society approach reverses the logic of the relations between the international and national realms, suggesting that states are the products of world culture (Meyer et al. 1997). Although international organizations facilitate the diffusion of world culture, however, in world society accounts they have little role in shaping the models that they help disseminate. Rather, these models originate from Western Europe and North America (Meyer et al. 1997: 165). In spite of significant differences, therefore, these three theories all agree that states' preferences and the relations among member states should be sufficient to explain policies that emerge out of international organizations.

The case of the WHO reveals, however, that the decisions made at international organizations are not simply the outcome of member states negotiating with each other. First, historical evidence shows that the WHO policies did not emerge out of unmediated debates and negotiations between member states holding competing positions. Interstate negotiations and compromises have certainly been part of the decision-making process. Yet WHO leadership and staff—those who planned the budget, ranked program priorities, authored position papers, formulated arguments, and advocated policies to its member states—have been active in influencing policies. Second, the WHO secretariat did not act as a neutral mediator, merely helping to find a workable compromise among competing member states or disseminating ideas developed elsewhere. Instead, the WHO secretariat acted as an interested, and therefore biased, actor: it incorporated its own goals and perceptions into the policies it formulated for the member states. As a result, the global health policies and programs that emerged did not simply reflect compromises member states could agree on, but compromises that were aligned with the preferences of the organization. Studies of other international organizations reveal a similar pattern (Barnett and Finnemore 2004). For example, in a masterful account of the negotiations over a global standard for bankruptcy law under the auspices of the UN Commission on International Trade Law (UNCITRAL), Halliday, Block-Lieb, and Carruthers (2009) show that the UNCITRAL secretariat incorporated its own goals when orchestrating the necessary compromises between the different parties.

The WHO bureaucracy's authorship of international health policies supports the views of the constructivist (Finnemore 1996, Barnett and Finnemore 2004, Weaver and Leiteritz 2005) and the principal-agent theories (Kiewiet and McCubbins 1991, Koremenos, Lipson, and Snidal 2001, Nielson and Tierney 2003) that international organizations are purposive agents, whose actions help shape the content of policies.[1] However, the case of the WHO also highlights the challenges international bureaucracies inevitably confront when attempting to act autonomously.

Constructivist theorists have convincingly argued that international organizations are actors, with capacity to develop and act according to independent interests and perceptions that cannot be reduced to the interests and perceptions of their member states. According to this theory, the capacity of international organizations for autonomous action stems from their (rational-legal, delegated, moral, and/or expert) authority, which provides them ability to exercise

---

1. Earlier international relations theories that regard international organizations as actors include the epistemic communities literature (Haas 1992) and the international organization decision-making literature (Cox 1969, Cox and Jacobson 1973).

(compulsory, institutional, or productive) power (Barnett and Finnemore 2005). General formulations of the constructivist view acknowledge and identify the external constraints imposed by states (Barnett and Finnemore 2004: 12). In most of the empirical analyses, however, the potential tension between the independent goals of the international organization and external demands is bypassed by choosing case studies in which international organizations act independently but in line with states' interests, or case studies in which international organizations act where states are indifferent. No special attention is paid to the cases that could result in much greater conflict, in which international organizations fail to carry out state demands or act in ways that run against states' interests (see Barnett and Finnemore 2004: 28). One of the outcomes of this empirical bias is that, in practice, many constructivist accounts tend to overstate the autonomy and power available to international organizations and downplay the influence of external pressures and constraints (Barnett and Finnemore 2004, Abdelal 2007, Chwieroth 2008a). For example, Rawi Abdelal's fascinating analysis of the IMF's promotion of capital account liberalization convincingly shows that initiatives came from "within the management of the Fund itself," but it avoids the need to explain how this type of autonomous action could survive external opposition because, according to his account, the U.S. Treasury Department was indifferent to, and Wall Street financial firms largely uninformed of, the IMF's initiatives (Abdelal 2007: chapter 6).

As Nielson and Tierney (2003: 244–245) have described with a colorful metaphor: "For organizational theorists . . . [international organizations] are like global Frankensteins terrorizing (or more often benefiting) the international countryside. Once [international organizations] have been created, they take on a life of their own and are largely beyond the control of their creators." Barnett and Coleman (2005: 594) conceded: "The virtue of a focus on the characteristics of the organization for explaining organizational change is also its vice: The emphasis on the organization can lead to the neglect of the environment." I suggest, however, that the oversight of constructivist accounts is not in overstating the autonomy of international organizations but in neglecting to explore the factors that enable international organizations to advance their interests even under conditions of external pressures. In other words, it is possible that international organizations do prevail in conflicts with member states or other actors, but because constructivists avoid analyzing actual conflicts, they cannot account for such cases.

The principal-agent approach shares with the constructivist theory lack of attention to how international organizations can exercise their partial autonomy and pursue their own agenda in the face of incongruous external demands. The principal-agent analysis holds that an international organization (the agent) "can exhibit significant independence" because member states (the principals) are impeded by the complications of "collective principal," "multiple principals," and "chain of delegation," which limit their effective supervision (Nielson and Tierney 2003). While this formulation reflects greater attentiveness to the necessary tensions between member states and international organizations than most constructivist accounts, the principal-agent literature has mostly focused on identifying the characteristics of principals that allowed for more or less effective supervision. As a result, by some scholars' own admission, the analysis "contains a remarkably thin view of agent behavior" (Hawkins and Jacoby 2006: 1999).

In short, both the constructivist and principal-agent theories have rightly identified the partial autonomy of international organizations. They have developed convincing arguments regarding the tendency of international organizations to develop autonomous interests and goals, but they have yet to develop a more complete understanding of the capacity of international organizations to protect those goals *when these clash with the preferences of member states*. To remedy this oversight, I describe the institutional factors that determine the level of autonomy of international bureaucracies and the types of strategic action that enable international bureaucracies to act on their partial autonomy and circumvent external controls.

The Institutional Origins of Agency and Dependence

To identify the institutional factors determining the partial autonomy of international organizations, it is useful to draw on insights from political sociology and organizational sociology (see also Barnett and Coleman 2005, Weaver 2008). Political sociology is useful for understanding the capacity of public bureaucracies to develop independent goals, preferences, and interests. Indeed, the debate over the nature of international organizations clearly parallels an earlier debate on the nature of the state, between society-centered and state-centered approaches. In this discussion, state-centered scholarship questioned the conceptualization of the state as a mere venue and developed a theory of the state that leaves room for the state to act relatively autonomously (Block 1977, Evans, Rueschemeyer, and Skocpol 1985, Skocpol 1992). The approach taken here similarly relies on the capacity of international bureaucracies to develop goals independently of member states. However, key differences between states and international organizations do not allow us to comfortably apply theories of the state to analyze the relations of international organizations to external forces. Specifically, the relations between the state and the capitalist class on which it depends are structurally different from the relations between international organizations and member states. According to the literature on the relative autonomy of the state, state managers are dependent on the maintenance of some reasonable level of economic activity and are therefore unlikely to act against the general interests of capital. This alignment of state managers with the interests of capital occurs independently of direct pressures by capitalists of state managers through means such as political contributions (Block 1977). Hence, the relative autonomy of the state is based on structural, rather than direct, relations of dependence. International organizations have no such relations of structural dependence: they do not have an impact on and cannot directly benefit from the well-being of their member states. Instead, their dependence is based on direct relations of dependence. To understand these relations of dependence it is useful to apply sociological theories of organizations, particularly the resource dependence approach (Pfeffer and Salancik 1978) and the neoinstitutionalist approach (DiMaggio and Powell 1991), which analyze the external constraints imposed on organizations and their capacity to act within such constraints.[2]

Based on sociological theories of states and of organizations, we can view international organizations as actors with independent goals. The ability of international organizations to pursue these goals, however, is bounded by their dependence on exogenous actors, particularly member states, for funds (resource dependence), majority of votes (procedural dependence), and legitimacy (normative dependence). The content of the independent goals and the scope of dependence reflect the institutional contours of the international organization. The discussion below identifies a number of factors that influence international organizations' independent goals and scope of vulnerability.

International organizations' material and ideational goals. Political sociologists have shown that elected officials and civil servants develop interests independently of their constituencies and donors, and that these interests go beyond sheer need of survival. Similarly, organizational sociologists have shown that organizations develop distinct identities: beliefs about what kind of organization it is, what it should look like, and how it should behave (Albert and Whetton 1985, Dutton and Dukerich 1991, Golden-Biddle and Rao 1997, Glynn 2000). International bureaucracies, too, develop autonomous material and ideational goals.

The material goals of international bureaucracies include possessing sufficient authority to act and having sufficient funds to act effectively. International bureaucracies also develop expansionary tendencies, attempting to attain

---

2. For early analyses of international organizations as organizations see Haas 1964, Cox 1969, Crane and Finkle 1981, Ascher 1983, Jonsson 1986, Ness and Brechin 1988. For the most systematic current articulations see Barnett and Finnemore 1999, 2004.

bigger mandates and bigger budgets. However, material goals are not absolute. Opportunities for expansion may be rejected, for example, if they threaten the autonomy of the organization or undermine its legitimacy (Barnett and Coleman 2005). Similarly, the amount of funds is hardly ever the sole consideration. International bureaucracies may want to maintain control over how resources are spent and therefore, for example, normally prefer mandatory to earmarked voluntary contributions. Like other international bureaucracies, the WHO secretariat has always been motivated by material goals. This has been particularly pronounced during the neoliberal era, when the WHO suffered severely from budget cuts and its authority was threatened by the rise of new international entities responsible for global health.

International bureaucracies also develop principles, preferences, and philosophies that guide their perception of the mission of the organization and their understanding of the best way to achieve that mission (Jepperson 1991, Barnett and Finnemore 2004, Barnett and Coleman 2005). Hence an organization's staff is not only concerned with material goals, the staff also wants the organization to function according to its principles and wants the organization's policies and programs to reflect those principles. Organizational principles have numerous potential origins, and although the sources that generate ideational goals and the perceptions drawn from those sources may change over time, there are two sources that are particularly important. First, an international bureaucracy is heavily influenced by the values and goals of the organization's founders, especially as these are expressed in the organization's foundational texts, such as its constitution (Harris and Ogbonna 1999, Johnson 2008). Second, if the bureaucracy is dominated by one profession, the organization's principles are strongly shaped by professional expertise and ethos (DiMaggio and Powell 1983, Glynn 2000, Weaver and Leiteritz 2005, Babb 2007, Chwieroth 2008a). These two sources—founding declarations and expert knowledge—are considered by staff and member states to be legitimate references and the reliance of international bureaucracies on such sources to justify preferences often ensures member states' normative support. Consistency with the constitution confirms that the organization functions within its mandate, and that it is apolitical; reliance on professional knowledge signifies impartiality and objectivity and creates the appearance of political neutrality (Barnett and Finnemore 1999: 708). At the WHO, the constitution and professional ethos have played a particularly central role in defining the organization's ideational preferences and principles and in legitimating them. The constitution has served as an enduring touchstone although the meaning granted to the principles declared in the constitution, and their relative priority, have changed over time. Public health expertise and ethos have also had great influence on WHO preferences and principles.

In short, international bureaucracies develop material goals and ideational perceptions that determine their positions on initiatives and other demands placed by member states. However, the capacity of international bureaucracies to act on their independent preferences is constrained by three main sources of dependence on exogenous actors: resource dependence, procedural dependence, and normative dependence.

Resource dependence. International organizations need financial resources to survive and accomplish their goals and are therefore heavily dependent on external actors who provide the funds. Resource allotment is probably the most effective form of control among the three identified here and the one most thoroughly analyzed in the literature (Pfeffer and Salancik 1978, see also Blau 1964, Thompson 1967, Babb 2009). The extent of resource dependence may vary depending on the institutional arrangements in place. A number of conditions are particularly relevant in determining the level of resource dependence of international organizations: (1) *The amount of external funds required for operation.* The greater the amount of funds required by an international organization for pursuing its mission, the more dependent it is on exogenous donors. The World Bank, for example, is especially vulnerable to donors because its operations require large amounts of funds. The World Trade Organization, in contrast, requires a small budget and therefore exogenous actors cannot influence its actions and policies simply by withholding resources or promising additional ones. The IMF, in turn, needs significant resources but is less vulnerable than the World Bank since it generates its own revenues (Chorev and Babb 2009). The WHO cannot generate its own revenue, and given its growing focus since the 1960s on operational rather than technical assistance, the organization was heavily dependent, like most UN agencies, on the resources granted by member states and other donors. The level of resource dependence was mostly contingent on how heavily the WHO's proposed programs relied on (expensive) technology and highly trained personnel. (2) *The differences in members' contributions.* The greater the amount of funds given by wealthy member states compared to the amount of funds given by poor member states the more international organizations are dependent on their wealthier members. International organizations like the World Bank, which only rely on contributions of rich countries, are particularly vulnerable. UN specialized agencies normally rely on a proportionate formula for assessing contributions, usually according to member states' capacity to pay, taking into account their gross domestic product and size of population. While clearly appropriate, this created disproportionate dependence of UN agencies, including the WHO, on the United States and other rich countries. A related condition is *the number of states that contribute significant funds to the organization and the coherence of their position.* The smaller the number of consequential contributors and the more homogeneous their position, the less leverage an international organization has. (3) *Mandatory versus voluntary contributions.* Mandatory contributions reduce the ability of wealthy member states to use their payments as a bargaining leverage, and in organizations that have a one-country/one-vote rule mandatory contributions increase the influence of poor countries, if they have the majority of votes. At the WHO, one component of the budget is the mandatory contributions of member states (the regular budgetary funds), which are suggested by the director-general and then discussed in the Executive Board and voted by the World Health Assembly. Another component is the voluntary contributions earmarked for specific purposes (the extrabudgetary funds), which are provided by wealthy donor nations, as well as international organizations such as the UN Development Programme and private foundations such as the Rockefeller Foundation. The balance between the regular and the extrabudgetary funds greatly affects the relative weight of resource dependence and procedural dependence (see below). (4) *Competition with other organizations for access to resources.* Resource dependence is greater when a number of institutions with overlapping mandates compete for the same funds. The WHO is the designated UN agency for international health policies and programs. At times, however, it had to compete for funds with other international organizations that initiated, within the scope of their own mandate, health-related programs.

Procedural dependence. When member states are represented in the governing body, international organizations are vulnerable not only to the power of states to withhold their funds but also to their power to withhold votes. To function properly, international organizations require a majority of member states to agree on policies and programs. If international bureaucracies were neutral, they would have little interest in the content of the policies and programs that are passed by a majority of members. However, since international bureaucracies are interested in the content of the policies and programs, their dependence on voting members is greatly heightened. As with resource dependence, the institutional arrangements in place shape the degree of procedural dependence. (1) *Voting arrangements.* Some international organizations follow one-country/one-vote rule, while others follow a "weighted" arrangement, in which the weight of a state's vote reflects its proportionate financial contribution to the organization. Arguably, procedural dependence has not attracted much attention in the literature because in the international organizations most often studied, the World Bank and the IMF, rich countries also have the majority of votes, which creates a close overlap between resource and procedural dependence. At most UN agencies, however, the one-country/one-vote rule has established dependence on voting members, independently of their financial contributions. Following decolonization, members from the developing world have become the majority and UN agencies have since been dependent on the votes of poor member states, which potentially restrains the monopoly of the rich minority. At the WHO, the Executive Board creates an additional layer of procedural dependence that is similarly divorced from resource dependence. Board members reflect the geographical and economic diversity of the WHO members, with poor countries again making the majority. The ability of rich countries to influence the board is further tempered by a rule that does not allow member states to be elected consecutively and by the expectation that board members will serve in their individual capacity and not as representatives of states. (2) *Location of decision-making authority.* Voting arrangements matter only as long as decisions are made by the assembly and are not diverted to other sites. We will see that one effective way for rich countries to reduce international organizations' dependence on the majority of votes has been providing voluntary contributions, which are earmarked. (3) *Coalition building.* Resource dependence allows member states that control resources to act unilaterally in an attempt to shape the behavior of international organizations (although a coalition of contributing members makes resource dependence even more effective). The effectiveness of procedural dependence, in contrast, depends on the capacity of a majority of member states to form a stable coalition. (4) *Structural dependence of poor countries on rich countries.* The leverage member states have over international organizations is not independent of their relations with other member states. Bloc voting of a majority of developing countries against the position of developed countries depends, among other conditions, on poor countries' shared perceptions of their economic and political dependence on developed countries (Kim and Russett 1996, Voeten 2000).

Normative dependence. As sociologists of organizations remind us, international organizations need symbolic resources in addition to material ones. To generate support, an organization's presentation of itself, its mission, and its programs have to be accepted as legitimate (Meyer and Rowan 1977, Suchman 1995, Hurd 2007). One effective way for member states to have leverage on an organization, therefore, is to present the organization's positions or actions as illegitimate. Both rich and poor countries, as well as health activists and multinational corporations, have tried to influence the position of the WHO by questioning the appropriateness of its decisions.[3] Most sources of legitimacy are internal (Barnett and Finnemore 2004: 166–170, Hurd 2007, Halliday

---

3. On the other hand, exogenous pressures for change, too, have to be viewed as legitimate; that is, they have to be viewed as compatible with the WHO's mandate.

and Carruthers 2009). To be considered internally legitimate, the policies and programs of international organizations need to be consistent with and not go beyond their original mandate. They also have to be seen as neutral: they cannot be seen as serving the interests of rich countries (or multinational corporations) or to be the mouthpiece of poor countries. Finally, international organizations have to show managerial competence. Competence and efficiency have often been related to the question of neutrality, as rich countries, in particular, blamed politicization for leading to organizational malfunction. Other sources of legitimacy are external. To attain external legitimacy, international organizations need to conform to global norms, rules, and principles as they are defined and redefined by dominant global actors (Meyer and Rowan 1977, Scott and Meyer 1983, DiMaggio and Powell 1983, Goodrick and Salancik 1996, Hurd 2007).

The degree and relative importance of each type of dependence, and therefore the balance of influence between rich and poor countries, may change over time, according to the conditions articulated above. In the 1970s, when developing countries established and were able to maintain a stable coalition, many WHO decisions were informed by its procedural dependence on developing countries. In the mid-1980s, however, the gradual move from mandatory to voluntary contributions and the increased number of competing international organizations with overlapping health programs led to the decline in procedural dependence and the intensification of resource dependence.

If describing the sources of dependence emphasizes the constraints within which international bureaucracies function, identifying the sources of agency explains the desire of international bureaucracies to influence policies in spite of such constraints. Although international bureaucracies are vulnerable to exogenous pressures, they are not neutral about them. Dependence prevents international bureaucracies from acting irrespective of exogenous demands, but when such demands clash with independent goals and principles, bureaucracies are motivated to avoid them. Notably, although the analytical focus on the dependence of international organizations on their member states maintains the significant influence of member states over policy outcomes, it shifts the source of this influence from relations purely among states, which is the focus of most theories of international relations, to relations between states and the international bureaucracy. Policy outcomes, according to the analysis here, do not depend only on the ability of member states to shape the position of other member states but also on their ability to control the international organization's leadership and staff who attempt to circumvent exogenous pressures they oppose by strategically adapting to them.

Strategic Adaptation to External Pressures

In contrast to what most theories of international organizations would predict, the WHO staff and leadership actively participated in forming and greatly influenced the policies, programs, and initiatives that were adopted by the organization's member states. Furthermore, the WHO bureaucracy was not a neutral mediator, simply seeking to facilitate a workable compromise between competing interests. Rather, as a mediator, the WHO secretariat often tried to defend its independent ideational and material goals. Weaver (2008: 5) identifies two sources of potential conflicts for international organizations: "When the demands imposed by the external . . . environment conflict with [the organization's] internal structures and culture" and when "demands [among various masters] clash." In both instances, the independent goals of the international organization are at stake. In the first case, acting neutrally would directly undermine the international organization's goals. Also in the second case, the mediating role of the secretariat would be motivated by its independent concerns, and it would support member states whose position is in line with its own goals and preferences (see also Halliday and Carruthers 2009). This is especially so in the surprisingly frequent cases where member states defend their position by targeting criticism not at other member states but at the organization, thereby undermining the organization's legitimacy. The history of the WHO shows that when the goals or preferences of the organization were threatened, the WHO secretariat was often able to protect these goals and preferences.

This raises an important question that has so far attracted little attention in the literature: given the heavy dependence of international organizations on external actors, how could they possibly influence policy outcomes when their interests explicitly clash with the external expectations? The literature that perceives international organizations as arenas has unsurprisingly little interest in this question. Constructivists and principal-agent scholars, as we have seen, have also for the most part neglected to address this issue. Constructivists have mostly studied international organizations' autonomous action in instances in which external forces were supportive, indifferent, or uninformed of the action. Principal-agent scholars have similarly ignored instances of actual clashes.

To understand the capacity of international organizations to protect their goals and preferences even in cases of a potential conflict with member states, we have to focus our analysis not on organizations' symbolic resources, such as authority or knowledge, but on their practices, particularly their capacity for strategic action. Constructivists and principal-agent theories identify the conditions under which autonomous action is possible—authority and incomplete supervision, respectively—but acknowledge that this autonomy is typically partial.

The analysis here relies on their insights to suggest that in conditions of partial autonomy, the success of international organizations to protect their goals depends on how they *use* their symbolic resources, that is, their choice of strategies.

My analysis of the strategic responses available to international bureaucracies when facing demands that threaten their goals builds on explorations that have begun both among principal-agent scholars and constructivists. In a study on the issue by principal-agent theorists, Hawkins and Jacoby atypically investigate not the agents' characteristics but the strategies they use to try to circumvent principals' controls (Hawkins and Jacoby 2006). Their analysis, however, is limited to strategies intended to influence the agent's level of autonomy, such as reinterpretation of mandates, and they do not discuss strategies used by agents within given levels of autonomy. In turn, some constructivist accounts have begun to investigate the possibility of autonomous action under conditions of existing pressures (Barnett and Coleman 2005, Weaver 2006). These studies rely on insights from organizational sociology, which identify the capacity of organizations to act strategically to protect their goals and preferences against incongruous demands.

In organizational sociology, the focus on strategic action came as scholars reconsidered early articulations of neoinstitutionalist theory that suggested that organizations conformed to the dictates of their environments (DiMaggio 1983, Powell 1988) and came to recognize the possibility for an organization of purposive action and strategic choice. Significantly, these studies began to highlight the extent to which exogenous dictates were susceptible to interpretation, manipulation, revision, and elaboration by those subject to them (Scott 2008: 430, see also DiMaggio 1991, Goodstein 1994, Goodrick and Salancik 1996). Most systematically, Christine Oliver (1991) has offered a list of five possible responses by organizational actors to exogenous pressures.[4] Briefly, the possible responses include: acquiescence (acceding to pressures); compromise (exacting concessions); avoidance (attempting to preclude the necessity of conformity); defiance (rejecting expectations); and manipulation (attempting to actively change the content of the expectations). Barnett and Coleman (2005) have argued that the same range of strategies was available to international organizations and suggested a sixth response, that of strategic social construction (tailoring the environment so that it is consistent with the organization's goals); Weaver (2008) has described in detail the use of avoidance (or "organized hypocrisy") as a central strategy of the World Bank.

In these works, scholars have analyzed the responses available to organizations as if they followed a linear logic, varying "from passive conformity to active

---

4. Oliver (1991) draws on earlier articulations of possible strategies, including Pfeffer and Salancik (1978) and Scott (1981: chapter 8).

resistance" (Oliver 1991: 146). But the two dichotomies—passive/active and conformity/resistance—do not neatly overlap. What makes a response "passive" or "active" is not whether it conforms to or resists the exogenous demands. Rather, it is whether the response includes an attempt to alter the meaning of those demands, be this part of either conforming to or resisting them. (What Oliver calls "active" responses I refer to from now on as "strategic.") For example, Oliver lists manipulation—the purposeful attempt to co-opt, influence, or control institutional pressures in order to change the content of the expectations—as resistance, because it is "the most active response to these pressures" (Oliver 1991: 157). If due to manipulation the organization is able to avoid compliance with the original demands, then manipulation should indeed be viewed as a strategy of resistance. However, if after manipulating the content of the demands the organization adheres to the altered expectations *in a way that satisfies the original demands,* manipulation should instead be viewed as a form of strategic compliance. Lumping the two dichotomies together prevents an independent assessment of passive and strategic responses as distinct from compliance and resistance, which, I suggest below, is fundamental for our understanding of international organizations' ability to successfully deviate from exogenous prescriptions.

Table 2.1 displays the different types of responses that emerge if we maintain a distinction between the two dichotomies, so that the categories are based on (1) whether the responses employed lead to changes that satisfy the exogenous forces (compliance) or whether the responses employed avoid changes or lead to changes that do not satisfy the exogenous forces (resistance), and (2) whether the organizations take the pressures "as a given constraint to be obeyed or defied" (passive) or whether they attempt to redefine—"alter, re-create, or control"—the meaning of the exogenous pressures (strategic) (Oliver 1991: 159).

This categorization creates four types of possible responses. Passive responses are those that accept the demands as given and include passive compliance, when the international bureaucracy adheres to the original expectations, and passive resistance, when the international bureaucracy explicitly disobeys the exogenous demands. The familiar dichotomy between compliance and resistance refers, in fact, to these "passive" categories. However, the more common responses to external demands are adaptive responses, of strategic compliance and strategic

TABLE 2.1 Types of response to exogenous pressures

	COMPLIANCE	RESISTANCE
Passive	Adherence to original expectations	Disobedience
Strategic	Adherence to *reinterpreted* expectations	Voidance

resistance. Both strategic responses involve altering the meaning of the demands but with different intentions. In the case of strategic compliance, the international bureaucracy alters the meaning of the demands before it adheres to them. In the case of strategic resistance, the international bureaucracy reframes the demands so that it is no longer expected to conform to them.

When strategically complying with exogenous demands, an international bureaucracy endorses the demands of member states but only after giving those demands a meaning that, while compatible with the original expectations, could be reconciled with the organization's independent goals. Importantly, reinterpreting expectations (altering the meaning of the demands) is not the same as changing expectations (altering the demands), which should be considered an act of resistance rather than compliance. Strategic compliance is not about making the exogenous forces change their demands so much as convincing those forces that the original demands were met. Such strategic compliance leads not to partial compliance, which is one expected outcome of passive compliance (for example, in compromise), but to distorted compliance, that is, a complete adherence to the requirements, once those requirements are reinterpreted. By offering an acceptable reframing of the dominant logic—the challenge is exactly in making such reframing acceptable—international bureaucracies make such a distorted compliance look complete.

When strategically resisting exogenous demands, an international bureaucracy accepts, but does not adhere to, the external principles. Strategic resistance involves directly confronting, rather than bypassing (as in avoidance), the exogenous demands. Unlike passive articulations of defiance, however, strategic resistance attempts to minimize the extent to which external forces would view the response as challenging the legitimacy of their expectations. An international bureaucracy that strategically resists external expectations does not reject the dominant logic, but rather relies on that very logic to legitimate its refusal to comply. Such justifications may allow an international bureaucracy to void the expectation to comply, thereby rendering what member states might have viewed as provocative (passive) resistance into an agreeable action.

The response of the WHO secretariat to exogenous pressures reveals that when conflict emerged between the external demands and the organization's preferences, the organization's leadership and staff often did not take the course of passive compliance, which would have required a sacrifice of their material and/or ideational goals, but they also did not take the course of passive resistance, which would have threatened resources, votes, and/or legitimacy. Similarly, when trying to reach a compromise between competing positions, the secretariat generally avoided siding (complying) with one coalition and opposing (resisting) the other coalition. Instead, the WHO secretariat took authorship over the organization's response, by reframing the external demands so that they could be more easily reconciled with its own position. By formulating policies according to altered expectations, the WHO leadership and staff were able, at times, to comply in a way less disagreeable to them, hence minimizing the cost of compliance, and at other times, to refuse compliance in a way that was not considered resistance, thereby minimizing the risk of sanctions. In both cases, the WHO secretariat granted a new meaning to the dominant logic that altered the existing logic without explicitly challenging it. The selective compatibility between the NIEO logic and the WHO policies in the 1970s–1980s, as well as between the neoliberal logic and the WHO policies in the 1990s–2000s, was the outcome of this strategic adaptation: WHO policies were not simply a reflection of exogenous imposition as much as a translation to that imposition.

The WHO secretariat strategically complied with exogenous demands when adhering to reinterpreted expectations, that is, when successfully giving the dominant logic a meaning that was easier to reconcile with the organization's material and/or ideational goals. In the 1970s–1980s, the WHO leadership successfully presented the organization's agenda of Health for All by the Year 2000 and the primary health care approach as adhering to the New International Economic Order by redefining NIEO principles: regarding development as social development, focusing on intrastate rather than interstate inequities, championing self-reliance while downplaying the duties of developed countries, and supporting the transfer only of appropriate technologies. In the 1990s–2000s, the WHO was able to successfully incorporate health into a neoliberal agenda by promising that investment in health would lead to economic development and making cost-effective calculations an element in its call for "new universalism."

The WHO secretariat strategically resisted exogenous demands when accepting the dominant logic while being able to nullify the expectation to comply by suggesting that compliance was incompatible with that logic. During the NIEO phase, the WHO leadership successfully opposed an international code of marketing practices of pharmaceutical products by drawing on NIEO principles of political and economic sovereignty. During the neoliberal era, the WHO leadership was able to present its antismoking campaign as a justifiable exception to its otherwise probusiness position. In a dispute over intellectual property protection, the WHO secretariat again resisted without challenging the dominant logic by claiming that intellectual property rules already contained the flexibilities that should be used for the manufacturing of generic versions of patented AIDS drugs.

The experience of the WHO suggests that while passive responses are the ones most often described in the literature, strategic responses are at least as common. The reason is risk avoidance: passive compliance undermines the organization's material and/or ideational goals and passive resistance threatens its resources, votes, and/or legitimacy. In contrast, altering the meaning of the demands reduces the extent to which an organization's principles and goals are sacrificed, and successfully justifying resistance lowers the risk of being penalized for it. This form of risk reduction, in turn, has important analytical implications regarding the limits of strategic responses and the conditions under which such responses are possible.

Conditions for Strategic Adaptation and the Question of Leadership

Both in the 1970s–1980s and 1990s–2000s, the WHO secretariat responded to a new dominant logic by strategically adapting to it. The experience of the WHO is not unique: other international bureaucracies have also often strategically complied with or strategically resisted exogenous demands. For example, during the NIEO era, the International Labor Organization (ILO) focused on manpower and productivity, which gave it an entry into issues of interest to developing countries, and avoided debates over labor standards and trade union freedom, which were not supported by them (Melanson 1979, Standing 2008). With the rise of neoliberal thought, the ILO strategically adapted to the probusiness environment by initiating, in 1998, the ILO Declaration on Fundamental Principles of Rights at Work, which committed member countries, and their employer and union bodies, to a small number of "core" labor standards. As Standing (2008) rightly maintains, these were only a few of the labor standards previously defended by the ILO and the least controversial from among them, but in this way the ILO secretariat was able to preserve some of its goals in a relatively hostile environment. The staff at the UN Children's Fund (UNICEF) also strategically adapted to the neoliberal environment: in the mid-1980s, the UNICEF secretariat endorsed some neoliberal-compatible initiatives, such as the selective primary health care approach (which the WHO leadership at the time still opposed; see chapter 3) and, following the World Bank's position, user fees (see chapter 6). However, UNICEF also launched a campaign for "adjustment with a human face" that called for the consideration of children's health in the World Bank structural adjustment programs (Jolly 1991, Banerji 1999).

In other cases, however, international organizations took a different path, whether passively complying with or passively resisting the expectations of their member states. The UN Educational, Scientific and Cultural Organization (UNESCO) in the 1970s, for example, passively complied with relatively radical demands of developing countries and initiated a controversial New International Information Order without attempting to alter the demands so to maintain the organization's legitimacy in the eyes of developed countries. The U.S. government argued that the proposed policies undermined independent journalism and ultimately withdrew from the organization. The WHO, too, at times employed passive responses. Indeed, the organization began to respond strategically to neoliberal demands only in the late 1990s. In addition, not all the strategic responses are equally effective. Under what conditions, then, do international bureaucracies engage in strategic rather than passive forms of response? When do they choose strategic compliance and when strategic resistance? And under what conditions are they more likely to succeed?

Scholars have argued that an organization's choice of response to exogenous pressures is determined by the perceived cost to the organizational goals that compliance would require compared to the cost to the organization if it resisted the exogenous demands (Oliver 1991, Barnett and Coleman 2005). However, strategic responses to exogenous demands lower the potential costs: altering the meaning of the demands that the organization complies with reduces the degree to which the organization's principles and goals are sacrificed, and being able to convincingly justify resistance reduces the risk of being penalized for it. The potential ability to reduce costs, by means of strategic compliance or resistance, means that costs alone cannot explain an organization's choice of action. Instead, we need to consider the factors that provide organizations capacity for reducing the potential costs, that is, capacity for adaptive strategies. The history of the WHO highlights three conditions that enable strategic responses: independent goals and preferences, scope of supervision, and leadership.

Independent goals and preferences. Strategic adaptation is called for only when there is a recognized clash between the demands made by the environment and the organization's material or ideational goals (Barnett and Coleman 2005: 595). For such a clash to occur the organization's goals have to develop independently of its political environment. This would normally be the case unless the dominant forces in the environment are able to co-opt the organization or its leadership. Co-optation by exogenous forces is more likely when an organization is dependent on the same parties both for votes and funds (for example, the World Bank) but can also occur without such an intentional design (for example, UNESCO during the NIEO era was arguably overcommitted to the NIEO at the expense of the organization's own goals). Without the presence of other conditions, however, independent goals and preferences could still lead to passive, rather than strategic, responses.

Scope of supervision. As principal-agent theorists rightly emphasize, the scope of supervision available to member states over the international bureaucracy affects the agent's capacity for strategic action. Principal-agent theories identify a number of likely imperfections of oversight mechanisms that lead to agency, including uncertainty, lack of information, and multiple principal problems. One potentially significant condition for effective supervision, not mentioned in the principal-agent analyses, is the position of the delegates representing and talking on behalf of member states at the international organization. States themselves are fragmented into partially autonomous bureaucracies, with officials often representing the position of their respective departments rather than of the government as a whole (Chorev 2007). Most delegates to the World Health Assembly come from health ministries and are likely to have their own reasons (such as competition for budget allocations at home) to support policies advocated by the WHO secretariat. These delegates also often share the professional ethos of WHO officials. The potential alliance of delegates with the international organization undermines effective supervision. This is all the more so when the delegates come from departments relatively marginalized in the government, such as health or education, rather than departments that are likely to be more influential in the government, such as finance or foreign affairs. This is one of the reasons wealthy states tend to send to the World Health Assembly also delegates from ministries of foreign affairs.

Scholars often suggest that a multiplicity of external demands, made by competing parties, decreases members' supervision and increases the organization's room for maneuvering (Oliver 1991, Nielson and Tierney 2003). The WHO's experience reveals that the opposite is the case, and that conflicting expectations—from wealthy countries, poor countries, health activists, pharmaceutical companies, and so on—have limited the secretariat's adaptive capacity. In such cases, especially when conflict between member states puts the reputation of the organization at risk, strategic adaptation is often used to reach a compromise agreeable to the competing exogenous interests at the cost of the marginalization of the organization's own position. This was illustrated in the modified position of the WHO bureaucracy regarding the model list of essential drugs, which reflected the bureaucracy's need to address both the expectations of developing countries and the fierce opposition of pharmaceutical companies to the way the WHO responded to those expectations (see chapter 4). The presence of a multiplicity of demands may also affect the choice among strategic responses: a multiplicity of demands limits the organization's interpretive flexibility while providing some external support for a defiant response, and so multiple demands often lead to strategic resistance rather than to strategic compliance, as was the case in the WHO bureaucracy's response to the code of conduct of marketing of pharmaceutical products (see chapter 4).

A third factor that determines the scope of supervision relates to the precision of the demands. Goodrick and Salancik (1996) have convincingly maintained that exogenous pressures are most influential—that is, most likely to lead to passive compliance—when they are certain, since uncertainty creates discretion, which allows organizations to use their own particularistic interests to guide their definition of appropriate action. When the exogenous expectations are imprecise, organizations can "generate variation in practice while conforming to their [political environment] by pursuing their strategic interests within the limits of the discretion permitted by the [environment] generating it" (Goodrick and Salancik 1996: 2, also Edelman 1992). The types of expectations, then, set the boundaries of permitted discretion and therefore the range of available strategies. Some organizations are more likely to face loose expectations while others more often receive tailored instructions: international organizations, due to their unique specialization and differentiated mandates, often face loose expectations, but this does not need to be the case.

The specificity of demands may also affect the choice between adaptive strategies and the likelihood of success. While loose expectations allow for strategic compliance, the possibility for creative interpretation is more restricted when demands are more concise, and organizations are therefore likely to resort to strategic resistance in such cases; when organizations resort to strategic compliance, their scope of maneuvering is limited. This is one reason for some differences in the WHO's strategic adaptation in the 1970s–1980s and the 1990s–2000s. The NIEO principles did not directly touch on health issues, which allowed for the creative interpretations provided by the WHO secretariat. In the 1990s–2000s, in contrast, partly due to the interest of the World Bank in global health policies, the exogenous pressures were, at times, uncharacteristically specific. This made it more difficult for the WHO bureaucracy to reinterpret the exogenous expectations in a way more compatible with its goals.

Leadership. Another reason why the same organization would choose strategic adaptation in some periods and not in others is the leadership in place. At the WHO, in particular, directors-general have greatly influenced the strategic capability of the organization. Both Halfdan Mahler, who was the director-general from 1974 until 1988, and Gro Harlem Brundtland, who was the director-general from 1998 until 2003, were essential in making strategic adaptation possible during the NIEO and the neoliberal eras, respectively. In contrast, toward the end of his tenure, Mahler failed to respond to neoliberal pressures when they first emerged at the international level and the WHO was all but inactive throughout the tenure of Hiroshi Nakajima, from 1988 to 1998.

How to explain the constitutive role of leadership in public bureaucracies? Traditionally, most of the literature on international relations concerned with the question of executive leadership followed a "great-man theory of international organization," which focused on the personal characteristics of the leader in question. The exception was the work by Ernst B. Haas (1964), which situated the leader within a given environment and emphasized the leader's capacity to manipulate that environment to expand the agency's authority. Robert Cox (1969), while agreeing with Haas, has criticized him for "an underestimation of the constraints which are inherent in the set of relationships of which the executive head is a part," particularly with the rest of the bureaucracy, member states, and the international system. Indeed, in just the way that the agency of international organizations is constrained by its environment, as analyzed in detail above, the agency of individuals in an international organization, including leaders, is also constrained by both the organization and the environment. We can think of it in terms of "nested agency," where individual agents act within the constraints of their organizations that act, in turn, within the constraints of their environments.

Here again, it is useful to draw from organizational sociology, which has similarly struggled with the "paradox of embedded agency" (Holm 1995), that is, with the possibility for human agency in conditions of organizational constraints. Scholars of organizations identified two types of conditions that enable "institutional entrepreneurship" (DiMaggio 1988), that is, agents capable of introducing changes that are "divergent with reference to the institutional environment in which they are embedded" (Battilana, Leca, and Boxenbaum 2009). The first type of enabling conditions includes "field-level" institutional characteristics (Battilana, Leca, and Boxenbaum 2009: 74) that determine the institutional scope of action. The two factors highlighted above, independent goals and imprecise expectations, are such field-level characteristics. However, as the example of the WHO clearly illustrates, "although field-level conditions . . . seem to play an important enabling role in institutional entrepreneurship, all actors embedded in the same field are not equally likely to act as institutional entrepreneurs" (Battilana, Leca, and Boxenbaum 2009: 75). The second type of enabling conditions emphasizes actors' specific characteristics. Particularly important here are an actor's institutional characteristics, including "the social position an actor occupies within an organizational field" (Battilana, Leca and Boxenbaum 2009: 75). A comparison of the WHO's divergent experiences under Mahler, Nakajima, and Brundtland suggests that an actor's position both in the organization and in the environment are important. In particular, institutional entrepreneurship in the form of strategic adaptation depends on three types of social position.

The first is social position in the organization. Strategic response is more likely to occur when the institutional conditions allow for strong, effective leadership. Institutional conditions for strong leadership provide the actor with the means to transform the organization without such attempts being paralyzed by external opposition or internal debates. Specialized agencies and programs in the UN have been unexpectedly conducive to strong leaders, such as Raul Prebisch at the UN Conference on Trade and Development (UNC-TAD) and James P. Grant at UNICEF. At the WHO, too, the institutional conditions have allowed directors-general to effectively shape the direction of the organization. For example, the director-general has control over the budget and therefore great influence over the organization's priorities.[5] In addition, directors-general can often create new divisions, hire new recruits to run those divisions, and in other ways "layer" (Schickler 2001, Streeck and Thelen 2005: 22–24) new priorities on top of old programs, while avoiding the conflicts that would emerge out of actively abandoning previous priorities. The authority that directors-general have over staffing is essential for strategic adaptation because, as Chwieroth (2008b) convincingly argues, while it is possible to change the position of existing staff, it is more common for organizations to change their perceptions through the entry into the organization of new recruits.

The second type is social position in the environment. Strategic response is more likely to occur when the leaders are partially embedded in the exogenous environment. The organizational literature on individual characteristics focuses mostly on actors' social position in their organization. In addition, however, and fundamental for understanding the differences between Mahler and Brundtland on the one hand and Nakajima on the other hand, we have to consider the social position of the actor in the environment (Thornton and Ocasio 1999). Specifically, institutional entrepreneurship is more likely when the actors can function as bridges between the organization and the broader environment. Both Mahler and Brundtland were familiar with and appreciative of the dominant logic that as directors-general they were expected to navigate. In each case, being part of the new logic meant that the incoming director-general could adopt, at least in part, the new exogenous principles and was in possession or able to gain sufficient knowledge of the new environment to be able to manipulate it. Mahler's experience as a WHO official in India led to a great fit between his position on public health matters and the New International Economic Order. Similarly, Brundtland's political background and experience, especially as the

---

5. As I describe in chapter 1, the WHO's Executive Board makes comments and recommendations regarding the program and budget estimates. However, this failed to translate to evident influence: "If he wishes, the Director General may ignore any such [Executive Board] recommendations. . . . This fact does tend to render discussions on the budget by the Board less effective than they might be." "Memorandum by the Ministry of Health," Paper to be submitted by France to the Geneva Group Meeting 6 and 7 April, 1967, World Health Organization, FCO 61/75 (Finances—Geneva Group). UK National Archives.

chair of the UN World Commission on Environment and Development, were compatible with the neoliberal world order. In both cases, member states respected the directors-general and trusted their agenda. In contrast, one explanation for the WHO's inaction during the 1980s was that the director-general during that time, Hiroshi Nakajima, was poorly positioned in the U.S.-dominant order: the U.S. government initially opposed the appointment of Nakajima, who was Japanese, and U.S. and many Western European delegates objected to his leadership style, complained about his communication skills, and the like. While partial embeddedness is an important condition, complete embeddedness— leading to greater loyalty to the environment than to the organization—may lead to passive compliance, which was the case with UNESCO in the NIEO era.

Third is a tendency for strategic capacity of leaders to decline over time. The institutional arrangements allowing for strong leadership are particularly useful for newly recruited leaders who can rethink the organization's position and introduce strategic changes that, if the leaders are also well positioned in the environment, are likely to be successfully accepted by member states. However, these policy changes, and the ideas that inform or legitimate them, then get institutionalized and become barriers when new exogenous conditions introduce themselves and require a response from the organization. Moreover, once the external environment changes, the leader may no longer be an effective bridge. Indeed, strategic responses to the NIEO and neoliberalism were launched at the WHO by Mahler and Brundtland, respectively, when they were both just appointed. Directors-general who were in charge of the organization before the environmental changes occurred are likely to find it difficult to respond effectively. Mahler was ineffective when neoliberalism emerged in the mid-1980s. In contrast, the UNICEF secretariat, which had a shift of leadership in 1980, was much quicker than the WHO to respond to the rise of a new order in this period.

In short, a number of conditions need to be in place for an international bureaucracy to engage in strategic response. In particular, strategic adaptation is more likely to occur when the organization has independent goals and preferences that clash with the new expectations; when external supervision is relatively loose; and when the organization has a strong, well positioned, and recently appointed leader.

Organizational Change and Strategic Limitations

Finally, how are international organizations affected by a strategic response to external demands? One of the consequences of considering strategic responses as a form of resistance is that it gives the impression that an altering of external demands will prevent compliance, and therefore the need for change. Supposedly, successful alteration of the original demands allows the organization to stay the way it was. In contrast, the distinction between compliance/resistance and passive/strategic responses highlights how significant changes are often called for even when strategic action is involved. Strategic compliance requires the international organization to adapt to the new demands, however much they are successfully altered. Change is also often the outcome of strategic resistance, since it requires the acceptance of the dominant logic even while resisting it.[6] In responding to new environments, the WHO secretariat changed the organization's priorities, the types of policies and programs advocated to address those priorities, and in the 1990s also its institutional structure. Strategic adaptation to the dominant logic—either by way of compliance or resistance—has forced the WHO to abandon old policies and adopt new ones, which, while protecting some of the organization's interests, have nonetheless been in line with the new environment. The need for change implies that while reinterpretation of demands allows better protection of an organization's goals, strategic compliance and resistance are not about "duping" the environment: to be effective, the reframing has to make sense to the exogenous forces and therefore cannot stray too far from the dominant logic.[7]

The likelihood of organizational change reflects the real constraints imposed by exogenous pressures even when these are successfully tamed. Hence, strategic adaptation demarcates not only the possibilities for international bureaucracies to preserve their goals in the midst of exogenous transformations, but also the *limits* to their abilities to do so, even when successful. The possible success of a strategic response is limited, even when the international bureaucracy is capable of strategic action, by the logical boundaries of the original demands. In some cases, it may also be limited by the ability of external forces to later co-opt the interpreted meanings provided by the international bureaucracy so that they fit more closely to their own interests (see, for example, the case of selective primary health care, in chapter 3).

In the remainder of the book I describe the WHO bureaucracy's strategic adaptation to external pressures. I show that when the WHO bureaucracy has faced exogenous pressures for change, the staff and leadership have responded by designing programs and policies that are compatible with reformulated demands,

---

6. Change may even be the result of passive resistance. In the case of avoidance, for example, DiMaggio and Powell (1983) suggest that "the fact that these changes may be largely ceremonial does not mean that they are inconsequential," and Hallett (2010) shows that myths do become incarnate.
    7. This was recognized by the "old" institutionalists in organizational sociology. Selznick (1949) stressed, for example, that the strategy of co-optation, which the Tennessee Valley Authority adopted, "decisively affected its capacity to uphold standards of environmental protection."

so that they can be reconciled with the organization's preferences and goals. Strategic compliance has minimized the sacrifice of the organization's goals, which passive compliance would have required, and strategic resistance has minimized the risk of costly sanctions, which passive resistance would have entailed. Using such strategies, the WHO has changed quite radically and has not always avoided the sacrifice of its goals or the dissatisfaction of at least some member states. Nonetheless, the gap between the dominant logic and the WHO programs in each era and the ability of the WHO bureaucracy to maintain, in spite of radical changes, a stable notion of its identity and its goals, attest to the ability of international organizations to transform the global regime and align it with their agendas and therefore to significantly contribute to the future of the international community.

A NEW INTERNATIONAL ORDER IN HEALTH

By the early 1970s, the global political-economic conditions that had informed the policies of the World Health Organization during its first decades had radically transformed. Decolonization led to the establishment of a large number of independent states, and Third World countries, as they were then called, soon became the majority in the United Nations and its specialized agencies, and therefore an influential force in shaping international policies. Cooperation among Latin American, Asian, and African countries resulted in a unified criticism of the relations of developed countries and transnational enterprises with the developing world, which, these developing countries now argued, had impeded poor countries' potential for economic growth. In 1974, these accusations led to a formal call at the UN General Assembly for a New International Economic Order (NIEO). The NIEO was based on a number of fundamental principles, including sovereign equity and justice, duties of developed states, economic and social development, economic sovereignty, universal international organizations, and collective self-reliance.

With decolonization, the WHO secretariat confronted new exogenous demands, as developing countries expected the organization to advance policies and projects that were compatible with NIEO principles. Some of the new issues raised at the World Health Assembly reflected developing countries' support of self-determination and political sovereignty; for example, concerns regarding health conditions under apartheid in South Africa and the Israeli occupation of Palestinian territories. In addition, and fundamental to the core mission of the organization, the WHO was asked to develop health programs that responded to the economic needs and aspirations of poor countries.

At the time, developing countries had an uncharacteristic leverage over the WHO secretariat. An unprecedented level of the WHO's dependence on poor countries was the outcome, first, of developing countries gaining the majority of votes at the World Health Assembly, which followed a one-country/one-vote rule. Additionally, at the time, developing countries were able to maintain an exceptionally stable coalition, so that they were consistently unified in how they voted. The economic theories informing the new international economic order were also essential for the willingness of developing countries to utilize their procedural leverage: holding that their economies could grow independently of the global north gave developing countries the confidence to consistently vote in defiance of rich countries' demands.[1]

The level of the WHO's resource dependence on rich countries during that period, in turn, was relatively low. This was largely because, at the time, the WHO's budget consisted mainly of mandatory (rather than voluntary) contributions, which were suggested by the director-general and determined by the World Health Assembly. As a result, the minority of rich countries did not have much impact on budget decisions. Under these institutional conditions, the only way for rich countries to utilize their resource leverage was to withdraw from the international organization. The WHO secretariat was certainly aware of this possibility, since during the same contentious period the United States did withdraw from the ILO and later UNESCO (Melanson 1979, Imber 1989), but given the extremity of such an "exit" measure, it was useless for most disagreements (Hirschman 1970). In an attempt to have a "voice" against the "rapid growth in the activities and budgets of the main Specialized Agencies and the accompanying decline in our influence,"[2] the countries that contributed significant funds to the WHO and other UN agencies established a forum for coordinating their strategies, the Geneva Group (see chapter 5). However, during the 1970s and the 1980s, Geneva Group members were too disjointed in their positions to maintain a coherent stand at the assembly. Finally, the WHO leadership's embrace of public health trends that favored community-based care, which could be pursued even in conditions of scarce resources, had the effect not only of preempting the

---

1. During that period, the U.S. administration complained of having only limited influence over developing countries and the Arab nations at the World Health Assembly: "We are often in the dark about G-77 or Arab League closed-door decisions in the course of the World Health Assembly until they suddenly appear as conference documents. Our ability . . . to influence the actions of those delegations once the caucus has reached a decision is limited." Memorandum, "Improved U.S. Participation in International Organizations and Programs—WHO," June 27, 1978, Box 53. Carter Presidential Library.
2. Note by the Foreign Office, "UN Specialized Agencies," October 2, 1964, OD 29/59. UK National Archives.

potential opposition of developed countries but also of reducing the resource dependence of the organization on them.

In short, the balance between procedural dependence on developing countries and resource dependence on rich countries was uncharacteristically tilted in favor of developing countries, and the WHO leadership, realizing that they were in no position to ignore "the imperatives of contemporary history,"[3] committed itself to the cause of a new international economic order. In the 1970s and early 1980s, the WHO put forth new priorities that were celebrated as loyal representations of the NIEO spirit. A WHO document, "Technical Discussions on The Contribution of Health to The New International Economic Order," contended that "the health sector is giving the lead in showing how the theory of the NIEO can be put into practice, and is providing models for other sectors" (WHO 1980a). However, the WHO secretariat's response to developing countries' expectations was often strategic. The decision to act strategically and the content of the strategic response were heavily informed by the WHO leadership's public health orientation and by the desire not to unnecessarily upset the rich countries.

Consequently, the WHO secretariat embraced principles and policies that were based on NIEO themes, but only after altering the meaning of these themes so they were compatible with WHO's core mission and public health understanding and more agreeable to Western countries than the original call for the NIEO had been. This chapter focuses on the WHO's central program and main contributions to the NIEO: a call for "Health for All by the Year 2000," to be achieved by primary health care. (In chapter 4, I examine a number of additional programs, which required the WHO to form a position on multinational corporations). The analysis of Health for All and of primary health care shows that the WHO secretariat shifted the NIEO call for "economic and social development" from the original focus on economic development, measured in terms of economic growth, to a focus on social development, which referred to individuals' quality of life and allowed for attention to be paid to conditions such as health and education. In addition, the WHO bureaucracy championed the NIEO call for greater equity, but altered the focus of concern from equity among states to equity within states, which reflected WHO's concern with those "most in need." The WHO secretariat also altered the NIEO principle of collective self-reliance. Self-reliance was used to encourage the full participation of developing countries in the decision-making process of the WHO but also to encourage the participation of communities at the local level, thereby expanding NIEO principles beyond

---

3. "The Political Struggle for Health," Address by Dr. H. Mahler, Director-General of the WHO, at the Twenty-Ninth Session of the Regional Committee for the Western Pacific, Manila, 21 August 1978. WHO Library.

their original intention. In other instances, self-reliance was used to justify a nation's reliance on its own economic resources, a principle integral to the primary health care approach and crucial for gaining the support of developed countries.

The WHO policies and priorities during the 1970s and 1980s—based on the principles of development, equity, and self-reliance—changed the organization quite radically, a transformation described as the end of "the technological explosion in public health" and the beginning of "a social revolution in community health."[4] This "social revolution," however, reflected a significant discrepancy between the NIEO and WHO policies. This chapter shows that this discrepancy was created through the maneuvering of the WHO leadership and staff rather than negotiations between North and South. By means of strategic adaptation, the WHO satisfied the expectations of developing countries while safeguarding the organization's material and ideational goals. Through its strategic response, the WHO bureaucracy did not simply reproduce the dominant logic, but significantly altered it.

The New International Economic Order

The Rise of "Young and Unsophisticated Countries"

The rapid wave of decolonization increased the number of UN member states from the 51 original members that had signed the Charter on the United Nations in 1945, to 126 members by 1968.[5] Western countries that had previously dominated the international stage soon realized the impact decolonization could have on the operations of the United Nations. A memo from Arthur Schlesinger, special assistant to President John F. Kennedy, warned of "an impending crisis of confidence in American attitudes toward the UN." The memo explained,

> The new apprehensions . . . rise in great part from the flow of new small nations into the UN, from the expectation that this will continue for some time to come, and from the proposed consequence that the General Assembly will be dominated in the future by untried people from young and unsophisticated countries.[6]

---

4. "Social Perspectives in Health," Address by Dr. H. Mahler, Director-General of the World Health Organization, in Presenting his Report for 1975 to the Twenty-Ninth World Health Assembly, Geneva, 4 May 1976. WHO Library.

5. A list of UN members, by the year of becoming a member, is published in http://www.un.org/en/members/growth.shtml#text.

6. Memorandum from Arthur Schlesinger, the President's Special Assistant, to President John F. Kennedy, January 19, 1962. Ford Presidential Library.

Indeed, a year before this exchange, an association of developing countries, the Nonaligned Movement (NAM), had emerged on the international scene with the number of its members growing rapidly from an original twenty-five in 1961 to eighty-five by 1976. "By non-alignment," explained the president of Tanzania Julius Kambarage Nyerere, "we are . . . asserting the right of small . . . nations to determine their own policies in their own interests, and to have an influence on world affairs" (cited in McMichael 2000: 54). The main objectives of the non-aligned countries were initially political, including decolonization, national self-determination, and noninterference in the internal affairs of states. But concerns with economic development were expressed at the NAM's first meeting, and they gained greater prominence as some of the political objectives were achieved or lost their urgency (Sauvant 1981: 7–9).

Concretely, Third World governments felt increasingly cheated out of the trade-induced economic growth that rich nations enjoyed. The economic-nationalist strategy of import substitution industrialization (ISI), which many developing countries had embraced, first in Latin America and then in Asia, Africa, and the Middle East, spurred impressive industrial development but translated to limited economic growth (Frieden 2006: 305).[7] The Third World comprised 70 percent of the world's population, but contributed no more than 12 percent of the world's production. The share of developing countries in world trade steadily declined, from 31 percent in 1950 to 18 percent in 1972, and the income gap between the North and the South failed to decrease. The rich industrial states also held almost 100 percent of the world's research facilities (Sauvant 1981, Doyle 1983). Trade restrictions under President Richard Nixon's New Economic Policy and the closing of the gold window in 1971 established new grievances against the United States and reaffirmed the perception that the international order operated to the detriment of all Third World states (Murphy 1984: 92–100).

Third World governments understood that their shared fate of poverty was the outcome of their common structural position in the world economy. As President Nyerere of Tanzania put it: "What we have in common is that we are all, in relation to the developed world, dependent (not interdependent) nations. Each of our economies has developed as a by-product and a subsidiary of development in the industrialized North, and is externally oriented" (cited in Doyle 1983: 430). The South became poor under colonialism and remained poor by being subject to the disadvantages of growth in a world economy dominated by

---

7. ISI consisted of policies aimed at reserving the domestic market of consumer nondurable goods for local industries, in attempt to shift away from specialization in primary product exports and to increase industrial production of goods. For that purpose, governments imposed high tariffs to exclude competing imports, manipulated the exchange rate, and provided public subsidies especially for "infant industries" (McMichael 2000: 36–38, Frieden 2006: 301–310).

the North in which the South was relegated to raw-material production (Doyle 1983: 430–431). Both the understanding of the international division of labor as a form of injustice and the articulation of the demands owed much to Raul Prebisch, an Argentine economist who had been the secretary-general of the UN Economic Commission for Latin America, ECLA (Murphy 1983, Sanders 1991).

These realizations led to fresh radicalization, reflected in statements such as those made by Dr. Mahbub ul Haq, a former finance minister of Pakistan, who described a "poverty curtain" that had descended across the face of the world, "dividing it materially and philosophically into two different worlds, two separate planets, two unequal humanities—one embarrassingly rich and the other desperately poor." The struggle against this unequal relationship, he warned, was "the most formidable challenge of our time" (ul Haq 1976: xv).

Lifting the "Poverty Curtain"

This overwhelming sense of injustice led to concrete political and economic demands. At the first Conference of Nonaligned Heads of State or Government, in 1961, the communiqué declared that the nonaligned countries "consider it necessary to close, through accelerated economic, industrial and agricultural development, the ever widening gap in the standard of living between the few economically advanced countries and the many economically less developed countries" (cited in Sanders 1991: 299). Developing countries' first organizational achievement was the UN Conference on Trade and Development (UNCTAD I), which convened in 1964 and was intended as an alternative forum to the North-dominated General Agreement on Tariffs and Trade (GATT) (Murphy 1984, Sanders 1991). During the conference, developing countries established the Group of 77 (G-77), which became a powerful coalition that represented the economic interests of developing countries in international organizations. The G-77, together with UNCTAD, was crucial in elaborating many of the individual elements of the NIEO and representing developing countries in the subsequent negotiations with the North (Sauvant 1981: 9). But UNCTAD I itself was not a great success, as Western developed countries opposed or abstained from many of the conference's sixty major resolutions. A patronizing memo by the U.S. undersecretary of state George Ball described the conference as "an organized pressure campaign designed to force a massive transfer of resources from the industrialized countries to the less-developed countries."[8] However, the conference did create, over the

---

8. Memorandum from George W. Ball, the Undersecretary of State, to President Lyndon B. Johnson, March 30, 1964. Ford Presidential Library.

objections of the developed countries, a permanent secretariat for the UNCTAD, and Raul Prebisch was appointed the founding secretary-general (Helleiner 1976, Sanders 1991). Under the leadership of Prebisch, the UNCTAD secretariat created special relations with the G-77, which were reflected in UNCTAD's ideological commitment to the developing world. The secretariat also gave much administrative help to the Third World: it produced papers, advised the G-77 on negotiating strategies against the Western states, made partisan alliances, and arbitrated disputes between developing countries (Sanders 1991).

In subsequent UNCTAD and other international conferences, the demands of developing countries extended beyond reform of the existing economic system (mostly, by removing inequitable terms of trade) to a call for the establishment of a *new* order.[9] This shift was greatly influenced by the provocative actions of the Organization of Petroleum Exporting Countries (OPEC). In response to the war that had broken out in the Middle East in October 1973, OPEC imposed an embargo on oil exports to the United States and other states and quadrupled oil prices, from $3.01 to $11.65 per barrel (Jankowitsch and Sauvant 1981). Developing countries that imported petroleum suffered severely as a consequence, but it made them realize that they, too, were not without effective means for applying pressure (Helleiner 1976, de Montbrial 1975: 61–62, Gosovic and Ruggie 1976: 316–319). A UK memo succinctly summarized the political effects the oil shock had on the G-77:

> It was the power demonstrated by the oil producers . . . which first suggested to developing countries as a whole that the economic dominance, so long resented, of the industrialized countries might not be inevitable or eternal. Many developing countries claimed, and perhaps believed, that this presaged a more general transfer of power to the developing world as a whole. . . . The objective of this campaign is the establishment of a "New International Economic Order."[10]

Soon thereafter, the UN General Assembly passed a number of resolutions that were to form the basis for this New Order. The Sixth Special Session of the General Assembly, which took place from April 9 to May 2, 1974, adopted two documents, the "Declaration on the Establishment of a New International

---

9. Conferences at which developing countries called for a new order included UNCTAD II in February 1968, the Third Conference of Heads of State or Government of Nonaligned Countries in Lusaka in September 1970, UNCTAD III in 1972, the Nonaligned Foreign Ministers Conference in Guyana in August 1972, and the Fourth Summit of Nonaligned Countries in Algiers in September 1973 (Sauvant 1981, Sanders 1991).

10. "The New International Economic Order," Undated, FCO 49/573, NIEO Planning paper. UK National Archives.

Economic Order," and "Programme of Action on the Establishment of a New International Economic Order."[11] The resolutions were adopted by consensus (without a vote) but "contained a great deal that was unacceptable to western countries."[12] Although more than two hundred reservations were expressed by the industrialized countries, this was a major triumph for the developing world as the resolutions covered all of the economic issues of concern to the G-77 (Murphy 1984: 114). Following the Sixth Special Session, on 12 December 1974 during the Twenty-Ninth Session of the UN General Assembly, the G-77 brought to vote a "Charter of Economic Rights and Duties of States," which stated the right of states to regulate foreign investment and activities of transnational corporations. The charter was adopted by majority vote rather than consensus, with most developed countries voting against or abstaining (Gosovic and Ruggie 1976: 314, Jankowitsch and Sauvant 1981). Finally, the Seventh Special Session introduced a much less controversial resolution, "Development and International Economic Cooperation."[13]

What's New in the New International Economic Order?

The resolutions supporting a New International Economic Order expressed a number of principles that intended to remedy the injustices of the existing system. These NIEO principles were broad in scope and potentially inconsistent, because the G-77 was composed of countries that were quite differently positioned in the world economy and therefore had diverse needs and priorities. While the more industrialized countries tended to be concerned with access to markets and debt relief, countries that heavily relied on a small number of export commodities looked for policies that would increase the purchasing power of their export revenues (Sanders 1991, Hart 1983). Unity among these diverse interests was often achieved by including every concern of any country (Sanders 1991, Hart 1983).

Sovereign equity. The UN resolutions committed member states to establish a new order that would "correct inequalities and redress existing injustices [and] make it possible to eliminate the widening gap between the developed and the

---

11. I describe the principles accepted in these and subsequent resolutions below. See also Murphy 1984: 114, Gosovic and Ruggie 1976, Jankowitsch and Sauvant 1981: 68–71.

12. Memorandum from J.A.L. Faint, "The 'New International Economic Order,'" 1 August 1975, FCO 61/1297 (UN and the New Economic Order). UK National Archives.

13. The resolution diluted most of the more radical principles the G-77 had put forward in the Sixth Special Session and was viewed by some as a "major diplomatic coup" for the United States (Berlin 1975). The resolution was adopted unanimously, with the United States and some other Western nations expressing a number of reservations (Gosovic and Ruggie 1976).

developing countries."[14] The New Order was to be based on equity among sovereign nations, "whereby the prevailing disparities in the world may be banished and prosperity secured for all."[15]

Duties of developed states. Inequalities among states were perceived as the doing of industrialized countries, which therefore had the duty to support poor countries in creating a new world order. Governments of the newer states, mostly African, explained the duties of developed states toward the world poor by the fact that they had once exploited their colonies (Murphy 1984: 82–83). Latin American dependency theories emphasized current relations of exploitation that linked the poverty of the underdeveloped nations to the wealth of the developed nations, thereby establishing the duties of developed states to all poor countries, not only the recently decolonized (Murphy 1984: 92).

Economic and social development. The objective of the Programme of Action was to strengthen "the role of the United Nations in the field of world-wide cooperation for economic and social development."[16] To "ensure steadily accelerating economic and social development,"[17] the G-77 focused on means to improve the position of developing countries within the global economic order. Given a tendency for declining terms of trade—prices of raw materials and agricultural products tended to decline over time while prices of manufactured products tended to rise (Frieden 2006: 310–311)—the G-77 called for increased industrialization, which was perceived as the only sustainable strategy for economic growth, and for improved access to foreign markets for their primary commodities.[18] Industrialization was to be achieved through the transfer of industrial production, mostly labor-intensive and low-technology, from industrialized countries.[19] To gain better access to foreign markets, the G-77 asked for reduced tariffs and nontariff barriers to trade.[20] To improve the terms of trade of their

---

14. "Declaration on the Establishment of a New International Economic Order," UN General Assembly, Sixth Special Session, 1 May 1974, A/RES/S-6/3201.

15. Ibid.

16. "Programme of Action on the Establishment of a New International Economic Order," UN General Assembly, Sixth Special Session, 1 May 1974, A/RES/S-6/3202.

17. "Declaration on the Establishment of a New International Economic Order," UN General Assembly, Sixth Special Session, 1 May 1974, A/RES/S-6/3201.

18. "Charter of Economic Rights and Duties of States," UN General Assembly, Twenty-ninth Session, 12 December 1974, A/RES/29/3281; Sauvant 1981.

19. To help promote industrial development in developing countries, the UN Industrial Development Organization (UNIDO) was established in 1967, over the objection of the West (Murphy 1984: 75, Wells 1991). In 1975, UNIDO adopted the "Lima Declaration Plan of Action on Industrial Development and Cooperation," which quantified the targets for the industrial development of developing countries, from 7 percent in 1974 to the goal of 25 percent of world industrial production by the year 2000 (Magarinos et al. 2001).

20. Developing countries pushed for a General System of Preferences (GSP) that would be nonreciprocal, permitting them access to markets in developed countries without the need to lower their

exports, developing countries also called for commodity agreements, a Common Fund to finance buffer stocks to stabilize commodity prices, and a system of indexation.[21] Invoking the duties of developed states, developing countries also asked for increased foreign aid and for debt relief (Sauvant 1981, Hart 1983).

Economic sovereignty. The call for a new international economic order extended the principles of self-determination and political sovereignty to the economic realm. A British official described the G-77 rejection of "economic neo-colonialism" and foreign influence in the following way:

> Economic neo-colonialism has replaced traditional colonialism and Western political influence as the new enemy and was increasingly regarded as a form of dominance. . . . . The growing discontent of the developing countries found expression first of all in a drive for greater control over their own economies. . . . . There was a trend in favor of the concept of national sovereignty and state control in the economic sphere. . . . . In many countries the prospects of economic growth offered by the introduction of foreign capital, enterprise and technology seemed to be too dearly purchased if the price was the acceptance of foreign influence.[22]

Concerns regarding "foreign influence" were often aimed at multinational corporations (MNCs). Developing countries initially viewed the operations of MNCs favorably, as they brought in capital, along with modern products, technologies, and management techniques (Frieden 2006, Marton 1986: 169), but concerns grew that reliance on transnational firms prevented real development and maintained a dependent position in the world economy (Murphy 1984: 107–108). Criticisms intensified when attempts to influence local politics were revealed, in particular the participation of the U.S.-headquartered International Telephone and Telegraph Corporation in plots to overthrow the socialist Salvador Allende

---

tariffs in turn. The G-77 wanted the GSP within UNCTAD, but Western developed countries unilaterally introduced it under the auspices of GATT (Sauvant 198, Sanders 1991).

21. Commodity agreements, planned for at least eighteen key commodities, could improve market conditions by providing price and quota regulations, purchase-guarantees, financing of surplus production, and automatic compensation for diminishing earnings. The main function of buffer stocks was to absorb common market fluctuations—caused by weather changes, cyclical overproduction, or fluctuations in industrial country demand—by stabilizing the prices of the products covered between lower and upper price margins, selling when the upper margins were reached, and buying at the lower ones. A key advantage of a *Common* Fund was that, as long as demand-supply patterns of the individual commodities did not move parallel to each other, costs for one stock could be offset by gains from the others (Sauvant 1981: 90, Jankowitsch and Sauvant 1981: 62–63). A system of indexation would link the prices of developing countries' commodity exports to the prices of developed countries' manufactured exports as a way to preserve the real purchasing power of their exports.

22. "The New International Economic Order," Undated, FCO 49/573, NIEO Planning paper. UK National Archives.

in Chile in 1972 (Broad and Heckscher 2003, Frieden 2006: 349). The G-77 outlined guidelines for MNC behavior, including that

> Transnational enterprises should be subject to the laws of the receiving (host) country and the exclusive jurisdiction of its courts; that they should abstain from all interference; that they should not serve as an instrument of the external policy of another state; that they should supply all pertinent information, should conduct their operations so as to result in net receipts of financial resources for the host nation, should contribute to development, should refrain from restrictive commercial practices, and should respect the socio-cultural identity of the host nation.[23]

The Sixth Special Session adopted the principle of national sovereignty of every state over its natural resources and all its economic activities (Sauvant 1981: 23, Gosovic and Ruggie 1976).[24] It reserved the right of states to nationalize natural resources and the production facilities associated with them, and the right of states to determine the amount and mode of possible compensation, dropping the common references to international law in case conflicts should occur (Jankowitsch and Sauvant 1981: 65).

Strengthening "universal" international organizations. A central contribution of Prebisch to the NIEO ideology was his political analysis of economic decision making. As Murphy (1983: 65) summarizes, "accepting Prebisch's ideas meant looking for ways to change institutions that structured and governed international trade by shifting the power over those institutions to the South." Hence, Third World countries tried to enhance their sovereign prerogatives not only by widening the scope of activities subject to the unilateral sovereign will of individual states but also by strengthening international organizations that followed the one-country/one-vote rule (Krasner 1985: 7, Murphy 1984). Seeking to reverse the uneven influence in the process of decision making at the international level, they rejected the legitimacy of the World Bank and the IMF, in which the Western powers enjoyed weighted voting; and they tried to shift authority from GATT, in which decisions were made by consensus, to UNCTAD (Sanders 1991, Murphy 1983). To address the requests of the G-77, the UN established new international entities, including the UN Industrial Development Organization (UNIDO) and the UN Center for Transnational Corporations (UNCTC). The G-77 also relied

---

23. Memo, Seymour J. Rubin, U.S. Representative to UNCTC, "Reflections concerning the United Nations Commission on Transnational Corporations," July 1975. Ford Presidential Library.

24. Developing countries did not completely reject foreign investment, and the Programme of Action called for "urgent measures" to promote foreign investment in developing countries but also insisted that transnational enterprises had to operate in the framework of the countries' development plans (Sauvant 1981: 127).

on the cooperation of existing UN agencies. These new and existing universal international organizations were expected to monitor interstate relations as well as state-MNC relations, the latter by means of international codes of conduct regarding, for example, restrictive business practices or transfer of technology.[25]

An international code of conduct on the transfer of technology was of particular interest to the developing world. Technological dependence on foreign companies was especially costly as it added a burden of financial payments and allowed for a widespread use of restrictive business practices (Sauvant 1981: 118–119). Developing countries therefore asked for access to Western technologies whose transfer was not subject to private decision (Murphy 1984: 143). The quest for technology transfer was justified based on the duties of developed states to help but also on the argument that technology was in the category of "common heritage," which granted all countries right of access.[26]

Collective self-reliance. Whereas most NIEO principles and demands accepted that economic growth in developing countries depended on engagement with the industrial world and therefore focused on attempts to change the distribution of profits coming out of that engagement, some developing countries considered their own national resources the only sure basis on which they could make development plans. Self-reliance symbolized that recognition. *Collective* self-reliance of Third World states suggested that aid and cooperation among developing countries was essential for success (Murphy 1984: 94–95, Mortimer 1984). The goal was to create conditions that would allow developing countries to move away from exclusive dependence on the demands of the industrialized countries for raw materials and cheap labor, and to instead create domestic markets where poor countries would trade with other poor countries (Sauvant 1981:18, Mortimer 1984). A moderate version of this principle called for South-South cooperation; a more radical version saw collective self-reliance as the successful delinking of the South from the North.

The concept of self-reliance, which served as an economic counterpart of the political theme of Third World solidarity, was introduced into the development debate by the president of Tanzania, Julius Kambarage Nyerere, in a speech before the Dar-es-Salaam Preparatory Conference of the Nonaligned Countries in 1970. In the subsequent Third Conference of Heads of State or Government of Nonaligned Countries at Lusaka in September that year, the concept became the main

---

25. "Charter of Economic Rights and Duties of States," UN General Assembly, Twenty-ninth Session, 12 December 1974, A/RES/29/3281.

26. Developing countries drew on the notion of common heritage also in the UN Conference on the Law of the Sea, where they claimed unknown natural resources as the collective property of the world's nation states, and in negotiations over the international control of resources on the moon and in outer space.

plank of the economic program of the nonaligned countries (Mortimer 1984, Sauvant 1981). In 1979, the G-77, in a conference in Arusha, Tanzania, resolved "to give the highest priority to implementing economic cooperation among developing countries . . . as an essential element in the establishment of the New International Economic Order" (cited in Mortimer 1984: 127). Fundamental economic elements of the collective self-reliance approach were integrated into international development programs under the title "cooperation among developing countries" (Sauvant 1981: 19).

Combined, these major NIEO principles contained some radical ideas but also many reformist programs. A memorandum to President Gerald Ford from his secretary of the treasury and his economic adviser warned that "the call for a new economic order . . . could imply a substantial rejection of the free market system,"[27] but others saw it as little more than confirmation of dependence insofar as most proposals depended on Northern concessions (McMichael 2000: 124). Whether the NIEO could replace exploitation with cooperation was to be determined in the process of implementation. Here, international organizations had a potentially important role to play.

"A New Health Order as Part of the New Social Order"

The WHO's Strategy: "Don't Adopt, Adapt"

To take full advantage of existing universal international organizations, in 1974 the General Assembly asked all specialized agencies to develop action plans for the NIEO (Murphy 1984: 131). A year later, a U.S. Central Intelligence Agency (CIA) report discussed the "concern that politicization has now spread from the General Assembly to the international technical and specialized organizations which the US has long valued as assemblies where the technical bases for broader international cooperation could be somewhat dispassionately established" (CIA 1975: 1). While the CIA report concluded that there was no basis for such a concern, the dominant view in the United States was that of a "growing threat of politicization of Specialized Agencies and consequent deterioration in their ability to concentrate on basic technical, economic, and social missions for which they were established."[28]

---

27. Memorandum from W. E. Simon, Secretary of Treasury, and L.W. Seidman, economic adviser, for President Gerald Ford, May 1975, Office of Economic Affairs. L. William Seidman, Box 72. Ford Presidential Library.

28. From U.S. Embassy in the UK to UN Department in the Foreign Office. "Geneva Group Consultation, February 4–6, Preventing Politicization of Specialized Agencies," January 1975, FCO 61/1328, Twelfth consultative level meeting of Geneva Group. UK National Archives.

Two contentious issues that were centrally featured in these charges of "politicization" were related to the G-77 concern with self-determination: apartheid in South Africa, and the Israeli occupation of Palestinian territories.[29] International organizations were also mobilized to promote economic issues. A UK official complained: "Since the Special Session, the Group of 77 has sought on every possible occasion to insert references to the Special Session resolutions in resolutions and decisions adopted by other bodies usually in a form calling for the unqualified implementation of the resolutions."[30] UN agencies and programs—including the newly established UNCTAD, UNCTC, and UNIDO, but also the ILO, the World Bank, UNESCO, the FAO, and the WHO among others—implemented programs in line with NIEO sensibilities. International organizations called for codes of conduct, such as the ILO Tripartite Declaration of Principles Concerning Multinational Enterprises and Social Policy (November 1977) and the FAO/WHO Code of Ethics for International Trade in Food (December 1979); the ILO and the World Bank developed "basic needs" programs; and UNESCO drew on NIEO principles to establish a controversial "New World Information and Communications Order" to address issues of news coverage in developing countries in the predominantly Western controlled global news media (Imber 1989, Wells 1991: 8).

At the forefront of this mobilization were expected to be those international organizations concerned with "disparities in the share of economic and social world outputs available for the population," including the WHO.[31] The "health situation in the world" was a serious cause for concern. A study comparing eighteen industrialized countries to thirty-seven low-income countries reported a twenty-one-year difference in life expectancy between industrialized and low-income countries (with sub-Saharan countries, the difference was twenty-nine years). Child and infant mortality were 13.5 and 8 times higher, respectively, in low-income countries than industrialized countries. There were 16 times more physicians per capita in industrialized countries, and 46 times more nurses.[32]

The World Health Organization, under the leadership of Director-General Halfdan T. Mahler, committed itself to address these disparities and in other

---

29. Most upsetting for the Americans were resolutions on these issues passed by the ILO and UNESCO, but resolutions passed in the Universal Postal Union, the International Telecommunications Union, the Food and Agriculture Organization (FAO), the International Atomic Energy Agency (IAEA), and the WHO also put pressure on South Africa and Israel (Buehrig 1976, Melanson 1979, Williams 1987, Imber 1989).

30. Political notes for the UK delegation to the 28th WHA, prepared by the UN Department in the Foreign and Commonwealth Office, 9 May 1975, FCO 61/1350 (28th WHA). UK National Archives.

31. "Health for All by the Year 2000," Summary of the Presentation Made on 30th October 1979, R8293, vol. 21, file 34. Canada National Archives.

32. Ibid.

ways contribute to the new order. Mahler genuinely believed that "the winds of history [had] shifted dramatically over the last decade," and he was "personally convinced that the next decade [would] see very significant steps towards introducing all the key elements of the New International Economic Order."[33] The WHO had a role to play in that historic moment.

The WHO report, "Technical Discussions on The Contribution of Health to The New International Economic Order," affirmed the WHO's allegiance to the NIEO.[34] The report forcefully argued that "the philosophy, policy, principles and practices recently adopted in the world health sector *correspond fully* with the aims of the NIEO and with the means for achieving them" (WHO 1980a, emphasis added). In describing this correspondence, the report asserted, "The objectives of the NIEO are not in question: the transfer of resources, to ensure their more equitable distribution and to provide poorer countries with better opportunities to participate in world trade; and the transfer of those countries of appropriate technologies, with the accent on self-reliance." The report continued: "The adoption of these features has been initiated in the health field, which therefore provides an example of the application and practice of the principles involved in the NIEO" (WHO 1980a). In referring to the WHO flagship programs, Health for All by the Year 2000 and primary health care, the report reiterated the affinity between NIEO principles and the WHO programs:

> The characteristics inherent in the strategy of health for all by the year 2000, based on primary health care . . . are precisely those demanded by the NIEO. Examples are: multisectoral coordination, with the mutual contribution to development of actions in the health and relevant socioeconomic sectors; the transfer of technology (as in the policy of appropriate technology for health); redistribution of resources on a more equitable basis, leading to universal accessibility of primary health care and its supporting services; increased self-reliance (as in the policy of technical cooperation among developing countries); and mass participation, ensuring involvement of the community in shaping its own health and socioeconomic future. (WHO 1980a)

---

33. "Rescue Mission for Tomorrow's Health," Interview with Director-General Dr. Halfdan Mahler, *People*, vol. 6, no. 2, pp. 25–28, 1979. WHO Library.

34. In May 1978, the Executive Board decided that the subject for the Technical Discussions at the Thirty-Third World Health Assembly should be "the Contribution of Health to the New International Economic Order." In preparation, Six Working Groups were established, with a total of 331 participants. A33/Technical Discussions/1 (WHO 1980a) was the Background Document that was sent to the six WHO Regional Offices to facilitate consideration of the subject. The views expressed at the Regional Committee meetings were subsequently included in the Background Document, which was then sent to all member states (WHO 1980b).

The assertions made in the report of the WHO's support of, and conformity with, the NIEO begin to indicate the means by which the WHO bureaucracy responded to the exogenous expectations.

First, the report proudly listed the radical changes in the agenda of the WHO, including new policies and programs that had been consciously designed to follow the principles of the NIEO and which amount to the making of "a new health order as part of the new social order" (WHO 1980a). According to the report, the WHO had loyally conformed to the NIEO logic and had fully addressed the expectations of developing countries. Second, the principles of the NIEO that the WHO conformed with had been modified. In the passage quoted above, for example, the report referred to the transfer of *appropriate* technology, to equitable distribution by way of *universal accessibility,* and it emphasized *self-reliance* rather than duties of developed states. This translation of the original principles allowed the WHO secretariat to promote "the philosophy, policy, principles and practices" that were acceptable to developing countries but were also compatible with the WHO's own goals.

Spearheading the WHO's response to the NIEO was Director-General Mahler, who was elected by the Executive Board in 1973 and served in that capacity between 1974 and 1988. Although an insider who had been the "chosen dauphin"[35] of the former director-general, Dr. Marcolino G. Candau, Mahler had a different background than his predecessor, which made him more suitable to carry the change that developing countries demanded. Candau was a malariologist who favored eradication programs, which were the WHO's signature initiatives in the 1950s and 1960s (Brown and Cueto 2011). Mahler, in contrast, was a tuberculosis specialist. Between 1950 and 1951, Mahler led an antituberculosis campaign for the Red Cross in Ecuador. Mahler then spent almost ten years in India as a senior officer of the WHO attached to the National Tuberculosis Program, which informed his skeptical position regarding vertical, or disease-specific, interventions. Later, as assistant director-general, Mahler was responsible for divisions and programs that were concerned with improving national capabilities in health planning. In this capacity, he presented the institutional *alternative* to the prevalent agenda of the time (Litsios 2004: 1885, Cueto 2004: 1865).

There were also important personality differences between Mahler and Candau. As I discuss in chapter 2, the institutional arrangements of the WHO afforded directors-general relatively easy influence over the direction of the organization. Mahler was still unique among other directors-general, as he was both

---

35. Telegram, from UK mission in Geneva to UN (E&S) Department, "World Health Organization," 4 February 1971, FCO 61/784 (Consideration of finances of WHO). UK National Archives.

ambitious in his plans for the organization and particularly charismatic. He was described by the Americans as "a strong idealist,"[36] and early in his tenure a UK memo reported: "[Mahler] is approaching his task with a vigor and missionary zeal which are bound to alter to some extent the character of the WHO and its work."[37] A lesser endorsement agreed that "Dr. Mahler is a very astute operator" but also remarked that "his effect on the Assembly itself is produced mainly through the two or three major speeches which he makes, and his committed eloquence, which in other fora may appear rather over-bearing."[38]

During Mahler's tenure, the secretariat relied heavily on the WHO Constitution as the source for the organization's principles, goals, and programs. In his first address before the World Health Assembly, in May 1974, Mahler reminded member states that the constitution had one objective only, namely, the attainment of all peoples of the highest possible level of health,[39] and in the following years the pursuit of this specific objective was made the central mission of the organization. Mahler also relied on the constitution's broad definition of health—"a state of complete physical, mental and social well-being and not merely the absence of disease or infirmity"—to move the organization away from its previous biomedical focus. This emphasis on the attainment of health by all peoples and the rejection of a biomedical focus were aligned with new public health sensibilities that favored comprehensive health care over curative programs. Given Mahler's experience in India, he was well positioned to endorse these public health trends.

While historical accounts often emphasize Mahler's idealism, he was also a pragmatist who was deeply concerned with the functionality of the WHO. Mahler's "missionary zeal"[40] was grounded in a very clear perception of what could and could not be achieved, and he had no interest in fighting losing battles. On numerous occasions he warned member states that "the Organization should have a clear vision of its goal, but unless it was pragmatic in its approach it would

36. Note, "Dr. Halfdan Mahler, DG of the UN WHO," Attached to a memorandum from Robert Emrey, International Health Assessment Staff at the White House, to Peter Bourne, Special Assistant to the President for Health Issues, 6 July 1977, Staff Offices, Peter Bourne, Box 34, International Health 7/1/77–7/31/77. Carter Presidential Library.

37. Report, Steering Committee on International Organizations, WHO, Report on the 27th WHA, Geneva, 7–23 May 1974, Department of Health and Social Security, 19 July 1974, FCO 61/1208. UK National Archives.

38. WHO, 28th WHA, Geneva, 13–30 May 1975, Department of Health and Social Security, 29 August 1975, FCO 61/1351. UK National Archives.

39. "The Constitutional Mission of the World Health Organization," Address by Dr. H. Mahler, Director-General of the WHO, in Presenting his Report for 1973 to the Twenty-Seventh World Health Assembly, 8 May 1974. WHO Library.

40. Report, Steering Committee on International Organizations, WHO, Report on the 27th WHA, Geneva, 7–23 May 1974, Department of Health and Social Security, 19 July 1974, FCO 61/1208. UK National Archives.

fail to achieve it."[41] In regard to resolutions condemning Israel or South Africa, for example, Mahler warned that such resolutions might "blow up our Organization," and pleaded with member states (albeit often unsuccessfully) not "to be lured astray into fields beyond our constitutional competence" (cited in Williams 1986: 63).[42] Mahler was also aware that developed countries were extremely reluctant to pay for advancing an international order that they did not support, and that NIEO-compatible programs that led to additional funds or expanded authority were especially likely to alienate the rich majority, on which the WHO was dependent for material and normative support.

It was this combination of idealism and pragmatism that enabled the WHO secretariat to guard its principles and material interests when faced with the expectation to conform to the NIEO principles. In one of his early speeches, Mahler argued against the tendency to seek solutions for the problems of underdeveloped countries by transplanting methods used in advanced countries. According to Mahler, the motto should have been: "don't adopt, adapt."[43] The same motto also applied to the WHO's response to those who wanted to transplant principles promoted by developing countries for economic issues under the NIEO to solve health issues. In adapting rather than adopting NIEO principles, the WHO leadership and staff found a way to make the NIEO principles compatible with the organization's independent goals before embracing them.

Health for All by the Year 2000

At the Twenty-Ninth World Health Assembly, in 1976, Mahler proposed a new and an all-encompassing goal for the organization, which he called "Health for All by the Year 2000." The following year, the assembly adopted Resolution WHA30.43, which had the same name and declared that "the main social target

---

41. WHO Document, January 1982, EB69/SR/15. WHO Library.

42. The U.S. government held the position that "introducing politically-charged issues in [a] technical meeting such as WHA is inappropriate, disruptive, irrelevant to [the] real business of [the] meeting, and should be opposed." At the same time, the U.S. Department of State chose not to hold the WHO leadership responsible for such resolutions, partly because of Mahler's explicit efforts to block them. As a note from the Department of State described, "Mahler has tried hard, and with some success, to keep the Israeli issue from boiling over. [But] he is not about to 'fight valiantly' to keep it out of the World Health Assembly. He takes the view that the Assembly is sovereign where he's concerned. He would resent our trying to stick him with the responsibility for keeping the Arabs and the G-77 in line on the Israeli issue." See Telegram, From Department of State, 13 January 1961, RG59 General Records of the Department of State, 1960–1963, Box 831. U.S. National Archives; Note, Department of State, "Mahler the Man," Undated, Staff Offices, Peter Bourne, Box 38, International Health—Undated Material [1]. Carter Presidential Library.

43. Report, Steering Committee on International Organizations, WHO, Report on the 27th WHA, Geneva 7–23 May 1974, Department of Health and Social Security, 19 July 1974, FCO 61/1208. UK National Archives.

of governments and WHO in the coming two decades should be the attainment by all citizens of the world by the year 2000 of a level of health that will permit them to lead a socially and economically productive life."

This resolution expressed a radical departure from the WHO concerns and programs in the previous two decades. During the 1950s and 1960s, programs that targeted specific diseases had been the preferred form of the WHO's operational assistance. Newly independent states had poor health infrastructure, but it was believed that such limited infrastructure could potentially be bypassed due to availability of new technologies: the discovery of effective chemotherapeutic agents against communicable diseases such as tuberculosis, leprosy, and syphilis, the use of insecticides against vector-transmitted diseases, and technical improvements such as jet injectors and bifurcated needles (Raviglione and Pio 2002). Hence, with the encouragement of donor countries, the WHO focused on such vertical interventions that relied on "magic bullets" for targeted diseases (Smith and Bryant 1988: 911, see also Packard 1997: 288, Armith 2004). During those years, the WHO launched mass campaigns against tuberculosis (1947–1951), malaria (1955–1970), yaws (1955–1970), and the exceptionally successful eradication program of smallpox (1967–1980) (Lee 2009: 48).[44] Each of these disease eradication programs operated vertically, which is to say, autonomously, with its own administration and budget and little integration into the larger health system, if one existed, or into other vertical programs (Smith and Bryant 1988: 911, Raviglione and Pio 2002). Health for All by the Year 2000 (combined with the primary health care approach, and see below) rejected this piecemeal attitude of targeting specific diseases based on available technological advances, and committed the WHO member states to a vision of *overall* improvements in health conditions, without discriminating among people based on their economic or social conditions or on the availability of medical solutions.

Health for All reflected an unprecedented attempt to redirect the WHO back to its constitutional commitments. According to Mahler, the goal of health for all by the year 2000 "embodied" the constitutional objective of the attainment by all people of the highest possible level of health.[45] An Executive Board member from Burma expressed a common view when he stated that the only innovative aspect of the goal of health for all, if compared to the constitution, was setting a deadline.[46] As importantly, Health for All was also celebrated as a faithful articulation

---

44. For detailed explorations of the WHO's vertical initiatives see Packard 1989 and Amrith 2002 on tuberculosis; Cleaver 1977, Litsios 1997, and Cueto 2007 on malaria; and Manela 2010 on smallpox.

45. WHO Document, January 1980, EB65/SR/6. WHO Library.

46. WHO Document, January 1979, EB63/SR/19, p. 4. WHO Library.

of the NIEO in the field of health. In 1975, when Mahler presented to member states, in a number of venues, the concept of health for all, he stated,

> I have chosen as my subject 'Health for *all* by the year 2000!' because it permits me to express my views on how you and your Organization might make a contribution to the New Economic Order.[47]

A report of a WHO expert committee similarly presented a genealogy that linked Health for All back to the NIEO:

> The commitment of the Member States of WHO to the goal of health for all by the year 2000 has been *presaged* by the General Assembly of the United Nations which proclaimed in 1974 . . . its united determination to work urgently for the establishment of a New International Economic Order. . . .
>
> The adoption of this resolution by the United Nations General Assembly was an important milestone in the age-old struggle for equity and justice. . . .
>
> Thus, when the Thirtieth World Health Assembly met in May 1977, *the way had been prepared* for a unanimous decision by the then 152 Member States of WHO.[48]

With Health for All, the World Health Organization responded to the NIEO by enthusiastically embracing two of its fundamental principles: development and equity. In doing so, however, the WHO secretariat reinterpreted these notions to better fit the values of the WHO Constitution. The WHO bureaucracy strategically complied with the NIEO by bridging the gap between economic and social development, and the gap between interstate and intrastate equity.

Economic and social development. The call for a new international economic order centered, as we saw, around developing countries' quest for economic and social development, and the WHO presented the objective of health for all as the organization's contribution to these efforts (Bryant 1980: 382). The WHO secretariat made the claim that "the recognition of the *close relationship between health and development . . . led* the Thirtieth World Health Assembly to decide in May 1977" on the Health for All goal (WHO 1980a, emphasis added). This "close

---

47. "Health for All by the Year 2000," Address delivered by Dr. H. Mahler, Director-General of the WHO to the Twenty-Sixth Session of the Regional Committee for the Western Pacific, Manila, 1 September 1975, the Twenty-Fifth Session of the Regional Committee for Africa, Yaoundé, 17 September 1975, and the Twenty-Third Meeting of the Directing Council of PAHO Twenty-Seventh Session of the WHO Regional Committee for the America, Washington, 29 September 1975. WHO Library.

48. "Health Manpower Requirements for the Achievement of Health for All by the Year 2000 through Primary Health Care," 1985, Report of a WHO Expert Committee, WHO Technical Report Series 717. WHO Library. Emphasis added.

relationship" was articulated in a number of ways, including that "the indicators of good health are also indicators of development," that "a healthy people [is] the most essential cause and effect of development," and, therefore, that "health development [is] a viable strategy for development planners to pursue" (WHO 1980a).

However, development here stood not for economic development but for social development. Economic development is defined as the quantitative change and restructuring in a country's economy, usually measured in terms of gross national product (GNP) per capita, which reflects an increase in the economic productivity and average material well-being of a country's population. Social development, in contrast, is defined as the qualitative change in human welfare, usually measured in terms of improved access to shelter, health, education, and productive employment. The NIEO resolutions made repeated references to economic and social development, but the focus was clearly on economic growth with an implicit assumption that social development would be achieved through economic development. The "Technical Discussions on the Contribution of Health to the New International Economic Order," however, defined development in social terms: "Development implies continuing improvements in the living conditions and quality of life of people" (WHO 1980a). Once the goal became social development, the central role of health emerged: "The quality of life depends directly upon the level of health. Health development is therefore essential for social and economic development" (WHO 1980a). In short, to integrate the WHO's policies into the new order in a way compatible with the organization's goals, the staff's statements, reports, and speeches played down the centrality of economic development and called for greater attention for social development, and hence to health development. This was not simply because the WHO's contribution could be more apparent if the concern was with social development. The references to social rather than economic development also allowed the WHO leadership to present its foremost objective of quality access to health as a goal that should and could be pursued independent of developing countries' success in promoting their economic goals. Promoting development in social rather than economic terms was also more agreeable to developed countries, exactly because the policies advocated by the WHO leadership to advance social development did not require change in the global economic hierarchy, and therefore served as a balancing formula that allowed the WHO to pursue policies in line with the NIEO without risking its material interests or normative stand.

In some reports and statements, the WHO presented Health for All as complying with the NIEO by suggesting that the NIEO principles were equally concerned with social development as with economic development. In other times, WHO reports and statements offered the organization's concern with social development as a welcome corrective to the focus on economic development that was predominant in the United Nations. In addressing the social aspects of development, the WHO joined a broader movement of critics who objected to the narrow view of development, including Dudley Seers, a British economist, who redefined development as realizing the potential of human personality and questioned the sole emphasis on quantitative growth targets, particularly GNP (Seers 1977, de Kadt 1985, also Murphy 1984: 132, McMichael 2000: 122–123). Mahler agreed: "Too often is development equated with economic growth instead of with the progressive wellbeing of people."[49] Hence, while confirming that "the purpose of the New International Economic Order is development," WHO reports asserted that "development cannot be equated with economic growth alone" (WHO 1980a).

Instead, the WHO emphasized the importance of non-quantitative measures that would address different aspects of "social poverty"—a combination, according to Mahler, of "unemployment and underemployment, economic poverty, scarcity of worldly goods, a low level of education, poor housing, poor sanitation, malnutrition, ill health, social apathy, and lack of the will and the initiative to make changes for the better" (cited in WHO 2008: 20). The goal was the "improvement in the living conditions and quality of life of the people . . . particularly the underprivileged" (WHO 1980a). Mahler told member states that he would "personally . . . prefer" to call the New Economic Order a "New Development Order,"[50] disclosing his displeasure with a narrowly economic emphasis.

Such statements successfully convinced developing countries that Health for All, in addressing social development, could contribute to the NIEO in significant ways. In 1980, a draft resolution, jointly sponsored by sixteen non-Western countries at the World Health Assembly, asserted, "The New International Economic Order . . . can only be effectively set in motion when due attention is paid to social as well as economic development, of which health is an integral part," and defined the aim of "development efforts" as "raising the quality of human life as an essential part of aspirations to achieve national and international social and economic justice."[51]

In short, in response to the NIEO, the WHO shifted its central attention to the issue of development, as developing countries demanded. By emphasizing social development, however, the WHO secretariat offered a notion of development that

---

49. "Health for All by the Year 2000," Address delivered by Dr. H. Mahler, Director-General of the WHO to the Twenty-Sixth Session of the Regional Committee for the Western Pacific, Manila, 1 September 1975, the Twenty-Fifth Session of the Regional Committee for Africa, Yaoundé, 17 September 1975, and the Twenty-Third Meeting of the Directing Council of PAHO Twenty-Seventh Session of the WHO Regional Committee for the America, Washington, 29 September 1975. WHO Library.
50. Ibid.
51. WHO Document, 1980, WHA33, Committee A: Fourth Meeting. WHO Library.

put health in the center of the development strategy rather than in its margins. As importantly, this was a development strategy that was in line with the WHO foundational text. As Mahler insisted, health for all was "both a basic human need and a fundamental human right, in keeping with the very principles of our far-sighted Constitution."[52] The WHO did not always try to obscure the fundamental differences between economic development and social development and at times explicitly criticized the NIEO for focusing on the "promotion of economic growth without specifying how this will lead to social improvement" (WHO 1980a). But by linking health for all to social development and social development to the fundamental interests of developing countries, the WHO could convincingly claim *compliance* with the NIEO logic, and Health for All had the unconditional backing of all WHO member states.

International and intranational equity. Health for All offered a selective interpretation not only of development, but also of equity. The main motivation behind Health for All, mirroring the concerns leading to the NIEO, came from a strong sense of injustice in the face of blatant inequalities. While in both cases these inequalities were attributed to a colonial past, for the WHO leadership, the inequities existing among populations in poor countries were even more disconcerting than inequities between poor countries and rich ones. One of the legacies of colonial medical services, which had emphasized costly high-technology, urban-based, and curative care, was a skewed resource allocation in the national health systems in many developing countries. In the 1970s, health care services in many poor countries were still limited to urban areas where there were doctors, pharmacists, and hospitals, while the majority of people living in suburban and rural areas had no access to health care resources (Roemer 1986, Unger and Killingsworth 1986: 1001, Mamdani 1992: 2). Behind Health *for All* was the desire to improve the access to and quality of health services to the very poor. According to Mahler, "The question of *social equity,* the possibility of realizing oneself as a fundamental right, was the most important concept in the goal of health for all by the year 2000."[53]

By insisting on the importance of intrastate equity, the WHO implied that the NIEO's sole focus on international equity was insufficient and offered Health for All as a model for bridging the two. The "Technical Discussions on the Contribution of Health to the New International Economic Order" (WHO 1980a) made the tension explicit:

---

52. "World Health Target for Basic Human Needs," Address by Dr. H. Mahler Director-General of the WHO, in Presenting his Report for 1976 to the Thirtieth World Health Assembly, 3 May 1977. WHO Library.

53. WHO Document, January 1980, EB65/SR/6. WHO Library. Emphasis added.

It is apparent from the texts of [the NIEO] resolutions that the steps to be taken to redress the economic imbalances which persist between North and South are devoid of a social dimension except by implication. In other words, social development is taken for granted to the extent that should all the measures foreseen within the Programme of Action be taken, thus leading to more affluent societies in the developing countries, there will automatically be a higher quality of life. As such, it is assumed that international justice, to be realized through the establishment of the New International Economic Order, will lead to *intra*national justice, implying a more equitable distribution of national resources in all sectors, including social sectors such as health.

The WHO staff challenged the assumption that the benefits of an international restructuring of the economic system would be automatically translated into social improvements, such as the health status of all people. For social improvements, the report argued, "there needs to be equity [also] in the intra-national distribution of resources" (WHO 1980a). Hence, in describing the principles of Health for All, Mahler emphasized that

the distribution of health resources is as important as their quality and quantity. Resources are all too often allocated to central institutions, become proportionately scantier in direct ration to the distance from the main cities, and are non-existent or almost non-existent in rural areas. . . . The time is now long overdue for a *reduction of the growing disparity in the distribution of health resources not only between counties but also within countries.*[54]

Similarly, a program committee of the Executive Board "recognized that economic development did not necessarily make a positive contribution to health, and that there was an urgent need to improve social justice and equity in many countries."[55]

The WHO's campaign against the injustice of intrastate inequity—"the disparities existing within countries between the few who had access to expensive hospital and medical care and the vast majority who were deprived of any type

54. "Health for All by the Year 2000," Address delivered by Dr. H. Mahler, Director-General of the WHO to the Twenty-Sixth Session of the Regional Committee for the Western Pacific, Manila, 1 September 1975, the Twenty-Fifth Session of the Regional Committee for Africa, Yaoundé, 17 September 1975, and the Twenty-Third Meeting of the Directing Council of PAHO Twenty-Seventh Session of the WHO Regional Committee for the America, Washington, 29 September 1975. WHO Library. Emphasis added.
55. WHO Document, January 1980, EB65/SR/5. WHO Library.

of care"—promised to complement the battle against interstate inequity.[56] Also in regard to equity, therefore, Health for All could be successfully presented not as undermining but as contributing to the NIEO. In a piece published in a WHO magazine, *World Health*, Mahler reiterated the affinity between the two: "For . . . governments do have responsibility for the health and socio-economic development of all their people, and not only of the elite in the main cities. This implies distributing resources for health more evenly, and to do so means giving top priority to the socially under-privileged." Mahler then added, "This applies within countries, but it also applies internationally, since the more fortunate countries have a double responsibility—to their own people and to those in countries in less fortunate circumstances."[57]

In short, by presenting Health for All as contributing to two fundamental principles of the NIEO, development and equity, the WHO leadership and staff were able to convincingly claim that the organization's new agenda was complying with the expectations of developing countries. At the same time, by insisting on the importance of *social* development and *intrastate* equities, they were also able to maintain the WHO's ideational commitment to the constitution and protect the organization's material goals by ensuring the support of developed countries. The success of this strategic compliance is manifested by the fact that the WHO received the support not only of representatives of member states at the World Health Assembly but also the endorsement of the UN General Assembly. In 1979, UN Resolution 34/58, entitled "Health as an Integral Part of Development," which recalled the UN resolutions calling for a new international economic order, welcomed "the important efforts of the World Health Organization . . . associated with the effort to attain the goal of 'health for all by the year 2000.'"[58]

Primary Health Care

The objective of health for all required a global strategy and the WHO selected primary health care (PHC) as "the KEY to achieving the target of health for all" in one generation (WHO 1980a). Mahler declared primary health care "a frontline activity that is the corner-stone to ensure essential health for all in any society."[59] The primary health care approach, like Health for All, was framed in terms that

56. WHO Document, January 1976, EB57/SR/15. WHO Library.

57. Mahler, Halfdan, 1981, "What Is Health for All?" *World Health*. WHO Library.

58. WHO Document, "Text of Resolution 34/58, Adopted by the United Nations General Assembly on 29 November 1979," A33/5, p. 11. PAHO Library.

59. "Blue Print for Health for All," Address by Dr. H. Mahler, Director-General of the WHO to the Thirteenth Session of the Regional Committee for South-East Asia, Bangkok, 2 August 1977. WHO Library.

reinterpreted NIEO principles, including development, equity and self-reliance, which allowed compatibility between the demands of developing countries for a new international order on the one hand and a public health perspective that offered an alternative to the failed vertical approach on the other.

The search for alternatives to vertical interventions was a response to the ultimate failure of the Malaria Eradication Program.[60] Initiated in 1955, in its first ten years the program successfully eliminated the infection from twenty-four countries and freed 1 billion people from malaria risk through the widespread application of insecticides including DDT and medications to combat parasitic infection (Okie 2008). Yet the emergence of mosquito resistance to DDT and parasite resistance to chloroquine led to epidemic resurgence of malaria in some of the countries where it had been nearly vanquished. In addition, the campaign never included the tropical African countries, where about 90 percent of malaria deaths occurred. By 1964, the Executive Board conceded that "the early hopes had been over-optimistic."[61] In 1968, the World Health Assembly recommended that in such areas were eradication was not feasible in the near future, malaria eradication programs be returned to malaria control programs.

Many reasons were given to explain the failure of the eradication program, including high costs and lack of consultation with local populations (Packard 1997: 286). But WHO discussions emphasized one main barrier: the lack of health service infrastructure, especially in rural areas, that could reach every household and *remain in place.*[62] The recognition of the need for basic health infrastructure had major implications since it acknowledged the potential futility of targeting specific diseases in isolation of overall health conditions and opened up the possibility for the integration of vertical programs into "the general public health services of the country."[63] The declaration abandoning the malaria eradication program, in 1968, emphasized the need to develop rural health systems and to integrate malaria control into general health services (Nájera 1989).

In other disease-specific programs, including tuberculosis, experts also began to appreciate reliance on existing health services. As had happened with other initiatives, a WHO expert committee on tuberculosis proposed a vertical program for less-developed countries, which imitated the strategies used in industrialized

---

60. The WHO *eradication* program replaced long-term *control* methods. Control stands for an unending program of limiting the danger of malaria, without any attempt to end it completely. Eradication stands for ending of the transmission of malaria and the elimination of the reservoir of infective cases (Siddiqi 1995: 126). On the WHO program and its failure see Nájera 1989, Packard 1997, Brown, Cueto, and Fee 2006, Cueto 2007, Okie 2008.

61. WHO Document, 1964, EB33/Min/3 Rev. 1, p. 89. WHO Library.

62. WHO Document, 1969, EB43/SR/10 Rev. 1, p. 156. WHO Library; Newell 1988: 903.

63. WHO Document, 1963, EB31/Min/8 Rev. 1, pp. 257–258. WHO Library.

countries and was based on mass case finding and specialized case management. But a series of research studies on tuberculosis in India, supported by the Indian Government, local WHO officials, and the British Medical Research Council promoted a much less costly program that was based on simplified technology delivered through the general health services (Raviglione and Pio 2002).

Starting in the late 1960s, then, the WHO greatly increased the number of projects related to the development of basic health services, from 85 in 1965 to 156 in 1971 (Cueto 2004: 1866). In 1971, the Executive Board chose basic health services as the subject for its organizational study. The ensuing debates on this report in the Executive Board and the World Health Assembly moved the discussions and subsequent policies from basic health services to the broader primary health care approach (Newell 1988: 904, Litsios 2002: 711–713).

The report "Organizational Study on Methods of Promoting the Development of Basic Health Services" (WHO 1973) was prepared by the newly established Division of Strengthening of Health Services. The head of this division was Kenneth N. Newell, who used his position to effectively promote primary health care at the center of the WHO's new approach.[64] In 1973, the World Health Assembly adopted the Organizational Study in Resolution WHA26.35, which stated that WHO activities should give high priority to the development of health services. The resolution also defined the type of health services needed, with a novel emphasis on local needs and capacities. Health services were to be "both accessible and acceptable to the total population, suited to its needs and to the socioeconomic conditions of the country, and at the level of health technology considered necessary to meet the problems of that country at a given time."[65] A year later, another resolution, WHA27.44, called on the director-general to report on steps undertaken by the WHO "to assist governments to direct their health service programs toward their major health objectives, with priority being given to the rapid and effective development of the health delivery system" (cited in Litsios 2004: 1891–1892). This report was Kenneth Newell's—as well as Mahler's—opportunity to introduce the primary health care approach in a comprehensive manner, drawing on the WHO's work over the previous two years.[66]

---

64. Prior to this appointment, Newell had been the director of the Division of Research in Epidemiology and Communications Science, which was under the responsibility of Mahler when he had been the assistant director-general (Cueto 2004).

65. WHO Document, A26/VR/15, Resolution WHA26.35, "Organizational Study on Methods of Promoting the Development of Basic Health Services." PAHO Library.

66. According to Litsios (2004), Newell and Mahler's support of the primary health care approach was greatly influenced by the Christian Medical Commission (CMC), an organization that had been created in the late 1960s by medical missionaries working in developing countries. The CMC moved from providing curative services in hospitals to giving priority to preventive services at the community level, and it was CMC that coined the term "comprehensive health care," which they defined as "a planned effort for delivering health and medical care attempting to meet as many

The document submitted to the Executive Board in 1975 in response to Resolution WHA27.44 argued that the prevailing approach to the development of
health services, namely, "the transfer of health technology from one context to
another—developed to developing as well as urban to rural," had failed and that
"a radical departure from conventional health services approach is required."
The document forcefully argued that developing primary health services at the
community level was the "only way in which the health services can develop rapidly and effectively." This alternative approach was based on the integration "of
preventive, curative and promotive services," which provided for all interventions to be undertaken "at the most peripheral practicable level of the health services" and "by the worker most simply trained for this activity." Other echelons
of health services were to be designed in support of the needs of the peripheral
level. Health care, in turn, was to be "fully integrated with the services of the other
sectors involved in community development."[67]

Two other important publications that shaped the WHO's ideas on primary
health care were published the same year. The first was "Alternative Approaches
to Meeting Basic Health Needs of Populations in Developing Countries" (Djukanovic and Mach 1975), which was commissioned by the UNICEF/WHO Joint
Committee on Health Policy to evaluate existing basic health services and was
edited by two WHO staff members who worked under Newell. The report challenged the assumption that the expansion of Western medical systems would
meet the needs of developing countries. The principal causes of morbidity in
poor countries were malnutrition and vector-borne, respiratory and diarrheal
diseases. Based on an examination of successful experiences in a number of
developing countries, the report suggested that the best approach to address
such conditions was not vertical programs but primary health care.[68] The other

---

of the defined needs as possible with available resources" (Litsios 2004: 1887–1888). In 1970, CMC
established the journal *Contact,* which used the term *primary health care,* probably for the first time.
Many of the intellectual voices supporting primary health care, including Carl Taylor, who edited a
book that offered Indian rural medicine as a general model, and John Bryant, whose book *Health
and the Developing World* questioned the transplantation of the hospital-based health care system to
developing countries, were linked to CMC (Cueto 2004: 1864–1865, Litsios 2004: 1887; see Bryant
1969, Taylor 1976). Litsios (2004) describes a number of particularly constructive meetings between
CMC and WHO staff, including Newell, during the period in which the WHO leadership established
its support of the primary health care approach.

67. "Promotion of National Health Services. Report by the Director-General," World Health Organization, 1974, EB55/9. PAHO Library; see also Litsios 2004.

68. Many newly independent countries adopted vertical programs, supported by American
foundations (Rockefeller, Ford), the U.S. military, and early WHO programs (Unger and Killing-
sworth 1986: 1001). However, beginning in the 1950s and 1960s other countries, including India,
China, Kenya, Indonesia, Nicaragua, Costa Rica, Guatemala, Honduras, Mexico, Bangladesh, and the
Philippines, implemented more comprehensive approaches to the provision of basic health services
(Smith and Bryant 1988: 911–912, Magnussen, Ehiri, and Jolly 2004: 168, Roemer 1986).

publication was "Health by the People" (WHO 1975), which was edited by Newell and celebrated the experience of medical auxiliaries in developing countries (Litsios 2004: 1886, Cueto 2004: 1864–1866). A paper for the World Health Assembly, "Promotion of National Health Services," summarized the accumulated sentiments by proclaiming that the development of "primary health care services at the community level is seen as the only way in which the health services can develop rapidly and effectively" (cited in Newell 1988: 904).

Delegates of both developing and developed countries at the World Health Assembly expressed support of the concept of primary health care, which they came to view as "the only way in which the health of people in rural areas could be improved."[69] The representative from Kuwait summarized: "WHO's policy on primary health care was one of the most important landmarks in the philosophy of the Organization. All delegates welcomed that endeavor."[70] Western industrial counties were similarly swayed, but insisted that the same principles should not be applied to their countries (Gish 1983). The Soviet Union did express strong skepticism, reflecting an ideological battle between communist countries (Cueto 2004: 1867). In contrast to the Chinese form of medical care, which inspired the notion of primary health care, the Soviet Union defended a medically oriented approach and considered primary health care a step backward in scientific and technological progress, which "could . . . condemn children in developing countries to inferior services from poorly qualified personnel."[71] The British thought that the "[Russian] motive may be dislike of the stress laid . . . on the merits of Chinese and Tanzanian methods and the lack of attention there to Soviet experience."[72]

When the Chinese delegation to the WHO suggested an international conference to exchange experience on the development of primary health care, the Soviet Union delegation initially opposed, but then offered to host the meeting (Cueto 2004: 1867). The WHO leadership was not convinced of the need for a conference, possibly because they believed more had to be done at the national and regional levels before the WHO could try to bring together those experiences. Also, it was clear that "[the] Soviet government will not miss this opportunity to show [the] rest of world [the] great success and superiority of Soviet approach

---

69. WHO Document, 1976, EB57/SR/15. WHO Library.

70. WHO Document, 1976, A29/SR/20, p. 20. WHO Library.

71. From UK Mission in New York to UK Delegation to WHA, "UNICEF Executive Board: WHO/UNICEF Joint Study on Basic Health Needs in Developing Countries," 19 May 1975, FCO 61/1351. UK National Archives; see also Tejada de Rivero 2003.

72. Ibid.

and health system," as the Canadian mission put it,[73] and Mahler, who disagreed with the Soviet Union's highly centralized and medicalized approach to the provision of health services, was therefore reluctant to have such a meeting in the Soviet Union (Litsios 2002: 718, Brown, Cueto, and Fee 2006: 67). Hence, even though the World Health Assembly in 1975 passed a resolution, WHA28.88, that considered an international meeting or conference on primary health care "desirable,"[74] at the Executive Board meeting in 1976 Newell still indicated that the director-general "was not convinced that the time was opportune" for an international conference (cited in Litsios 2002: 715). Eventually, however, the WHO leadership accepted the Soviet offer to host the conference in the capital of the Soviet Republic of Kazakhstan, Alma-Ata. The International Conference on Primary Health Care took place from September 6 to 12, 1978, and became *the* landmark event for primary health care (Cueto, 2004: 1866, Brown, Cueto, and Fee 2006: 67).

Three thousand delegates from 134 governments, mostly represented by delegates from the ministries of health, and 67 international organizations attended the conference. Nongovernmental organizations, religious movements, and political movements were also present (Cueto 2004: 1867). By the end of the week-long conference, the delegates adopted the "Declaration of Alma-Ata International Conference on Primary Health Care" (WHO 1978), which made the primary health care approach the central overarching logic of national, regional, and WHO health programs.

The declaration provided its central tenet in section V, which affirmed that "the attainment by all peoples of the world by the year 2000 of a level of health that will permit them to lead a socially and economically productive life" was a "main social target." The section declared that "primary health care is the key to attaining this target."

Sections VI and VII defined the primary health care approach and described its main elements in a way that closely resembled previous WHO documents and reports. According to the declaration, the most important aspect of primary health care was universal access (while giving priority to those most in need) to essential health care, which was scientifically sound, socially acceptable, and at a cost that the community and country could afford to maintain. The primary health care approach relied on health workers, "including physicians, nurses, midwives, auxiliaries and community workers as applicable" (WHO 1978).[75]

---

73. Telegram, from Canadian Mission in Geneva, 1 September 1978, RG25, vol. 14977, file 46–4-WHO-1, part 8. Canada National Archives.

74. WHO Document, A28/VR/13, Resolution WHA28.88, "Promotion of National Health Services Relating to Primary Health Care." PAHO Library.

75. Drawing on the principle of national self-reliance, Mahler stressed "the capital significance of training national health personnel, so that countries can as quickly as possible become self-reliant

The approach also acknowledged the need to involve related sectors, including agriculture, animal husbandry, food, industry, education, housing, public works, and communications.

Section VII identified a number of provisions that were essential for primary health care, including "education concerning prevailing health problems and the methods of preventing and controlling them; promotion of food supply and proper nutrition; an adequate supply of safe water and basic sanitation; maternal and child health care, including family planning; immunization against the major infectious diseases; prevention and control of locally endemic diseases; appropriate treatment of common diseases and injuries; and provision of essential drugs" (WHO 1978). Combined, these three sections provided a clear roadmap of the types of programs and initiatives that would be needed if governments were to follow the primary health care approach.

The declaration made explicit references to the principles of the WHO Constitution as well as of the NIEO. Section I declared a commitment to the broad definition of health as defined in the constitution and to health as a fundamental human right, and reiterated the constitution's definition of the WHO's objective. In reflecting on the association between the constitution and the Alma-Ata Declaration, member states later agreed that the "strategies for health for all by the year 2000 [were] in perfect conformity with the spirit of the Constitution of WHO."[76] Mahler suggested that the Alma-Ata Declaration was a contemporary roadmap for the constitution:

> Alma-Ata articulated page 1 of the Constitution in such a way that, rich or poor, developed or developing, no country could escape the challenge of reexamination, an agonizing reappraisal for most, of what it had been doing to fulfill the Constitution.[77]

Sections II and III, in turn, echoed the language of the NIEO in regard to the two issues also at the heart of Health for All: equity and development. As in

---

in the conduct of their own health programmes." But since "it is most unlikely that the less developed countries will have enough traditionally trained health professionals within a reasonable period of time, solutions hitherto considered unorthodox will have to be adopted." In particular, he called for "increased training and use of auxiliary health personnel, traditional midwives and healers." Mahler conceded that reliance on auxiliary health personnel "may be unpopular with some policy-makers," but he argued that "the Organization should take the stand that their adoption would be in the best interest of the people and therefore politically wise in the long run, and in no way the expedient acceptance of an inferior solution." See "The Constitutional Mission of the World Health Organization," Address by Dr. H. Mahler, Director-General of the WHO, in Presenting his Report for 1973 to the Twenty-Seventh World Health Assembly, 8 May 1974. WHO Library.

76. WHO Document, 1979, WHA32, Committee A: Fifteenth Meeting. WHO Library.

77. WHO Document, January 1980, EB65/SR/6. WHO Library.

discussions on Health for All, the bridge between the NIEO and the primary health care approach was made possible by emphasizing inequities both across and within countries and then making the claim that the primary health care approach was fundamental for reducing such inequities. Section II declared that "the existing gross inequality in the health status of the people particularly between developed and developing countries as well as within countries is . . . unacceptable." Section III declared,

> Economic and social development, based on a New International Economic Order, is of basic importance to the fullest attainment of health for all and to the reduction of the gap between the health status of the developing and developed countries. The promotion and protection of the health of the people is essential to sustained economic and social development and contributes to a better quality of life and to world peace.[78]

References to inequality and the unequal distribution of resources were also made in other WHO documents on primary health care. In his speeches, Mahler often argued that "in the field of health, the most important measure for reducing some of the *cross national and international differences* that separate human beings is, perhaps, the promotion of primary health care."[79]

The primary health care approach offered a concrete program for promoting intrastate equity. Primary health care was based on the notion that to address "cross national . . . differences" the most important population to care for was, as the Alma-Ata Declaration announced, those "most in need." While referring to primary health care as universal, therefore, there was a strict distinction between the haves and the have-nots, with the WHO policies and programs targeting the latter. According to Mahler, "Priority in ensuring [primary health] care must clearly be given to those on the social periphery, and the total health system . . . must be reoriented to support the process."[80] At the same time, it was not always clear who was considered most in need. At times, the WHO leadership referred to those who did not "belong to a privileged 10 or 20 percent," thereby including the entire rural

---

78. References to "a" (rather than "the") New International Economic Order was due to the insistence of Western countries. "Report on International Conference on Primary Health Care," by the Head of the Canadian Delegation, RG25, vol. 14977, file 46–4-WHO-1, part 8. Canada National Archives.

79. Mahler, Halfdan T, 1980, "Primary Health Care—An Analysis of Some Constraints," An Address Delivered to the Special Congregation For the Conferment of An Honorary Degree on Dr. Halfdan T. Mahler at the University of Lagos on Saturday, 20 October 1979, University of Lagos Press. WHO Library. Emphasis added.

80. "Rescue Mission for Tomorrow's Health," Interview with Director-General, Dr. Halfdan Mahler, *People* 6, no. 2, pp. 25–28. 1979. WHO Library.

population in the developing world.[81] In other cases, however, those "most in need" were referred more narrowly as those "most urgently requiring care" (WHO 1980a).

The reference to those most in need, as well as to "basic health needs," echoed the concept of "basic needs," which was embraced by the same development scholars, like Seers, who were worried that economic development and growth would be achieved without affecting the quality of life of a large part of the population (Sauvant 1981: 19). The concept of basic needs offered a remedy, by focusing, as the direct objective of development, on satisfying the basic needs of the entire population, including for primary consumption goods (food, clothing, shelter), services (water, health, education, transport), and employment. Primary health care was an actualization of the basic needs approach in the realm of health. Primary health care, appropriate technology, and essential drugs (see chapter 4) were all concepts based on the philosophy of basic needs.

The basic needs approach was a central component of the NIEO programs at the International Labor Organization and the World Bank, and they were both endorsed by developed countries.[82] These countries also supported a basic needs approach for health services. Under the Carter administration, a five-hundred-page report on international health, written by the special assistant to the president for health issues, Peter G. Bourne, confirmed that "the United States interests in International Health involve . . . the provision of access to a basic minimum level of health care for people everywhere."[83] Developing countries, in turn, found rich countries' enthusiasm a cause for concern. Indeed, a memorandum to the U.S. delegates suggested that in "speak[ing] out in support of the new [primary health care] policies in WHO governing bodies," they need "not to upstage the DG or to foster any impression among developing countries that the DG is the mouthpiece of the developed countries."[84] On the one hand, developing countries were concerned with social development themselves; for example, a document adopted at the 1970 Preparatory Conference of the Nonaligned

81. "WHO's Mission Revisited," Address by Dr. H. Mahler, Director-General of the WHO, in Presenting his Report for 1974 to the Twenty-Eighth World Health Assembly, 15 May 1975. WHO Library.

82. The concept of basic needs was referenced in a number of specialized UN world conferences, including the 1972 Stockholm Conference on the Human Environment, the 1974 Rome World Food Conference, the 1974 Bucharest World Population Conference, the 1975 Mexico World Conference of the International Women's Year, the 1976 World Employment Conference, the 1976 Vancouver Conference on Human Settlements, the 1977 Mar del Plata Water Conference, and the 1978 Alma-Ata Conference (Sauvant 1981: 21; on the World Bank see Murphy 1984: 75, 131, McMichael 2000: 55).

83. Memorandum, "International Health," from Peter Bourne to President Jimmy Carter, January 9, 1977, Staff Offices, Peter Bourne, Box 34. Carter Presidential Library.

84. Memorandum, From Robert Andrew, IO/HDC, "Improved U.S. Participation in International Organizations and Programs—WHO," June 27, 1978, Staff Offices, Peter Bourne, Box 53. Carter Presidential Library.

Countries, declared that "the ultimate purpose of development is to provide opportunities for a better life to all sections of their population by *inter alia* removing glaring inequalities in the distribution of income and wealth, eliminating
mass poverty and social injustice, creating new employment opportunities and
providing better education and health facilities" (cited in Sauvant 1981: 20–21).
On the other hand, some developing countries were deeply concerned that the
question of basic needs was used as an excuse to digress from the fundamental task of restructuring the international economic order. In their view, basic
needs strategies were attempts to change the focus of global debate and escape
responsibilities (Sauvant 1981: 21, Gish 1983: 217, Murphy 1984: 131, 140). The
assistant director for international affairs in the Carter administration reported,

> A number of people raised issue with our government's stress on basic
> human needs, believing that it was . . . ignoring other legitimate de-
> velopment goals such as the need for infrastructure and capital devel-
> opment. The faster growing developing countries do not support the
> basic human needs approach since they feel that income distribution
> will change and improve with development.[85]

A particularly critical passage articulating developing countries' concern is
found in a draft text, at the Ministerial Meeting of the G-77, in Arusha, Tanzania, in 1979.

> While the satisfaction of basic human needs of the people and the
> eradication of mass poverty must have a high priority in economic and
> social development, the idea is unacceptable and erroneous that these
> goals can be achieved without the all around and comprehensive eco-
> nomic development of the developing countries and the establishment
> of the New International Economic Order. It is necessary for develop-
> ing countries to guard against the introduction of new concepts by de-
> veloped countries . . . which are being suggested but are in fact totally
> incompatible with the development requirements and aspirations of
> developing countries. (cited in Gish 1983: 216)

In spite of developing countries' reservations, the WHO leadership successfully defended the appropriateness of the term. According to a U.S. account from
1977, "To 'meet the basic needs' philosophy has been one of Mahler's most passionately expressed beliefs. . . . It is the main theme of every major speech he

---

85. Memorandum from Robert T. Angarola, Assistant Director for International Affairs, to Peter
G. Bourne, Special Assistant to the President for Health Issues, "Geneva Visit, June 11–15, 1978," 21
June 1978, Staff Offices, Peter Bourne, Box 28. Carter Presidential Library.

makes and he is determined that WHO member countries put it into practice at home rather than just pay lip service to it."[86] Mahler's address before the World Health Assembly in 1977 was titled "World Health Target for Basic Human Needs."[87] In that speech, Mahler defended the focus on noneconomic needs.

> Man does not live by per capita income alone. Among the most funda-mental of his needs and desires is a yearning for a longer life and less illness, and for greater social opportunity so that he may have his proper enjoyment of these things. It is this that makes health improvement so powerful a lever for the genuine development of the person, the fam-ily, and the community. . . . The essential health improvements can be achieved at such a low relative cost . . . that I cannot help wondering why primary health care continues to be dismissed by the politicians of so many countries with an indifferent shrug of the shoulders.[88]

Ultimately, by insisting on the compatibility of the WHO programs with devel-oping countries' national aspirations, the WHO successfully mobilized delegates from developing countries to support the WHO secretariat's concern with intra-national inequities and the WHO's call to resolve these inequities by addressing people's basic needs.

In addition to development and equity, the Alma-Ata Declaration made use of a third NIEO principle, making the claim that primary health care was "in the spirit of self-reliance and self-determination" (WHO 1978). References to self-reliance were also common in other WHO statements and documents. In an early broad policy statement, Mahler celebrated a new relationship among member states that emerged out of the NIEO:

> I . . . sense a beginning of a general awareness in all of us being in the same global spaceship and [a general awareness] that if we are to pre-vent mutiny we must muster the conscience and will it takes to tackle the social indecencies prevailing on board. There are hopeful signs of, on the one hand, the most disfavored in our spaceship realizing that self-reliance is the indispensable physical and moral quality to bet-ter their own lot and, on the other hand, the most favored on board

---

86. Note, Department of State, "Mahler the Man," Undated, Staff Offices, Peter Bourne, Box 38, International Health—Undated Material [1]. Carter Presidential Library.
87. Address by Dr. H. Mahler, Director-General of the WHO, in Presenting his Report for 1976 to the Thirtieth World Health Assembly, 3 May 1977. WHO Library.
88. Ibid.

equally realizing that paternalism carries the seed within it of ultimate self-destruction.[89]

Speeches and programs suggest two ways by which the WHO secretariat drew on the concept of self-reliance to integrate health programs into the logic of the NIEO. In some cases, self-reliance stood for reliance on a nation's own economic resources, while in other cases, self-reliance stood for self-determination and sovereignty. Both forms were fundamental to the construction of the primary health care approach.

The notion of reliance on a nation's own economic resources was also central to the primary health care approach, appropriate technology, and essential drugs (see chapter 4). In all these programs, an emphasis was given on choosing services "at a cost that the community and country can afford to maintain" (WHO 1978). In his first address, Mahler suggested that "quite clearly, the resources [to be used for applying the appropriate solutions] are first and foremost those of the countries themselves."[90] As a U.S. report approvingly described: "One of Mahler's favorite themes is that developing countries themselves must provide 90 percent of the effort and resources needed for attaining WHO's goals. By overlooking this factor, we make developing countries look like passive recipients of largesse. . . . Mahler sees [least-developed countries] as active participants in a process leading toward self-reliance."[91] For the WHO leadership, the attractiveness of primary health care was closely linked with the possibility of economic self-reliance, that is, the promise of improving health under conditions of scarce resources and therefore independently of the need for economic growth. At the same time, Mahler insisted that "maximum national self-reliance in health matters" should not be confused with self-sufficiency.[92] Without shedding the responsibility of developing countries for financing their own programs, Mahler still assigned moral duty on developed countries.[93] In that way, developing countries could maintain their prerogative of designing those programs, which was the second, and more central, meaning of self-reliance.

---

89. Provisional Agenda Item 5, Statement by the Director-General Dr. H. Mahler, Regional Committee for Europe, Twenty-Third Session, 11–15 September 1973, FCO 61/1060. UK National Archives.

90. "The Constitutional Mission of the World Health Organization," Address by Dr. H. Mahler, Director-General of the WHO, in Presenting his Report for 1973 to the Twenty-Seventh World Health Assembly, 8 May 1974. WHO Library.

91. Note, Department of State, "Mahler the Man," Undated, Staff Offices, Peter Bourne, Box 38, International Health—Undated Material [1]. Carter Presidential Library.

92. "World Health Target for Basic Human Needs," Address by Dr. H. Mahler, Director-General of the WHO, in Presenting his Report for 1976 to the Thirtieth World Health Assembly, 3 May 1977. WHO Library.

93. See text of note 57 in this chapter. On negotiations over budget during the 1970s, see chapter 5.

During his tenure, Mahler commonly referred to self-reliance to motivate the formulation of policies and programs "from below," giving it a meaning of self-governance that was in line with the NIEO support for sovereign will.[94] Mahler's prime aim was to "open up the Organization to all member States." He wanted the WHO to be a "participatory democracy, acting on behalf of member States' own wishes and aspirations."[95] A British official reported, "Dr. Mahler's . . . message is . . . coming over loud and clear that it is the member States who have the key formative role in WHO's development."[96] In a speech before the World Health Assembly, Mahler presented self-reliance as self-governance in the following way:

> The Organization has embarked on an ambitious developmental function known as country health programming. The ambitiousness lies not in its methodology, which is as unsophisticated as can be, but rather in its ultimate aims. These, in keeping with the principle of attaining early national self-reliance, are to develop the capacities within countries to clarify for themselves the reasons for their health underdevelopment and decide by themselves, through a process that is both rational and consonant with their culture, on the most appropriate policies and programmes for developing the health of all their peoples.[97]

Self-reliance was one of the WHO's responses to the failure of vertical interventions of the 1950s, in which decisions were imposed from above with little consideration of the specific needs of countries, and Mahler explicitly contrasted the two approaches: "I emphasize the word 'collaboration' because that is the essence of the Organization's new relationship with its Member States. The provision of external experts to solve specific national problems is rapidly becoming outmoded."[98] Instead, "the starting-point [for technical cooperation programs] must be the Member States themselves. Only they can decide what is socially

---

94. In chapter 4 I show that self-reliance and sovereign will were also used to oppose the strengthening of WHO's regulative capacities.

95. WHO, Twenty-eighth WHA, Geneva, 13–30 May 1975, Department of Health and Social Security, 29 August 1975, FCO 61/1351. UK National Archives.

96. Ibid.

97. "WHO's Mission Revisited," Address by Dr. H. Mahler, Director-General of the WHO, in Presenting his Report for 1974 to the Twenty-Eighth World Health Assembly, 15 May 1975. WHO Library.

98. "Health for All by the Year 2000," Address delivered by Dr. H. Mahler, Director-General of the WHO, to the Twenty-Sixth Session of the Regional Committee for the Western Pacific, Manila, 1 September 1975, the Twenty-Fifth Session of the Regional Committee for Africa, Yaoundé, 17 September 1975, and the Twenty-Third Meeting of the Directing Council of PAHO, Twenty-Seventh Session of the WHO Regional Committee for the America, Washington, 29 September 1975. WHO Library.

relevant for them, and what methods they can apply at a political and economic cost they can afford."[99] The "Organizational Study on Methods of Promoting the Development of Basic Health Services" (WHO 1973) echoed the same sentiments. The report concluded that, "Each country will have to possess the national ability to consider its own position (problems and resources), assess the alternatives available to it, decide upon its resource allocation and priorities, and implement its own decisions." The WHO, the report said, should only serve as a "world health conscience," thereby providing a forum where new ideas could be discussed.[100]

The primary health care approach attached the meaning of self-governance to the principle of self-reliance and, in addition, shifted the focus from the country level to the community level. Participation was no longer of national governments at the international forum, but of communities and individuals at the national forum. The Alma-Ata Declaration called for "maximum community and individual self-reliance," which was defined as "participation in the planning, organization, operation and control of primary health care," and required services to "respond to the expressed health needs of the community" (WHO 1978). As with concerns regarding equity, therefore, to gain support to the primary health care approach, the WHO secretariat utilized principles central to the NIEO while providing them with a somewhat different meaning.

In short, primary health care was a radical shift in the WHO trajectory, moving from vertical interventions, which were based on Western technology and Western contributions, to a focus on health care services at the community level, which promised the universal provision of the most essential, "basic" services at affordable cost. The support for primary health care came from senior WHO leadership, most notably Newell and Mahler, who considered the primary health care approach a loyal application of WHO's constitutional mandate. They also believed primary health care served the interests of developing countries as described in the NIEO. This bridging between the primary health care approach and NIEO was achieved, as we have seen, by utilizing interpreted notions of development, equity, and self-reliance.

99. "World Health Target for Basic Human Needs," Address by Dr. H. Mahler, Director-General of the WHO, in Presenting his Report for 1976 to the Thirtieth World Health Assembly, 3 May 1977. WHO Library.

100. As I discuss in the conclusion of this chapter, the role of the WHO bureaucracy in advocating Health for All and primary health care among other policies reveals, of course, that the WHO nonetheless maintained a key and proactive position.

Countering the WHO's Strategic Adaptation: Selective Primary Health Care

The primary health care approach that was accepted in the Alma-Ata Conference and by the World Health Assembly was devoid of its original revolutionary potential, at least in the eyes of the approach's most salient advocates (Cueto 2004: 1871). Newell later tried to explain the inability of the primary health care approach to redirect national health services from particular programs to a comprehensive program:

> Large, formal international meetings of national representatives have their own peculiar needs. It is difficult for a representative to return home and report on an ideology. What is wanted is a programme. At Alma-Ata, almost inevitably the emphasis moved from what is wrong, and why, to what can health services do, and how can success be measured. Lists started to appear of health status problems which needed to be dealt with and they included the expected, including maternal and child mortality, water and sanitation, health education, fertility, and the communicable diseases. It can fairly be said that it would be surprising if such widespread horrors were not on such a list. However, the risk of such an activity is that when you start with *any* list, the entire reasoning starts to change and the list becomes the objective. (Newell 1988: 904)

For others, primary health care proved too radical. Despite initial enthusiasm, some member states soon criticized the Alma-Ata Declaration for being too broad and idealistic (Cueto 2004: 1868), and the impossibility of achieving anything so grandiose ("health for all") by a fixed date ("by the year 2000") was ridiculed (Litsios 2002: 308). Developing countries were deterred by the emphasis on "from below" devoid of concrete instructions. A representative of Botswana, for example, admitted that "her delegation had been overwhelmed by the responsibilities outlined and daunted by the absence of any tangible or quantitative aim."[101]

The section in the Alma-Ata Declaration specifying provisions, such as maternal health, that were essential for primary health care, combined with members' concerns that the primary health care approach was too broad, explains Newell's conclusion that "It can be said that 'selective primary health care' may possibly have started from the lists of Alma Ata" (Newell 1988: 904). This counterrevolution took an even sharper form following a conference in Bellagio, Italy, in 1979, which was sponsored by the Rockefeller Foundation, with the support of the World Bank,

---

101. WHO Document, 1979, WHA32/A/SR/15, p. 204. WHO Library.

and attended by heads of the World Bank, the Ford Foundation, the U.S. Agency for International Development (USAID), and the Canadian International Development and Research Center among others (Cueto 2004: 1868, Brown, Cueto, and Fee 2006: 67). In that meeting, wealthy countries managed to express support of the primary health care approach, while co-opting the language of the WHO's approach to create programs more closely aligned with their concerns.

The Bellagio Conference was organized around a paper entitled "Selective Primary Health Care: An Interim Strategy for Disease Control in Developing Countries," published that year by Kenneth S. Warren, the director of health services at the Rockefeller Foundation, and Julia Walsh, an assistant professor of medicine at New York University and a visiting research fellow of the Rockefeller Foundation (Walsh and Warren 1979). In the paper, the authors calculated the feasibility of controlling the "major" infectious diseases of the Global South (based on prevalence, mortality, and morbidity) in terms of the effectiveness and cost of available interventions. The paper then identified four interventions that, the authors claimed, should be at the core of a global program to improve health in many parts of the developing world: immunization, oral rehydration, breastfeeding, and the use of antimalarial drugs (Warren 1988: 891). In other words, the paper offered a strategic response to the WHO's primary health care approach by endorsing the principles of the approach in order to advocate a program that, in effect, contradicted those very principles by recommending that resources again be directed into programs that sought quick technical solutions rather than integrated programs that addressed a wider range of development issues over the longer term.

By the mid-1980s, several donor agencies had adopted policies in line with the argument put forward by Walsh and Warren and endorsed in the Bellagio Conference (Unger and Killingsworth 1986: 1002–1003). UNICEF, too, soon backed away from a holistic approach to primary health care. Under James Grant, who was appointed executive director in January 1980, UNICEF proposed a "children's revolution" that reduced the number of recommended interventions to four: growth monitoring of infants and proper nutrition, oral rehydration techniques to control infant diarrheal diseases, breast-feeding, and immunization (GOBI). Other agencies added food supplementation, female literacy, and family planning (FFF) to the interventions under GOBI (Warren 1988: 893, Cueto 2004: 1869). Eventually, selective primary health care (SPHC) came to replace primary health care as the dominant approach.

The WHO leadership and other early supporters of the primary health care approach refused to accept the changes adopted by others. They warned that SPHC involved heavy reliance on technology, that it was essentially a vertical program with a management structure very different from the horizontal decentralization advocated by PHC, and that it did not respond directly to the concerns of the people (Warren 1988: 892). They also claimed that the selective interventions did not tackle the real issues. Oral rehydration solutions, for example, were unsuitable in places where safe water and sewage systems did not exist (Cueto 2004: 1870–1872). According to Newell (1988: 904),

> SPHC proposals are not PHC at all but are the antithesis of it. They are disease control programmes which are ideologically similar to the malaria eradication disaster and are a regression to the very qualities of imposed systems. . . . In no way do they share the objectives of PHC.

Mahler, too, opposed the retreat from the original PHC concept. He also resented the consideration of health issues by bodies other than the WHO. In an address to the World Health Assembly, in 1983, Mahler presented the debate as one between the collective position of WHO delegates on the one hand, and "people outside developing countries" and "foreign agents," on the other.

> Honorable delegates, while we have been striking ahead with singleness of purpose in WHO based on your collective decisions, others appear to have little patience for such systematic efforts, however democratically they are applied. There are unfortunate signs that negative impatience is looming on the horizon and some of it is already peeping over and gaining superficial visibility. . . . I am referring to such initiatives as the selection by people outside the developing countries of a few isolated elements of primary health care for implementation in these countries; or the parachuting of foreign agents into these countries to immunize them from above; or the concentration on only one aspect of diarrheal disease control without thought for the others. Initiatives such as these are red herrings. . . . Without building up health infrastructures based on primary health care, valuable energy will only be wasted, and you will be deflected from your path. (cited in Unger and Killingsworth 1986: 1003)

In the following years, Mahler continued his crusade for more holistic primary health care in different forums. By then, however, he no longer had the full support of the WHO's bureaucracy. As I describe in chapter 5, selective primary health care reflected a general movement, which gained power in the mid-1980s, against many of the principles and programs informing the New International Economic Order, and Mahler's opposition to the new trends reflected his overall inability to adapt to the post-NIEO era (Cueto 2004: 1871).

Discussion

In his address before the World Health Assembly, in May 1978, just a couple of months before the Alma-Ata Conference, Mahler had passionately declared,

> I am taking the unusual step of appealing directly from the platform of this Health Assembly to the political leaders of the world. . . . I know that many of you have doubts about a New International Order; I do not share them. I know that many of you will have equal doubts about attaining health for all by the year 2000; again, I do not share them. I also know that others among you will fear that my proposal is a social smokescreen to hide the world's unwillingness to bring about the New International Economic Order. It is not; and I see no cause for fear. If you are vigilant and we are steadfast, the two will complement each other. . . .
>
> Political leaders of the world, use the neutral ground of health to promote global development dialogue! . . . Use health as a lever for social and economic development! More than that, use it as a platform for peace![102]

In this address and elsewhere, Health for All and primary health care were effectively presented as the contribution of the World Health Organization to the call for a new international economic order. The Alma-Ata Declaration concluded with a call "for urgent and effective . . . action to develop and implement primary health care throughout the world and particularly in developing countries . . . in keeping with a New International Economic Order." In his address to the World Health Assembly the following year, Mahler referred to the Alma-Ata Declaration as "the New International Economic Order in the field of health, or—if you prefer—a new international order in health."[103] However, the WHO secretariat's response to the demands of developing countries, which could control WHO programs with a stable coalition of votes, was not a passive compliance with NIEO principles, in spite of the WHO leadership's support of the cause of developing countries. Instead, the WHO leadership altered the meaning of central NIEO principles, including development, equity, and self-reliance, to introduce programs that reflected the mission of the organization as declared in the constitution and that echoed the new interest of public health experts in basic health infrastructure. In addition, given the minimal emphasis on economic issues, inequities among states, and external resources, the WHO leadership was

---

102. "World Health is Indivisible," Address by Dr. H. Mahler, Director-General of the WHO, to the Thirty-First World Health Assembly, 9 May 1978. WHO Library.
103. "Action for Health," Address by Dr. H. Mahler, Director-General of the WHO, to the Thirty-Second World Health Assembly, 8 May 1979. WHO Library.

able to recruit also the support of developed countries to these initiatives. The WHO secretariat did not always conceal the gaps and tensions between the NIEO and the WHO approach—between economic and social development, between inter- and intranational inequality, and between local self-reliance and national self-reliance—but it successfully legitimated those gaps, and thereby gained the support of developing countries.

As this chapter clearly shows, the call for Health for All by the Year 2000 and primary health care as the strategy to achieve it were informed by reports, documents, and studies written by or on behalf of the secretariat, who also formulated and actively promoted those programs. Clearly, specific formulations were the outcome of extensive negotiations among member states. The final wording of the Alma-Ata Declaration, for example, was somewhat different from the original drafts.[104] However, the core agenda and the reasoning used to justify it were the making of the WHO bureaucracy. This is not to suggest that the WHO staff acted autonomously. After all, much consideration was given to exogenous pressures. But these initiatives confirm the perception of an international bureaucracy as an agency, with the potential for holding and defending independent goals.

At the same time, WHO documents reveal a complex interplay between external pressures and the organization's understanding of its goals. While the NIEO logic was altered to fit better with the WHO principles, those principles were seen in the light of that external logic. Mahler insisted that Health for All reflected the truthful meaning of the constitution, but he knew that this meaning could have only developed in the particular context of the NIEO. Hence, while criticizing member states for until then reducing health to "questions of morbidity and mortality," and for turning the responsibility of the WHO to nothing more than "fragmented scientific groups and technical assistance projects," Mahler also conceded that the reappraisal of the organization's activities in the late 1970s occurred as a result of historical developments in the world. An Alma-Ata Conference could not have been held in the 1950s.[105]

Finally, there were important limits to the ability of the WHO to manipulate the environment. Health for All and primary health care revealed the capacity of an international bureaucracy to strategically adapt to exogenous pressures. Selective primary health care, in turn, showed the equal capacity of member states and

104. International Conference on Primary Health Care, Annotated Agenda, 15 May 1978, WHO/UNICEF, ICPHC/ALA/78.1, RG25, vol. 14977, file 46–4-WHO-1, part 8. Canada National Archives.
105. WHO Document, January 1980, EB65/SR/6. WHO Library.

other external forces to strategically adapt to the WHO's strategically adapted initiatives. In the next chapter, I describe the WHO policies that attempted to regulate the behavior of multinational corporations in developing countries. These attempts involved both strategic compliance and strategic resistance, and reveal further limitations in the ability of international organizations to act.

APPROPRIATE TECHNOLOGY, INAPPROPRIATE MARKETING

Medicines which may be of the utmost value to poorer countries can be bought by us only at exorbitant prices, since we are unable to have adequate independent bases of research and production. . . . Sometimes dangerous new drugs are tried out on populations of weaker countries although their use is prohibited within the countries of manufacture. It also happens that publicity makes us victims of habits and practices which are economically wasteful or wholly contrary to good health. . . . My idea of a better ordered world is one in which . . . there would be no profiteering from life or death.

—Indira Ghandi, prime minister of India, addressing the Thirty-Fourth World Health Assembly, 1981

The New International Economic Order intended to transform not only the relations between developing and developed countries, but also between developing countries and multinational companies. As examined in chapter 3, a central tenet of the NIEO was that of economic sovereignty, which promoted independence in economic affairs among developing countries, without interference from developed countries and multinational companies. To allow governments greater control over economic activities under their jurisdiction, the G-77 advocated the principles of national control over natural resources and private foreign investment. The G-77 also wanted UN member states to collectively monitor the behavior of multinational corporations in developing countries, for example, by regulating restrictive business practices. In addition, in an attempt to improve industrialization while lessening their dependence on multinational corporations, developing countries called for an international code of conduct on the transfer of technology that would commit Western governments to share their technologies with the South.

Developing countries directed some of their most pointed criticisms of multinational companies at the pharmaceutical sector. As forcefully expressed by the prime minister of India, Indira Ghandi, in the epigraph above, drug manufacturers were accused of selling unsafe products to uninformed, vulnerable, and poor populations in the developing world. In the new "ordered world" that Ghandi envisioned, in contrast, "there would be no profiteering from life or death" (cited in Patel 1983: 165). Developing countries asked UN agencies for guidance in manufacturing drugs locally. They also asked for assistance in their attempts to lower the prices of imported drugs and medical equipment and to curtail unethical marketing and pressure exerted by drug companies on governments to purchase drugs.

The focus on the pharmaceutical sector put the WHO at the center of the debate. The WHO staff shared developing countries' criticisms of the pharmaceutical sector. WHO reports confirmed the accusations that pharmaceutical companies had been exporting unnecessary or unsafe drugs to developing countries and had manipulated uninformed governments and vulnerable populations in other ways. Turning these criticisms into antipharmaceutical initiatives, however, would have been costly for the WHO. Transnational companies responded to threats to their commercial interests with little empathy and actively lobbied against proposed initiatives and against the UN agencies supporting them. Western governments, where big business had powerful lobbies and political interests, were also disinclined to respond to the demands of developing countries. Concerned that multinational companies would be successful in their attempts to undermine WHO legitimacy and authority, the WHO staff and leadership acted cautiously when assisting developing countries with the purchasing and local manufacturing of drugs.

By preparing (and, later, periodically updating) a model list of essential drugs—namely, affordable drugs that experts deemed of acceptable quality, safety, and efficacy and that were indispensable for the health needs of a given population—the WHO staff intended to help governments in their drug purchasing decisions.[1] The purchasing of essential drugs for the poor was considered a crucial aspect of primary health care and Health for All strategies, but like these initiatives, it was not obviously compatible with the NIEO. To reconcile the two, the WHO bureaucracy reframed the NIEO call for transfer of technologies to mean transfer of *appropriate* technology. However, the model list of essential drugs, which was presented as a tool to counter misinformation and pressure, was a provocative challenge against the pharmaceutical sector. When counterpressures coming from the pharmaceutical industry

---

1. WHO Document, 1975, "Prophylactic and Therapeutic Substances. Report by the Director-General," A28/11. PAHO Library.

threatened the legitimacy of the model list, the WHO secretariat was willing to relinquish some of its ideational goals and, in order to make it more agreeable to the industry, to limit the scope of applicability of the list. Hence, the model list of essential drugs was the outcome, first, of the WHO secretariat strategically complying with developing countries' expectations in a way that was compatible with the organization's ideational concerns with appropriate technology and equity, and second, of the WHO leadership then modifying the provisions in attempt to make the policy agreeable also to the pharmaceutical industry.

The list of essential drugs was a provocative experiment, but its prioritization reflected a neglect of developing countries' expectation that UN agencies would actively help in improving access to essential drugs through local manufacturing. The WHO bureaucracy initially supported other UN agencies' initiatives for transferring pharmaceutical technology to the South but later, in attempt to avoid a reputation of "amateurism and indecision," played down the importance of local production in favor of affordable imports.[2]

The WHO leadership's most explicit strategic resistance to developing countries' demands occurred when Mahler and others urged member states *not* to initiate an international code of marketing of pharmaceutical products. The very negative (although successful) experience of negotiating an international code of marketing of infant formula, which the WHO secretariat supported, convinced Mahler that a conflict over a similar code for the pharmaceutical sector would greatly undermine the WHO's legitimacy. Mahler used two arguments to dissuade developing countries from supporting an international code, both of which utilized the tension between international codes and NIEO principles. First, alluding to the principles of political and economic sovereignty (and disregarding the NIEO competing principle of strengthening universal international organizations), Mahler insisted that the organization was an international organization, not a "supranational" one, and that it should therefore not be involved in domestic regulation. Second, Mahler utilized the WHO's stated responsibility for the poor rather than the rich—the notion of equity—to suggest that the marketing of pharmaceuticals, which would have protected consumers who could afford to buy them, should not be a priority of the organization. In this way, while still resisting the demands of developing countries, the WHO avoided a seemingly inevitable confrontation that passive resistance would have led to.

---

2. WHO Document, 1980, EB66/SR/2. WHO Library.

Appropriate Technology
Against the "Technological Distortion of Social Relevance"

The primary health care approach was an explicit rejection of curative, urban-based, and high-technology care that many developing countries had inherited from colonial times (see chapter 3). As part of the skewed resource allocation typical of those health systems, developing countries spent most of their health budget on expensive imported medical technology and expensive imported drugs (Melrose 1983:182). This was what Mahler referred to as "placebo technology," namely, "the use of many drugs in vogue [and] expensive equipment which is often applied in an unselective manner."[3] In contrast, the primary health care approach focused on preventive care, rural populations, and importantly, on what Mahler termed *appropriate* technology. Implicitly criticizing transfer of *inappropriate* technology "in such areas as essential drugs, medical equipment, and spare parts for such equipment" (WHO 1980a), the Alma-Ata Declaration stated that one of the principles of primary health care was reliance on "scientifically sound and socially acceptable ... technology" (WHO 1978).

The suggestion that Western technology was likely not to be appropriate for developing countries reflected a rejection of the "magic bullet" approach of the 1950s, which Mahler attributed, in turn, to the relations between the North and South preceding the call for a New International Economic Order.

> We are still over-conscious of our past, with its successes and failures all related to a world context that is no more—one that was created by a postwar surge partly of international social awareness in technically advancing countries, and partly of national technical awareness in socially advancing countries that had just graduated from colonialism. In this situation, it was perhaps inevitable that the [World Health] Organization should give rather too much emphasis to an unselective transfer of technologies from the more technically developed to the less technically developed countries. This process . . . proved to be too uniform for our pluralistic world, and even in some cases counter-productive. That this technology transfer was not as neutral as it appeared, and that it was permeated by the consumer-culture of the civilization from which it stemmed were questions rarely raised. The time is now over-ripe to raise them. . . . We increasingly realize that technological advance will not of itself ensure its social application. . . . Indeed, the

---

3. "Social Perspectives in Health," Address by Dr. H. Mahler, Director-General of the World Health Organization, in Presenting his Report for 1975 to the Twenty-Ninth World Health Assembly, Geneva, 4 May 1976. WHO Library.

very under-development of health . . . is intimately connected with this technological distortion of social relevance.[4]

A criticism of transfer of inappropriate technology could be seen by developing countries as a rejection of the NIEO's central tenet of promoting technology transfer, which did not differentiate between appropriate and inappropriate technology. For different reasons, Western countries and the Soviet Union were also unenthusiastic about that principle. Western countries were concerned that it would be used for regulating multinational corporations, including the pharmaceutical sector. The Soviet Union, in turn, was a strong supporter of technology-based health systems (see chapter 3). Indeed, some of Mahler's statements were intended specifically at the Soviets. As a British delegate described at the time:

> [Mahler's] key message this year . . . was that there was a very real danger that technical knowledge was advancing and spreading so rapidly in the health field that it would be at the expense of the application of known basic health techniques. This was a scantily camouflaged reference to the ideological battle between the vast majority of member States who place great emphasis on primary health care in under-developed countries, and the minority, led by the USSR, who insist that a full-scale Soviet style health service is the only road to salvation. It was not difficult to see whose side the DG is on when he spoke of the danger of advanced health technology becoming a mockery when viewed from the Third World.[5]

In spite of these potential tensions, the WHO bureaucracy was able to effectively frame the notion of appropriate technology around NIEO principles. The WHO staff even presented it as an *exemplar* for how to turn NIEO into programs. As with primary health care, the WHO secretariat relied on the notions of equity, economic sovereignty, and self-reliance to translate the demand for transfer of technology into policies promoting appropriate technology.

Stressing the importance of equity, Mahler reminded member states that "we must always bear in mind the practical application of existing and new scientific knowledge *for the benefit of the masses* of the world's population."[6] And his criti-

---

4. "WHO's Mission Revisited," Address by Dr. H. Mahler, Director-General of the WHO in Presenting his Report for 1974 to the Twenty-Eighth World Health Assembly, 15 May 1975. WHO Library.

5. WHO, 28th WHA, Geneva, 13–30 May 1975, Department of Health and Social Security, 29 August 1975, FCO 61/1351. UK National Archives.

6. "Social Perspectives in Health," Address by Dr. H. Mahler, Director-General of the World Health Organization, in Presenting his Report for 1975 to the Twenty-Ninth World Health Assembly, Geneva, 4 May 1976. WHO Library. Emphasis added.

cism against the "very strong tendency to transfer to developing countries health technologies that have taken root in the industrialized countries" was that it exacerbated inequities by reaching those who already had access to such technologies and failing to reach those who did not have such access.[7]

> For all the speed with which disease technology has been flourishing in recent years, it has been failing in its purpose. . . . The extension and refinement of this technology on the one hand and its increased complexity and cost on the other have led to a contradiction between the technical potential and the socioeconomic ability to apply it to all who need it.[8]

Primary health care was not about granting the masses access to complex technology. Instead, "whenever possible, attempts should be made to devise simple yet effective health technologies that can be applied by auxiliary personnel to assist in meeting the needs of those hundreds of millions of people who today have no access to more sophisticated health care."[9]

Here and elsewhere, the WHO secretariat's focus was less on the prohibition of inappropriate technology, which could have been seen as blocking the development of poor countries and would have been opposed by poor and rich countries alike. To assure member states that the call for "appropriate" or "simple" technology was not an indiscriminate rejection of "modern" technology, Mahler reiterated that "it is not health technology per se that is being questioned. WHO will continue to collaborate in the transfer of so-called modern technology wherever it seems reasonable and significantly useful."[10] Instead, speeches, reports, and policies focused to a much greater extent on encouraging the use of, and improving access to, suitable or appropriate technology.

---

7. "The Constitutional Mission of the World Health Organization," Address by Dr. H. Mahler, Director-General of the WHO, in Presenting his Report for 1973 to the Twenty-Seventh World Health Assembly, 8 May 1974. WHO Library.

8. "Social Perspectives in Health," Address by Dr. H. Mahler, Director-General of the World Health Organization, in Presenting his Report for 1975 to the Twenty-Ninth World Health Assembly, Geneva, 4 May 1976. WHO Library.

9. "The Constitutional Mission of the World Health Organization," Address by Dr. H. Mahler, Director-General of the WHO, in Presenting his Report for 1973 to the Twenty-Seventh World Health Assembly, 8 May 1974. WHO Library.

10. "Health for All by the Year 2000." Address delivered by Dr. H. Mahler, Director-General of the WHO to the Twenty-sixth Session of the regional committee for the Western Pacific, Manila, 1 September 1975, the Twenty-Seventh Session of the regional committee for Africa, Yaoundé, 17 September 1975, and the Twenty-Third meeting of the directing council of PAHO, Twenty-seventh session of the WHO regional committee for the America, Washington, 29 September 1975. WHO Library.

Examples of appropriate technology, in the context of health, included "provision of potable water and the adequate disposal of sewage, the elimination of disease vectors, the prevention of environmental pollution at the source, immunization against specific infectious diseases, specific chemotherapy including the use of antibiotics, some forms of surgery, and certain family planning methods."[11] Mahler regarded the successful smallpox eradication program as a particularly useful illustration of such technology, which was highly scientific but free of corporate manipulation.

> Technical realism [in the smallpox eradication program] led to the development and use of the right action—surveillance, containment, selective vaccination facilitated by freeze-dried vaccine, the use of the bifurcated needle and, above all, adequate community involvement. The development of all these tools demanded research of a highly scientific, technical and operational nature, whose results were put to immediate use wherever needed, without any commercial hindrance.[12]

Mahler then suggested that programs such as smallpox eradication were at the core of a successful New International Economic Order: "Add to this the international transfer of resources in kind and in cash, and you have all the ingredients of a success story that . . . truly can act as a shining example to any field of endeavor within the New International Economic Order."[13]

In addition to equity, more provocatively, the WHO staff also relied on the NIEO themes of self-determination and economic sovereignty to support the concept of appropriate technology. WHO reports declared that "the transfer of inappropriate technology can be viewed as a form of foreign occupation or of technological neo-colonialism" and that, in contrast, "appropriate technology is a principal stepping stone to self-reliance, and self-reliance, in turn, is at the heart of NIEO and primary health care" (WHO 1980a). In the same report, the "transfer of appropriate technology for health to developing countries" was described in the following way:

> The aim is to promote the development within countries of simple but scientifically sound health technologies, adapted to local needs,

---

11. "Social Perspectives in Health," Address by Dr. H. Mahler, Director-General of the World Health Organization, in Presenting his Report for 1975 to the Twenty-Ninth World Health Assembly, Geneva, 4 May 1976. WHO Library.

12. "Action for Health," Address by Dr. H. Mahler, Director-General of the WHO to the Thirty-Second World Health Assembly, 8 May 1979. WHO Library.

13. In the same speech, Mahler appealed to the governments of developed countries for funds: "You are already making huge savings by being absolved from the need to vaccinate your people against smallpox. Please do plough that money back into health in the developing world! It will bring you social and economic dividend as your investment in smallpox did." "Action for Health," Address by Dr. H. Mahler, Director-General of the WHO to the Thirty-Second World Health Assembly, 8 May 1979. WHO Library.

acceptable to those who apply them and to those for whom they are used, and able to be maintained by the people themselves, in keeping with the principle of self-reliance, with resources that the community and the country can afford. . . . Emphasis is laid on the development of the right kind of health technologies by Third World countries themselves. . . . By diminishing the influence of the socially irrelevant health technologies of the affluent countries and their high import costs for developing countries this type of programme could be one of the bases of a NIEO. (WHO 1980a)

In short, by suggesting that only the transfer of appropriate technology was compatible with the NIEO principles of equity, economic sovereignty, and self-reliance, the WHO secretariat was able to justify its position and make it acceptable to developing countries. Applying the logic of appropriate technology to the issue of drugs in a way that would also make it acceptable to the pharmaceutical sector, however, proved to be more challenging, as the WHO staff discovered when developing the concept of essential drugs.

Model List of Essential Drugs

The WHO's criticisms of inappropriate technology coincided with the experience of developing countries in regard to the distribution and marketing of drugs (Mamdani 1992: 12). In discussions on the need of Third World countries to gain access to drugs, some damning accusations were made against the business practices of transnational pharmaceutical companies, including charges of product dumping and of unethical marketing. Studies showed that drug companies produced medicines for exports in the Third World that did not meet the same standards of safety and efficacy as those intended for sale in the West, and they sold to the Third World harmful or ineffective drugs that had been withdrawn from the market in industrialized countries. Drug companies also used misleading labeling and information and failed to warn against serious and possibly fatal side effects. For example, a study for the International Organization of Consumers Unions examined the labeling of fifty-five packs of chloramphenicol from twenty-one countries and found that not a single one warned against all the conditions for which the use of chloramphenicol was contraindicated, and many packs failed to warn against serious and possibly fatal side-effects (Fazal 1983: 266). A popular publication on the unethical practices of the multinational drug industry, *The Drugging of the Americas*, showed that the information attached to drugs distributed in Latin America differed considerably from the information provided in the United States, that indications for use of the drugs were far more numerous, and that contraindications were fewer (Silverman 1976). Drug companies also utilized ruthless methods of promotion in an attempt to artificially create a demand for the most profitable of their patented drugs, with a limited relation to actual needs (Mamdani 1992: 6–7, also Melrose 1983: 183–185). An executive board member from Bangladesh complained, "Demand had been created more by the promotional activities of the manufacturers than by the genuine needs of the population, and consequently many unnecessary drugs had come on the market, resulting in much wasteful expenditure."[14] The prices of these drugs, in turn, were out of proportion to the purchasing power of the poor and often out of proportion to their effectiveness (Mamdani 1992: 2). Price manipulations and aggressive marketing meant that drugs represented a disproportionate percentage of the overall national health budgets in poor countries. For example, Thailand spent 30.4 percent of its government health budget in 1976 on drugs, while Bangladesh spent 63.7 percent of its health budget on drugs (Mamdani 1992: 2). In addition, the common problem of skewed allocation of resources applied also to the allocation of drugs, which were distributed mostly in urban areas (Melrose 1983: 182). Inadequate social infrastructure—including a lack of government policy, implementation difficulties, poorly trained physicians and pharmacists, and ineffective management capacity—exacerbated the problem (Reich 1987: 40, Mamdani 1992: 6).

Unlike Health for All and Primary Health Care, the impetus for a WHO action on drugs came not from the secretariat but the developing countries themselves, who were quite explicit in their criticisms. In expressing their anger with the misconduct of transnational pharmaceutical companies, Third World governments drew on themes from the New International Economic Order, juxtaposing the current situation of dependence and exploitation with a desired future of self-reliance.[15] Following the prevailing sentiments among poor countries, discussions at the WHO centered around two types of "national drug policies aiming at self-reliance":[16] the selection of essential drugs "to meet [developing countries'] real needs" and the local production of drugs "wherever feasible." These solutions drew on existing policies in several Third World countries, including Costa Rica, Cuba, Egypt, India, Mexico, Mozambique, Pakistan, Peru, and Sri Lanka. Governments in these countries had stepped up local production of drugs, purchased a bulk

---

14. WHO Document, 1978, EB61/SR/2, p. 10. WHO Library.

15. "Record of Meeting of Commonwealth Representatives, Prior to the Thirty-first World Health Assembly," Geneva, 7 May 1978, RG25, vol. 14977, file 46–4-WHO-1, part 7. Canada National Archives.

16. WHO Document, 1978, Background Document for reference and use at the Technical Discussions on "National Policies and Practices in Regard to Medicinal Products, and Related International Problems," A31/Technical Discussions/1. PAHO Library.

supply of essential drugs in generic forms, and established limited lists of essential drugs for the public sector (Mamdani and Walker 1986: 190, Mamdani 1992: 8).

The idea that the WHO could help guide governments in procurement strategies and the notion of "essential" drugs came from a meeting of experts in 1975 on the difficulties of developing countries in meeting the cost of the medicines needed for their health programs.[17] The experts prepared a report that confirmed the use of unethical practices by drug companies in developing countries:

> Drugs not authorized for sale in the country of origin—or withdrawn from the market for reasons of safety or lack of efficacy—are sometimes exported and marketed in developing countries; other drugs are promoted and advertised in those countries for indications that are not approved by regulatory agencies of the countries of origin. Products not meeting the quality requirements of the exporting country, including products beyond their expiry date, may be exported to developing countries that are not in a position to carry out quality control measures.[18]

The report argued that "while these practices may conform to legal requirements, they are unethical and detrimental to health." The report also blamed the international pharmaceutical industry for overproducing nonessential drugs for undeveloped and developing countries: "The development and marketing of a non-essential product for the symptomatic relief of trivial conditions may take precedence . . . [over] a new, essential drug for the control of a serious disease affecting millions of people in the least developing countries." The report concluded that "there is an urgent need to ensure that the most essential drugs are available at a reasonable price and to stimulate research and development to produce new drugs adapted to the real health requirements of developing countries." Relating it to NIEO principles, the report continued, "This calls for the development of national drug policies . . . formulated within the context of social and economic development."[19]

The report defined essential drugs as "those considered to be of the utmost importance and hence basic, indispensable, and necessary for the health needs of the population. They should be available at all times, in the proper dosage forms, to all segments of society." The report then recommended that the WHO draw up a model list of essential drugs.[20]

---

17. UNICEF and PAHO had used limited lists of drugs in supplying countries and assistance programs already prior to the 1970s (Reich 1986: 45–46). WHO Document, "Summary by the Chairman of the Ad Hoc Committee on Drug Policies," 1984, EB73/SR/13, p. 179. WHO Library.

18. WHO Document, 1975, "Prophylactic and Therapeutic Substances: Report by the Director-General," A28/11. PAHO Library.

19. Ibid.

20. Ibid.; see also Reich 1987: 40.

The expert report was presented to the Executive Board and the World Health Assembly. In Resolution WHA28.66, the assembly endorsed the report and requested that the director-general "develop means by which the Organization can be of greater direct assistance to Member States in advising on the selection and procurement, at reasonable cost, of essential drugs of established quality corresponding to their national health needs." At the Fifth Nonaligned Conference in Colombo, Sri Lanka, in 1976, developing countries formally endorsed the plan, calling for "the preparation of a list of priority pharmaceutical needs of each developing country and the formulation of a basic model list of such needs as a general guideline for action by the developing countries" (cited in Lall 1978: 29–30).

In 1977, the WHO established a new unit under the Division of Diagnostic, Prophylactic and Therapeutic Substances, called Drug Policies and Management (DPM). The DPM's first activity was to convene an expert panel to develop a model essential drugs list that would provide a template for countries seeking to establish their own national lists of priority medicines (Walt and Harnmeijer 1992: 27, Laing et al. 2003: 1723). The same year, the expert panel published a technical report, "WHO Expert Committee on the Selection of Essential Drugs,"[21] which included a model list of 224 essential drugs and vaccines as well as guidelines for preparing such a list at the national level that would depend on each country's morbidity patterns, available financial resources, and local preferences. The process for selecting the drugs was critical for the acceptance of the list by member states, and the Expert Committee carefully described the criteria it considered in the selection process. Drugs were selected based on benefit and safety evaluations obtained in clinical trials and/or epidemiological studies; generic names were used whenever possible; regulations and facilities had to be available to ensure that the quality of selected medicinal products met adequate quality control standards, including stability and, when necessary, bioavailability; cost (of the total treatment, not only the unit cost) represented a major selection criterion; preference was given to therapeutically equivalent products for which local, reliable manufacturing facilities existed; and, in future evaluations, new drugs were to be introduced only if they offered distinct advantages over existing ones.[22] By 1984, the WHO could proudly state that thanks to both the original model list, which was periodically updated, and to the guidelines, "More than 80, perhaps as many as 100, countries have already developed a list of essential drugs based on the WHO model list."[23]

---

21. WHO Document, 1977, Technical Report Series, No. 615. WHO Library.

22. WHO Document, 1978, Background Document for reference and use at the Technical Discussions on "National Policies and Practices in Regard to Medicinal Products; and Related International Problems," A31/Technical Discussions/1, p. 18. PAHO Library.

23. WHO Document, DAP Comments on ACC Task Force Project Proposal No. 3, 24 May 1984. WHO Library.

In introducing the model list in 1978, the chairman of the Executive Board stated, "The concept of an essential drug introduced a new dimension into the Organization's programme. Drugs were no longer viewed purely from the scientific or technical point of view but, above all, in the light of health priorities and of the delivery of health care to the population as a whole. It was thus a social approach that formed the basis of that concept."[24] Essential drugs were also a central aspect of Health for All and of the primary health care approach. A report by the director-general asserted, "There is no question that essential drugs are a major entry point into the community as part of the primary health care. . . . At all levels of health care delivery they are an essential part of the health-for-all strategy."[25] A report by the UN Conference on Trade and Development (UNCTAD) on the pharmaceutical industry, agreed: "The basic objective of every nation . . . is to provide at least an adequate supply of essential drugs and vaccines to meet the basic health needs of its people" (UNCTAD 1979: 2). The Alma-Ata Declaration identified the provision of essential medicines as one of eight key components of primary health care.

A model list of essential drugs was a radical endeavor. In effect, the WHO suggested that governments, following the advice of experts, should have the power to restrict the drugs available in the market or, at a minimum, prioritize the purchasing of drugs essential to the population over other drugs, including not only those deemed unsafe, but those that were considered too expensive or that were for treating "nonbasic" medical needs. This move went beyond the criticisms of most developing countries, and it challenged a long-held notion in the medical profession that persons should have the right to any drugs that would improve their health.

This move also threatened the commercial interests of drug companies. Indeed, the drug industry saw in the essential drugs list an unprecedented attempt to curtail its freedom of action in the production and marketing of drugs and was explicitly hostile in its response (Reich 1987: 49–50, Mamdani 1992: 19, Walt and Harnmeijer 1992: 30). When the list was published, a formal statement adopted by the Council of the International Federation of Pharmaceutical Manufacturers and Associations (IFPMA) expressed "serious reservations about the drug policies recommended in the . . . Report," and the industry's trade journal, SCRIP, declared that the list was "completely unacceptable to the pharmaceutical industry" (cited in Mamdani 1992: 19). The industry asserted that there was no "shred of evidence" to the assertions made in the report that "the number of necessary

---

24. WHO Document, 1978, EB61/SR/2, p. 8. WHO Library.
25. WHO Document, 1981, EB69/22, Action Programme on Essential Drugs, Report by the Director-General. PAHO Library.

drugs is relatively small" or that "promotional activities of the manufacturers have created a demand greater than [actual needs]."[26] The industry warned that "adoption of the Report's recommendations would result in suboptimal medical care and might reduce health standards already attained," and it threatened that the report "would discourage investment by the pharmaceutical industry in research."[27]

The objections of the pharmaceutical sector focused on two issues. First, the industry was worried that by creating a list of essential drugs, the WHO was arguing that all other drugs not included in the list were *non*essential.[28] An IFPMA note stated, "It is particularly unfortunate if the inference is drawn from the use of the word "essential" that all other drugs not so designated are unnecessary."[29] At least one American official believed that changing the name of the list from "essential" to "basic" drugs "would remove an impediment to support of the concept by the drug industry."[30] The WHO kept the term "essential" but, to mitigate the industry's antagonism, statements made by the WHO secretariat became intentionally ambiguous on whether essential drug policies were designed to promote essential drugs or to *exclude* certain nonessential drugs (Reich 1987: 49). The president of the International Organization of Consumers Unions (IOCU), Anwar Fazal, complained that "the WHO's programme on essential drugs originally referred to the need to restrict the supply of conspicuously inessential drugs. . . . It no longer does" (Fazal 1983: 267). In turn, Michael Peretz, executive vice president of IFPMA, was "glad to say that WHO . . . made it clear that . . . it was not indicating that drugs not included in the list were Non-Essential" (Peretz 1983: 131).

The second objection of the pharmaceutical sector was the list's universal application. The industry insisted that if the model list was to be used at all, it should apply only for the least developed countries (LDC). An IFPMA statement made this explicit:

---

26. IFPMA, "Statement as Adopted by the IFPMA Council on The Selection of Essential Drugs," Report of a WHO Expert Committee Technical Report Series No. 615, WHO, Geneva, 1977, April 1978. WHO Library.

27. Ibid.

28. Airmail from J. Richard Court, Director of Bureau of Drugs, Department of Health, Education and Welfare, USA, to the Director, Division of Prophylactic, Diagnostic and Therapeutic Substances, WHO, 9 February 1978. WHO Library.

29. A note from Imperial Chemical Industries Limited, Pharmaceuticals Division, to Dr. Kilgour, Department of Health and Social Security, 4 January 1978, MH 148/1050. UK National Archives.

30. Airmail from J. Richard Court, Director of Bureau of Drugs, Department of Health, Education and Welfare, USA, to the Director, Division of Prophylactic, Diagnostic and Therapeutic Substances, WHO, 9 February 1978. WHO Library.

Although the pharmaceutical industry questions the need for WHO to develop a "guiding" list for LDC use, the industry can understand the practical, if regrettable, decision of some developing countries, with severely limited financial resources and foreign exchange shortages, to curtail the importation of medicines and thus limit therapy available to their populations. . . . Where the decision is made to limit the number of available drugs it can be justified only by short-term economic necessity, and the resulting retardation of medical care is a situation to be lamented, not emulated and promoted as the WHO appears to be doing. Further to encourage the curtailment of the drugs available in *developed* countries with claims that such a measure would result in both savings and improvements in medical care is a disservice to the advancement of medical science.[31]

Drug companies were not only "trying to pass the idea that this concept was for developing countries," but also that "in developing countries [it was] for the poor people."[32] At the World Health Assembly, member states were divided between those that supported universal applicability and those that found the concept relevant only for the needs of developing countries. A board member from Tunisia, for example, asserted that "the question of the restriction of drugs . . . was not peculiar to the developing world,"[33] and a board member from the Nordic countries stated that "the principles involved were of equal importance for industrialized and non-industrialized countries."[34] In contrast, a member from the United Kingdom argued that "the report . . . would be particularly important for developing countries,"[35] and a member from Bangladesh claimed that "the concept of a basic list of essential drugs . . . would undoubtedly be of more benefit to the developing than to the developed world."[36] In response, the WHO secretariat continued to support the universality of the concept but avoided statements that were disagreeable to the IFPMA.[37] The IFPMA could therefore state approvingly that "WHO has clarified . . . that the concept is 'directed primarily to the needs of developing countries' although they go on to say that it does 'have values in

---

31. IFPMA, "Statement as Adopted by the IFPMA Council on The Selection of Essential Drugs," Report of a WHO Expert Committee Technical Report Series No. 615, WHO, Geneva, 1977, April 1978, WHO Library.

32. Interview by the author with Germán Velásquez, Drug Action Programme, World Health Organization, Geneva, Switzerland, 3 June 2008.

33. WHO Document, 1978, EB61/SR/2, p. 11. WHO Library.

34. Ibid., p. 10.

35. Ibid., p. 9.

36. Ibid., p. 10.

37. Interview by the author with Germán Velásquez, Drug Action Programme, World Health Organization, Geneva, Switzerland, 3 June 2008.

other contexts'" (Peretz 1983: 131). These modifications successfully defused the objection of the pharmaceutical sector. By 1982, according to the chairman of the Ad Hoc Committee on Drug Policies, "the manufacturers' associations . . . appeared not only to accept but to support the concept of essential drugs."[38]

The content and scope of the WHO's model list of essential drugs was, then, the result of a two-stage response to external pressures. In the first stage, the WHO secretariat strategically complied with developing countries' expectations in a way that was compatible with the organization's ideational concerns with appropriate technology and equity. In the second stage, however, the WHO secretariat modified two elements opposed by the pharmaceutical industry. In making these two concessions, the WHO staff chose pragmatic considerations over ideational principles: since the proposed policies were too contentious, the WHO bureaucracy sought a formula that would be agreeable to all parties, even at the expense of the organization's preferences. Notably, in agreeing to substantially narrow the scope of potential transformation, the WHO secretariat compromised not so much the interests of developing countries as much as the organization's own principles, particularly its commitment to equity. WHO policies on essential drugs, as well as primary health care, now applied only to the have-nots, thereby giving up on the original understanding that Health for All would require changes in the health services available to the haves as well. While this compromise did not undermine the WHO's central concern with those most in need, the distinction now made between health services to the poor and those to the nonpoor opened the door to concerns about substandard health care, and accusations that the primary health care approach focused on providing of "poor drugs to poor people."[39] These accusations were later used in justifying a move away from primary (or "primitive") health care to a broader principle of universalism (see chapter 6).

The Local Production of Essential Drugs

The model list of essential drugs was strongly supported by developing countries, but they made it clear that "establishing the list of essential drugs was not the main difficulty. . . . The main problem was to ensure the supply of drugs at reasonable prices for primary health care."[40] A report by the Executive Board Ad Hoc Committee on Drug Policies, from 1982, warned of an "unacceptable state of affairs whereby [essential] drugs are scarcely accessible to the vast majority of

---

38. WHO Document, 1982, EB69/SR/14. WHO Library.
39. WHO Document, 1978, EB61/SR/3, p. 5. WHO Library; WHO Document, 1980, EB66/SR/2. WHO Library.
40. WHO Document, 1982, EB69/SR/15. WHO Library.

the world's people."[41] In line with the broader NIEO goal of economic independence through industrialization, developing countries believed the most effective
solution to the problem of access to essential drugs was "progress towards self-
reliance in the production of drugs."[42]

The "crux of the problem," as a representative of India in a Commonwealth
meeting argued, was the unequal distribution of industrial capacity, which gave
the pharmaceutical companies unlimited scope of exploitation: 90 percent of
the drugs were produced in developed countries, 5 percent in three developing countries—Brazil, India and Mexico—and the remaining 5 percent in other
developing countries.[43] Following resolutions passed by the Fifth Conference of
Heads of State or Government Summit Meeting of Nonaligned Countries at
Colombo, Sri Lanka, in August 1976, and later by the G-77 in Mexico, a special
task force was established that included representatives from the United Nations
Industrial Development Organization (UNIDO), UNCTAD, the WHO, and
other UN bodies.[44] The task force prepared a project, "Economic and Technical
Cooperation among Developing Countries in the Pharmaceutical Sector," which
the United Nations Development Programme then approved for funding. The
Sixth Nonaligned Conference in Havana, Cuba, in 1979, endorsed the task force's
recommendations. The resolutions of the Havana Conference reiterated the importance of new initiatives that would enable developing countries to achieve
national and collective self-reliance in the pharmaceutical sector. The resolutions
emphasized the part to be played by relevant UN organizations, including the
WHO, in helping developing countries achieve the objectives they had outlined
(Lall 1978: 3, Patel 1983, Mamdani 1992: 16).

At the Executive Board meetings and World Health Assemblies, as in other
venues, developing countries claimed that "the long-term solution clearly rested
with local production of essential drugs at a favorable price and of a satisfactory
quality."[45] In Resolution WHA31.32, the World Health Assembly declared that the

---

41. WHO Document, 1982, "Report by the Executive Board Ad Hoc Committee on Drug Policies
on Behalf of the Executive Board," p. 99. WHO Library.
42. WHO Document, 1982, WHA35/A/6, p. 71. WHO Library.
43. "Record of Meeting of Commonwealth Representatives, Prior to the Thirty-first World
Health Assembly, Geneva, 7 May 1978," RG25, vol. 14977, file 46–4-WHO-1, part 7. Canada National
Archives.
44. In 1975 UNIDO looked at the possibility of promoting an industrialization policy for pharmaceutical production, and set a very ambitious target: by the year 2000, 25 percent of the world's
pharmaceuticals should be produced in developing countries. From 1976 onward, UNIDO concentrated on conducting feasibility studies and giving technical assistance to the numerous countries
trying to start up local production of finished essential drugs. UNIDO also promoted the idea that
groups of developing countries engage in cooperative production (Mamdani 1992: 15; see also Lall
1976, Reich 1986: 44, Wells 1991: 319).
45. WHO Document, 1978, EB61/SR/2, p. 8. WHO Library.

local production of essential drugs and vaccines was a "legitimate aspiration" of developing countries. The WHO's initial reports on access to drugs confirmed the significance of local production. A report by the Ad Hoc Committee on Drug Policies boldly stated, "This objective [to ensure that all people had regular access to safe and effective drugs] will be accomplished through programmes which ... emphasize the development and strengthening of national capabilities and infrastructures towards achievement of greater self-reliance in the pharmaceutical sector through national endeavors and inter-country cooperation."[46] Moreover, WHO reports suggested that the goal of local production of drugs could be attainable. In 1979, the director of the Division of Prophylactic, Diagnostic, and Therapeutic Substances, Dr. Fattorusso, assured member states that local drug production "could be started out almost anywhere using very simple methods."[47] The regional director for the Western Pacific, Dr. Nakajima, further promised, "Production technology for essential drugs was not as complicated as might be feared."[48] In 1981, the WHO established the Action Programme on Essential Drugs and Vaccines (known as DAP, or Drugs Action Programme).[49] The objective of the DAP was "to ensure the regular supply to all people of safe and effective drugs of acceptable quality at lowest possible cost, in order to reach the overall objective of health for all by the year 2000 through health systems based on primary health care."[50]

However, the call for WHO's involvement in local production and distribution was criticized by some member states as going beyond the WHO's ability and mandate. The executive board member from the United States argued,

> The need of the poorer countries for essential drugs called for a broad series of actions requiring a variety of competences. Many of these were well within WHO's current capabilities. . . . In other fields, WHO was generally not so well equipped: for example, drug pricing and procurement, drug supply infrastructure and quality assurance.[51]

The American board member argued that some actions, including drug manufacturing, laid outside the scope of the UN agencies and should be left to "industry and relevant agencies in the industrialized countries."[52]

---

46. WHO Document, 1982, "Report by the Executive Board Ad Hoc Committee on Drug Policies on Behalf of the Executive Board," p. 102. WHO Library.

47. WHO Document, 1979, EB63/SR/21, p. 14. WHO Library.

48. WHO Document, 1980, EB66/SR/2. WHO Library.

49. DAP replaced the Drug Policies and Management Division (DPM), which, among other things, had been responsible for the model list of essential drugs (Walt and Harnmeijer 1992: 28).

50. WHO Document, 1982, "Report by the Executive Board Ad Hoc Committee on Drug Policies on Behalf of the Executive Board," p. 102. WHO Library.

51. WHO Document, 1982, EB69/SR/13. WHO Library.

52. Ibid.

The WHO leadership did not welcome the pressures put on the WHO to steer clear of issues that industrial countries disapproved, but they chose to avoid a direct confrontation. In his speeches, Mahler began to warn member states against endeavors that would lead to conflicts with commercial interests and would therefore fail.

> Beyond [accepted] spheres of WHO's competence . . . lay areas in which the Organization was exposed to criticism on grounds of amateurism and indecision. Those were the areas in which giant multinational commercial interests operated and it was a very big question how . . . the Organization should attempt to venture into that field. . . . To suggest collective purchasing, storing or local production of drugs, let alone to suggest that some drugs were so essential that they should be taken out of the ordinary commodity market, was a most ambitious undertaking, but it was important not to generate expectations that went beyond what the Organization could in fact deliver.[53]

Mahler congratulated member states for what had already been achieved, thereby implicitly closing the door on the possibility of more ambitious goals: "There was still a long way to go, but WHO had been very courageous in even daring to promote that whole concept of essential drugs."[54]

Gradually, the WHO withdrew from initiatives involving local production. This was justified not only by the necessity of protecting the organization's reputation but also by the argument that the local production of drugs was not economically rational.[55] A DAP report argued:

> Few, if any, drugs can be produced locally if pure economic justification is the only justification. Prices on generic drugs are now so low

---

53. WHO Document, 1980, EB66/SR/2. WHO Library.
54. WHO Document, 1983, EB72/SR/1, p. 53. WHO Library.
55. In 1978 UNIDO, which was responsible for providing the technological capability to produce essential drugs in the developing countries themselves, started warning about challenges in the production of drugs:

> The difficulties that developing countries encounter in the development of pharmaceuticals are far more complex and widespread than those associated with the growth of most other industries. They ranged from the strictly technological problem common to most industries of obtaining know-how held by companies in developed countries and of fostering indigenous innovation to the economic difficulties of reducing the costs of buying technology and products in highly imperfect and oligopolistic markets, the medical difficulties of ensuring rational and effective therapeutic practice, the social difficulties of providing for the basic health needs of large numbers of poor people, the legal difficulties of defining property right contracts and obligations in the context of the international operations of private firms, and the political difficulties of countering abuses in the present system, with its entrenched interests, by careful and well-directed policies. Consequently the task of pharmaceutical development is formidable. (cited in Lall 1978: 1)

internationally that the least developed countries can face difficulties in formulating these at prices as low or lower than what can be obtained by international competitive tender. . . . We agree that there is a need to develop strategies for industrialization in the field of pharmaceuticals, but we believe that such strategies should emerge from careful studies of country needs and the related technical and economic feasibility.[56]

Without much discussion among member states, then, the WHO staff shifted its attention, in searching for improved access to drugs, from local production to affordable imports, which required cooperation with, rather than independence from, pharmaceutical manufacturers. Hence, while initially endorsing developing countries' call for the local production of drugs, the leadership reversed its position when this support threatened to undermine the WHO's reputation as a competent organization. In this case, given the relatively minor role of the WHO in the original initiative and the organization's continued interest in the question of access to drugs, it was possible for the bureaucracy to "passively" (rather than strategically) resist the expectations of developing countries.

Also in considering the regulation of pharmaceutical marketing, which followed bitter negotiations over the regulation of the marketing of infant formula, the WHO leadership chose cooperation over conflict, but this time clearly employing strategic resistance.

Inappropriate Marketing

Regulating Infant Formula

The WHO, a firm supporter of breast-feeding, became involved in the issue of breast-milk substitutes in the mid-1960s. In 1966, the WHO had published a pamphlet, "Child Nutrition in Developing Countries," which called attention to the dangers of formula feeding (Newton 1999). In 1970, the Pan-American Health Organization (PAHO) and UNICEF cosponsored a meeting on breast-feeding, and PAHO subsequently formulated guidelines for infant feeding in the Caribbean, which called, among other things, for the prohibition of questionable marketing practices (Jayasuriya, Griffiths, and Rigoni 1984: 7). In 1974, the World Health Assembly passed a resolution, WHA27.43, that noted "the general decline in breast-feeding, related to socio-cultural and environmental factors, including the mistaken idea caused by misleading sales promotion that breast-feeding is

---

56. WHO Document, DAP Comments on ACC Task Force Project Proposal No. 3, 24 May 1984. WHO Library.

inferior to feeding with manufactured breast-milk substitutes." The resolution urged member countries "to review sales promotion activities on baby foods and to introduce appropriate remedial measures, including advertisement codes and legislation where necessary." In 1978, the assembly passed another resolution, WHA31.47, which recommended member governments take measures to promote breast-feeding and to regulate "inappropriate sales promotion of infant foods that can be used to replace breast milk" (Reich 1987: 47, Shubber 1998). These resolutions, however, maintained a focus on regulation at the national level. That changed at the Joint WHO/UNICEF Meeting on Infant and Young Child Feeding, which took place in October 1979.

Paradoxically, it was the infant formula industry that initiated the international conference, erroneously believing that an international forum might be easier to manipulate than the national forums it had dealt with until then. Beginning in 1973, manufacturers of infant formula faced increasingly effective public criticism, due in part to two articles, entitled "Action Now on Baby Foods" and "Milk and Murder," which were published in the *New Internationalist,* in England. The articles criticized the promotional activities of Nestlé, which accounted for approximately 40 percent of infant formula sales in developing countries, as well as other companies (Jayasuriya, Griffiths, and Rigoni 1984, Sikkink 1986: 821). The content of the articles was taken up by War on Want, a British grassroots organization concerned with development and consumer issues. This organization commissioned a study, the results of which it published under the title "The Baby Killer." The study described the hazards of using infant formula in settings challenged by high levels of illiteracy, poverty, contaminated water, and limited health care systems (Jayasuriya, Griffiths, and Rigoni 1984: 6). These and other studies showed that contaminated water that formula was mixed with led to disease in infants, and furthermore, that poverty made mothers use less formula powder than was necessary, leading to malnutrition. Moreover, groups such as the IOCU, the Baby Foods Action Groups in the United Kingdom, and the Interfaith Center on Corporate Responsibility (ICCR) in the United States began to collect materials demonstrating that the infant formula companies were promoting their product in poor countries by using unethical and indiscriminate marketing strategies. Nestlé inadvertently provided the activists with a prominent public forum when it sued the Swiss-based Third World Action Group for defamation and libel after the group had translated the War on Want pamphlet into German and had retitled it, "Nestlé Kills Babies" (Sikkink 1986: 821). In July 1977, a recently formed U.S. group, the Infant Formula Action Coalition (INFACT) launched a boycott against Nestlé. A coalition of INFACT, ICCR, IOCU, and other groups also leafleted churches, demonstrated in front of Nestlé headquarters, and in other ways raised public awareness of the issue.

INFACT and its allies persuaded Senator Edward Kennedy, who was at the time chairman of the U.S. Senate Subcommittee on Health and Scientific Research, to hold public hearings on the issue of "The Marketing and Promotion of Infant Formula in the Developing Nations." The hearings took place in May 1978, and for Nestlé they were a public relations disaster (Sikkink 1986: 822, Newton 1999: 374–375). The chairman of Nestlé's Brazilian affiliate, Dr. Oswaldo Ballarin, questioned the legitimacy of the claims against Nestlé by suggesting that the campaign against them was run by "a worldwide church organization, with the stated purpose of undermining . . . the free world's economic system." Even more damaging to the reputation of Nestlé, Ballarin stated that it was beyond Nestlé's responsibility to find out how their products were being used: "You go into a region and they are not all literate—there are some who are. How can you control that the product goes to one rather than to the other?" Ballarin added: "In those places where there are high birth rates and you have many children in the same house, these children, anyhow, are infected by poor water, whatever they do, and, that, we cannot—we cannot cope with that" (cited in Sethi 1994: 75–80, also Jayasuriya, Griffiths, and Rigoni 1984: 8–9).

In an attempt to depoliticize the issue after these unsuccessful hearings, Nestlé asked Senator Kennedy to refer the issue to the WHO. Kennedy then wrote to Mahler and suggested that the organization sponsor an international conference to discuss the infant formula issue and come up with recommendations for marketing infant formula in the Third World (Sethi 1994: 91, Newton 1999: 376).

Nestlé favored an international conference under the auspices of the WHO because it believed the infant formula industry could more easily influence the course of events in international forums than it could in the United States (Sethi 1994: 91), especially since the industry had just appointed Dr. Stanislas Flasche, a former deputy director-general of the WHO, to be the executive director of the International Council of Infant Food Industries. For the same reasons, industry critics were initially skeptical of the WHO process. They also criticized Nestlé for using its support of the international conference to claim that the boycott was no longer necessary, and they denounced Nestlé's about-face, as the company first committed to follow any recommendation that would come out of the meeting, but then suggested it would abide only by those recommendations that were accepted by national governments (Sethi 1994: 171–172).

Both the infant formula industry and its critics were invited to the conference. Other participants included member governments, UN agencies, other intergovernmental organizations, and professional experts (Sethi 1994: 173–174). The outcome of the conference did not meet the industry's expectations. Instead, the Conference Statement considered infant feeding within the larger context of the call for a New International Economic Order and affirmed the right of member states to collectively regulate the practices of multinational corporations. The statement declared that "the problem [of poor infant-feeding practices] is part of the wider issues of poverty, lack of resources, social injustice and ecological degradation; it cannot be considered apart from social and economic development and the need for a new international economic order. It is also a basic issue for health care systems and its solution must be seen in the context of Health for All by the Year 2000."[57] The conference recommendations called for an international code of marketing of breast-milk substitutes. The World Health Assembly subsequently passed a consensus resolution, WHA33.32, requesting that the director-general prepare such an international code (Sikkink 1986: 831, Sethi 1994: 182).

An American suggestion that the code would be developed by an intergovernmental group of member states instead of a secretariat task force was dismissed by the secretariat (Sethi 1994: 182). Hence, it was the WHO staff that prepared the draft declarations, which were then circulated among the interested parties. The drafts triggered contentious debates among member states. In addition to heated disagreements regarding the substantive provisions, member states also debated whether the code should be adopted as a regulation, which would have a binding effect without the need for ratification at the national level, or whether it should take the form of nonbinding recommendation for governments to follow on a voluntary basis.[58] The U.S. government insisted on a nonbinding resolution and threatened that a binding resolution would not pass Congress.[59] Many other developed countries also preferred the voluntary option, which would have allowed them to avoid confrontation over obligations that they considered extreme or unsuitable to their countries. The Canadians, for example, found the draft code "unrealistically extreme" and therefore supported "a Code that is voluntary in its application."[60]

In the face of an explicit divide between North and South, the WHO leadership initially thought that to protect the organization's interests it would be best not to take a position. According to a Canadian report, "the Director-General gave to his officials instructions . . . to remain as neutral as possible [on whether the code

57. "Statement and Recommendations of the Joint WHO/UNICEF Meeting on Infant and Young Child Feeding," in http://www.unu.edu/Unupress/food/8F023e/8F023E04.htm.

58. Memorandum, "Draft International Code of Marketing of Breastmilk Substitutes," External Affairs, Economic Law and Treaty Division, 14 July 1980, RG25, vol. 14977, file 46–4-WHO-1, part 9. Canada National Archives.

59. Telegram from Canadian Mission in Geneva, "WHO: International Code of Marketing Breastmilk Substitutes," 9 September 1980, RG25, vol. 14977, file 46–4-WHO-1, part 9. Canada National Archives. In fact, after the U.S. delegation had voted against the code, the House approved by a 3-to-1 ratio a nonbinding resolution condemning the administration's vote. The joint resolution also urged the formula industry to abide by the code's guidelines (Hornblower and Hilts 1981).

60. Memorandum, "Draft International Code of Marketing of Breastmilk Substitutes," External Affairs, 15 July 1980, RG25, vol. 14977, file 46–4-WHO-1, part 9. Canada National Archives.

should be recommendation or regulation] as 'he does not want to appear as taking side the more so because he does not have mandate to take such a decision.'"[61] Behind the scenes, however, Mahler, who became increasingly concerned that the debate undermined the organization's reputation, expressed opposition to the adoption of a mandatory code and sought ways to prevent that outcome. For example, according to one account, Mahler tried to keep the decision on the format of the code to the secretariat, rather than to the World Health Assembly, where he believed the majority of members would vote in favor of a mandatory code.[62]

When the U.S. government warned that it would vote against the code if it were not strictly voluntary, which other developed countries were also expected to do (Anderson 1981), the WHO leadership abandoned its neutral position and expressed its preference for a nonbinding code. Although an attempt to reach a compromise on this issue was motivated by concern for the WHO's reputation, in public it was also justified by arguing that a unanimously voted code, even if nonbinding, would be more effective than a binding code that did not receive unanimous support. Mahler told the Executive Board that "the conclusion he drew was that the intensity of the moral *tour de force* of the initiative would depend not on a weak consensus, but on a unanimous backing."[63] Alluding to the need for unanimous support served to implicitly warn developing countries not to utilize their procedural leverage irresponsibly and to respect the WHO's dependence on the cooperation of developed countries. In that meeting, the Executive Board decided to advise the World Health Assembly that the draft code should be adopted as a voluntary code. In explaining that recommendation, the Executive Board underscored the importance of a unanimous decision. It also reasoned that a nonbinding code would preserve the national sovereignty of member countries in applying the code at the national level.[64] Members of the assembly agreed to make the code voluntary.

Partly thanks to the WHO leadership's attempts for mediation, the final code, "The International Code of Marketing for Breast-Milk Substitutes," was supported by all developing and developed countries, with the solitary exception of the United States, the only member that voted against the code.[65] The code

61. Telegram from Canadian Mission in Geneva, "WHO: International Code of Marketing Breastmilk Substitutes," 18 November 1980, RG25, vol. 14977, file 46–4-WHO-1, part 9. Canada National Archives.

62. Ibid.

63. WHO Document, 1981, EB67/SR/24. WHO Library.

64. WHO Document, 1981, WHA34/A/13. WHO Library; Hardon 1992: 55.

65. The U.S. position was strongly influenced by a joint campaign that the three American manufacturers of infant formula—Bristol-Myers, Abbott Laboratories, and American Home Products—had launched against the proposed code (Mintz 1981a, Mintz 1981b, Sikkink 1986: 830, Sethi 1994: 207–212). The Reagan administration also had principled objections to economic regulation by UN

restricted aggressive forms of marketing and advertising of baby foods. It called for a prohibition on the use of nurses to promote formula, banned direct advertising of breast-milk substitutes, prohibited distribution of free samples to mothers, and required product labels to acknowledge the superiority of breast-feeding and warn about the dangers of improper preparation. The code forbade the use of health care facilities for the promotion of baby food and limited company donations and gifts to hospitals and health care personnel. In addition, it specified that companies should not pay employees any commissions or bonuses on sales of infant formula (Sikkink 1986: 822).

The code demonstrated developing countries' ability to set the agenda in international organizations and, some significant concessions notwithstanding, their willingness to do so against the opposition of the U.S. government and powerful international companies. For the WHO leadership, however, the outcome was not considered a success. The very explicit conflict between developing and developed countries put the WHO's reputation and legitimacy at stake, as the organization was accused by developed countries of dealing with matters outside the scope of its constitutional authority. Mahler found it necessary, in a number of occasions, to publicly defend the secretariat by reminding member states that it was merely following the assembly resolutions. The minutes of Committee A at the Thirty-Third Assembly describe Mahler's protestation:

> The Director-General said that he had come to the Committee meeting particularly because of accusations that he had been making the Organization play a role it should not be playing and that he had gone beyond his mandate. He thought that two World Health Assemblies had instructed the Director-General in unambiguous resolutions to deal with all problems having to do with infant feeding, and particularly the role of breastfeeding. He invited the members of the Committee to read resolutions WHA27.43 and WHA31.47 and decide whether, in

---

agencies, especially regulations calling for greater state intervention. Elliott Abrams, the assistant secretary of state for international organization affairs, wrote in an op-ed at the *Washington Post*:

   The code seeks to ban advertising of infant formula to the public, no matter how truthful the information in the advertising. As in the case of UNESCO's effort to control the free flow of press information, the United States is very much opposed to such regulation of information by UN bodies. The code in addition interferes with the role of health professionals in dealing with their patients by assigning to government—not doctors—the central role in informing families about infant feeding. Once again, assigning more and more tasks to the state is a practice favored by many nations but not one that the United States wishes to encourage by a yes vote (Abrams 1981).

   Expressing similar sentiments, Secretary of Health and Human Services Richard S. Schweiker said that the WHO's code could not be enforced in the United States because it "runs contrary to the Constitution on the First Amendment" and would violate the antitrust laws, but he also stated that "the administration honestly doesn't believe the WHO should be an international Federal Trade Commission" (Rich 1981).

the light of these resolutions, it had not been a perfectly logical and necessary step to convene the joint WHO/UNICEF Meeting, to which had been invited not only the developing and developed countries, nongovernmental organizations, and the United Nations organizations most directly involved but also industries. He knew of no other meeting which had shown a greater degree of democracy and openness by the Organization than the one in question. It had clearly been within the instructions of the Health Assemblies to the Director-General.[66]

In describing the processes following the WHO/UNICEF Meeting, Mahler hinted at unwelcomed pressures coming from interested parties:

He had mobilized expertise to start drafting a code which would serve, through a continuous negotiating process, as a basis for every Member State to deal with what he considered to be a vital problem. . . . [He] was not to be envied for the letters he had received. Nevertheless, it was part of his job to expect such attacks. . . . The Organization believed that breastfeeding was a vital concept; if Member States did not think so they should not have passed their previous resolutions on the subject.[67]

Another comment by Mahler to the Executive Committee in January 1981 conveyed an even greater sense of distress.

Throughout what was called the free press the Secretariat had been labeled as secretive United Nations bureaucrats marching under the banner of WHO. He had hoped, however, that the Board would defend the Secretariat and see the proposals not as the Secretariat's policy but as the high degree of participatory democracy for which the Organization had been able to provide a platform in developing protection for children throughout the world.

Mahler concluded that talk "by saying that the experience had not been pleasant for the Secretariat," and that "it had been a difficult climate in which to maneuver and keep its vision straight."[68]

Mahler's statements expressed the secretariat's sense that the success of having a code of conduct for the infant formula industry was overshadowed by the price the bureaucracy had to pay in reputation and legitimacy. To avoid repeating the

---

66. WHO Document, 1980, WHA33/A/7. WHO Library.
67. Ibid.
68. WHO Document, 1981, EB67/SR/24. WHO Library.

same experience in debates over a similar code for the pharmaceutical industry, the WHO bureaucracy strategically resisted developing countries' demands.

Regulating Pharmaceuticals

As described earlier in the chapter, essential drugs were initially part of a broader discussion in which the main issue was helping Third World governments to avoid purchasing nonessential drugs. One of the difficulties for governments in developing countries was lack of information, which the model list of essential drugs helped to combat, but more urgent complaints referred to pressures exerted by drug companies on governments in developing countries to purchase drugs. At the Executive Board discussions, in January 1975, Mahler reiterated the problem of sales pressure from drug manufacturers as had been described by member states, and called the Health Assembly to consider ways of offering protection (WHO 2008: 245). At the World Health Assembly the following year, Mahler was explicit: "A specific health goal might be to ensure the availability of essential drugs to all those who need them. . . . To attain this goal it might be necessary in some countries to control the production or the import of drugs, or both, even if that entails limiting the free choice of drugs by individual practitioners."[69] One measure to limit nonessential drugs that was considered by the assembly was the regulation of marketing of pharmaceutical products. In 1978, Resolution WHA31.32 noted the risk of uncontrolled promotional activity by drug manufacturers, particularly in developing countries, and authorized the WHO to study strategies for reducing the prices of pharmaceuticals, "including the development of a code of marketing practices" (Reich 1987: 41). Such regulation was supported by the passionate group of activists that had also been behind the mobilization for a code for infant formula, including IOCU, Social Audit of the UK, Oxfam, and a West German coalition of development action groups, BUKO (Reich 1987: 46). Soon after the infant formula code was adopted by the WHO, consumer activists from twenty-seven countries formed an international coalition, Health Action International (HAI), to "resist the ill-treatment of consumers by multinational drug companies" (Walt and Harnmeijer 1992: 37).

A code of conduct for the marketing of pharmaceutical products seemed likely, especially after the WHO member states had voted in favor of regulating the marketing practices of the infant formula industry. Kenneth L. Adelman, deputy representative of the United States to the United Nations, wrote, "It appears that the

---

69. "Social Perspectives in Health," Address by Dr. H. Mahler, Director-General of the World Health Organization, in Presenting his Report for 1975 to the Twenty-Ninth World Health Assembly, Geneva, 4 May 1976. WHO Library.

infant formula drive was just the opening skirmish in a much larger campaign" (Adelman 1982: 16). A piece in the *Food Drug Cosmetic Law Journal* asserted, "The issues in this controversy are being framed within the context of the New International Economic Order . . . [and] it appears that the pharmaceutical industry is destined to be a testing ground on which the future of this UN program will be decided" (Phelps 1982: 2000). The *Pharmaceutical Executive* warned of "a coming WHO effort to impose unacceptable controls over all pharmaceutical commerce in the Third World" (Schwartz 1981). In response to the threat of an international code of conduct, but also to the essential drugs list and the WHO's interest in local production, the pharmaceutical sector first offered discounts on its drugs and, later, formulated a voluntary code.

Discounts. From 1977 onward, pharmaceutical companies wrote to the WHO leadership offering to provide drugs, most of which appeared on the essential drugs list, at "favorable prices" to the poorest countries (Mamdani and Walker 1986: 192, Walt and Harnmeijer 1992: 30). The offer of discounts was clearly an attempt by drug firms to "head off international restrictions with ideas of their own," as a headline in *Business International* put it.[70] The same article went on to say:

> Swift action by . . . pharmaceutical firms blunted the LDC drive towards a brave new world of supranational drug regulation. An industry-sponsored proposal to accommodate the needs of the poorest LDCs for essential drugs . . . is gaining plaudits from the WHO. The case illustrates how criticism of MNCs can be deflected before it reaches the stage of confrontation. . . . Over the long term, companies hope to gain a handsome quid pro quo from WHO in the form of a more conciliatory attitude on such sensitive topics as transfer pricing and advertising in third world markets.[71]

HAI warned that "any such drug supply scheme would involve substantial direct and indirect costs," including "the complete dependence on a small number of major foreign suppliers." They argued that "the scheme will inhibit development of local pharmaceutical industry; and will undermine the possibility of regional cooperation in drug purchasing." They were also worried that improved relations between the WHO and drug companies could compromise the independence of the WHO staff and might inhibit "the WHO from taking steps . . . to control harmful marketing practices."[72] Similar concerns were echoed by some member

---

70. Cited in Health Action International, May 1982, "The WHO and the Pharmaceutical Industry," HAI briefing paper for the 35th World Health Assembly. WHO Library.
71. Ibid.
72. Ibid.

states. At the World Health Assembly, the Dutch delegate warned against the industry's offer of discounts.

> Industry had its own goals, which were not those of the primary health care strategy. There were many potential problems that could not be ignored. WHO would have to know how to cope with problems such as misinformation, incorrect advertisement, defective product, the introduction of inappropriate technologies and the possible move from essential to non-essential drugs in the programme.[73]

In spite of these potential difficulties, the WHO secretariat began extended negotiations with the IFPMA. The possibility of collaboration between the pharmaceutical industry and the WHO was brought up formally for the first time in a meeting of the president of IFPMA, Dr. Vischer, with Mahler.[74] The meeting was followed by an exchange of letters, in which Vischer suggested "to begin in a modest way with the very minimum number of basic drugs and/or vaccines."[75] Regarding the choice of countries, Vischer preferred to "limit the scheme initially to only those least developed countries . . . who have both the need for the drugs and also some sort of health infrastructure which would allow them to make efficient use of the drugs."[76] Mahler agreed to "start the collaboration in a modest way," and invited the IFPMA to present "some concrete suggestions for collaboration."[77] But in follow-up meetings, "no concrete proposals were presented by IFPMA,"[78] and presentations and letters from the IFPMA repeated their elusive offer to sell their drugs to the WHO under favorable conditions, with no further specifications.[79]

When more concrete offers were finally made public, in 1982, they were stricter than could have been expected from earlier statements. A letter from Michael Peretz of the IFPMA to the Office of the Director-General listed their demands. The IFPMA wanted recipient countries to contribute financially to the scheme and to provide assurances that trained staff were available, that the drugs would be distributed to the population at need, and that guards would be in place against leakages of drugs to unauthorized sources.[80] The IFPMA "hoped that the

---

73. WHO Document, WHA35/A/SR/5. WHO Library.
74. WHO Document, "Note for the Record," 24 February 1981. WHO Library.
75. Letter from Vischer to Mahler, 9 January 1981. WHO Library.
76. Ibid.
77. Letter from Mahler to Vischer, 28 January 1981. WHO Library.
78. WHO Document, "Note for the Record," 24 February 1981. WHO Library.
79. Letter from Michael Peretz, IFPMA, to Dr. Ch'en Wen-Chieh, Assistant Director-General, 1 April 1981. WHO Library.
80. The IFPMA was concerned that discounted drugs would be sold for profit to neighboring countries or reexported to the country from where they were sourced.

cost of the drugs will be met from three sources: the countries themselves; international aid agencies, [and] national aid agencies."[81] The letter did not make any concrete offers in return: "The offers of support by individual companies should be seen as a preparedness to negotiate non-commercial prices with the country or countries concerned. Until their requirements have been quantified in terms of quantities, pack sizes, delivery schedules and dates, labeling, etc., I do not think that the companies will wish to be any more specific."[82]

A memorandum of the PAHO/WHO Interoffice reflected growing frustration in response to the IFPMA's letter: "The conditions of the offer continue to be vague. . . . Though *industry* conditions are not known, the IFPMA has defined relatively detailed conditions which the countries must meet."[83] The memorandum also expressed concerns that "most countries in need of assistance would have difficulty in completely satisfying some of the conditions listed."[84] While continuing to support collaboration with the pharmaceutical sector, the WHO leadership started expressing its discontent more publicly. When the IFPMA complained that WHO reports had failed to mention their willingness to supply essential drugs to developing countries under favorable conditions, Mahler insisted that the IFPMA had not yet given detailed information about the offer and that, "due appreciation could be expressed only when the Health Assembly fully understood the extent of the offer and its effect in practical terms."[85]

The negotiations, which were intended to increase confidence in the pharmaceutical industry, probably had the opposite effect. Nonetheless, U.S. delegates maintained their position that the offer of discounts should quiet the drive for international regulation. An Executive Board member from the United States announced that he "did not think it would be constructive to give that matter [the question of a WHO code] any further consideration, particularly in view of the fact that the Director-General was shortly to be engaging in consultations with the representatives of the IFPMA. It was important not to take any steps which might jeopardize the outcome of those consultations."[86] At the World Health Assembly, a U.S. delegate "hoped the assembly would take no action that might damage that cooperative relationship [between the WHO and the pharmaceutical

81. Letter from Peretz, IFPMA, to Dr. J. Cohen, Director-General Office, 7 April 1982. WHO Library.

82. Letter from Peretz, IFPMA, to Dr. Sankaran, Director, Division of Diagnostic, Therapeutic and Rehabilitative Technology, WHO, 27 April 1982, WHO Library.

83. PAHO/WHO Interoffice Memorandum, From Dr. Jorge Litvak, Chief, DPC to Dr. Mahler, "IFPMA Offer," 27 September 1982. WHO Library.

84. Ibid.

85. WHO Document, 1982, WHA35/SR/4. WHO Library.

86. WHO Document, 1982, EB69/SR/15. WHO Library.

industry] and prove counterproductive regarding the supply of essential drugs to countries where they were most needed."[87]

Ultimately, however, the negotiations between the WHO and the pharmaceutical industry came to a halt. Three factors contributed to the failure. First, the industry rejected a formal request by Rwanda for the supply of drugs under the scheme and the WHO staff felt that the industry's reasons for turning down the request were spurious. Second, the WHO staff was unhappy about the industry's package approach, in which drugs were supplied only if technical services were provided as well, since the WHO's primary concern was the price of actual drugs; and finally, the WHO staff considered some of the industry's conditions to be unduly restrictive.[88]

Voluntary code. In March 1981, just two months before the World Health Assembly approved the infant formula code, the IFPMA announced a voluntary "Code of Pharmaceutical Marketing Practices," which it approved in September 1981 (Peretz 1983: 262–263, Starrels 1985: 27). A year later, the IFPMA issued a supplementary statement that stressed the industry's commitment to observe and monitor the code and laid down procedures for dealing with any breaches of it (Hardon 1992: 50).

Consumer groups considered the voluntary code nothing but "an attempt to deflect criticism and forestall external regulation."[89] They charged that the industry proposal lacked specificity, monitoring procedures, and enforcement mechanisms (Starrels 1985: 28). The code was limited to marketing, and its lack of attention to issues such as the transfer of technology and controls on trading, prescriptions, and distribution was severely criticized by the nonaligned countries as well as the IOCU (Fazal 1983: 267). The G-77, in an UNCTAD meeting in Belgrade, expressed concern about the usefulness of the IFPMA code.[90] The representative of Tanzania stated before the World Health Assembly,

> The voluntary nature of the code betrayed the claims being made for it. How should those claims be viewed in the light of the increasing marketing of potency drugs in African countries, including his own? The effectiveness of the Code left much to be desired. Further, it applied only to marketing practices and not to production. . . . Besides being inadequate, the IFPMA Code only served to delay the establishment of a WHO code that would set required international standards

---

87. WHO Document, 1982, WHA35/A/SR/5, p. 60. WHO Library.
88. Health Action International, May 1982, "The WHO and the Pharmaceutical Industry," HAI briefing paper for the 35th World Health Assembly. WHO Library.
89. "Int'l Consumerists Target Drug Bans," 8 June 1981, *Advertising Age.* WHO Library.
90. WHO Document, 12 July 1983, "Note for the Record, Meeting with UNCTAD Technology Division." WHO Library.

for marketing, production and transfer of technology, as well as other key areas. . . . The IFPMA Code was no substitute for an appropriate and unbiased WHO code.[91]

Others, however, including the Dutch delegate who a year earlier had argued in favor of a WHO code, now suggested that a voluntary, self-disciplining approach was to be preferred to the long and arduous process of international regulatory action (Hardon 1992: 51–52). The WHO secretariat, too, welcomed the voluntary code and "reportedly decided to follow closely the implementation of the IFPMA Code, and refrain from pursuing vigorously the promotion of its own code during a trial, but unspecified period" (cited in Mamdani and Walker 1986: 191).

An international code of conduct. In spite of discount offers and the voluntary code, member states, including Chile, Cuba, Romania, Sudan, Ghana and Samoa, among others, emphasized the importance of WHO controls that would enable developing countries to defend themselves against marketing and high drug prices (Hardon 1992: 51). In 1984, the Ad Hoc Committee on Drug Policies declared, "Where the WHO was concerned, the ultimate goal was the elaboration and application of a code which would govern the manufacture, marketing and handling of drugs in such a way as to be consistent with the attainment of the goal of health for all." The Ad Hoc Committee also concluded that the IFPMA voluntary code "fell far short of WHO's aspiration."[92] Also in 1984, the Health Assembly passed Resolution WHA37.33, which requested the director-general to convene a meeting of experts of the concerned parties, including governments, pharmaceutical industries, and patients' and consumers' organizations, to "discuss the means and methods of ensuring the rational use of drugs, in particular through improved knowledge and flow of information, and to discuss the role of marketing practices in this respect, especially in developing countries." The planned meeting was clearly meant to resemble the expert meeting that had preceded the WHO/UNICEF code effort in 1979 (Sikkink 1986: 837).

In the heated debate preceding the voting on the resolution, member states expressed particularly hostile views toward the pharmaceutical sector. The representative of Tanzania, for example, stated,

> The developing countries were concerned that the attainment of health for all was being hampered by the malpractices found throughout the drug supply chain. . . . Sometimes, such malpractices were not only a violation of human rights but were a serious crime against humanity

---

91. WHO Document, 1984, WHA37/A/SR/10, pp. 139–140. WHO Library.
92. WHO Document, 1984, EB73/SR/15, p. 195. WHO Library.

and it was the moral duty of the Health Assembly to see that they ceased. It was not enough to gather annually to hear reports of such malpractices, practical action was required.[93]

The decision to convene an expert conference obtained support of an impressively broad coalition. However, the United States voted against, and West Germany and Japan (two other countries with powerful pharmaceutical companies) abstained (Laing et al. 2003: 1724).[94]

The WHO leadership was not enthusiastic about the conference. A debate among member states over a code of pharmaceutical marketing was inevitable, and it invited confrontation that, like the negotiations over the code on marketing of infant formula, could greatly damage the reputation of the WHO. Already in 1982, during discussions preceding Resolution WHA31.32, Mahler argued that "on the question of codes of practice, it was important to move forward in a spirit of cooperation, and not deliberately to seek confrontation, because to do so would be counterproductive."[95] And in 1984, speaking before the Executive Board, Mahler insisted that "WHO should, for all its major operational programmes, operate on the basis not of vote nor even of consensus, but of virtual unanimity."[96] Again, therefore, the WHO secretariat tried to negate their procedural dependence on developing countries by questioning the legitimacy of their majority vote. The desire to avoid confrontation was particularly acute after Ronald Reagan had been reelected president and the U.S. government warned that it would stop paying its 25 percent share of the WHO budget if a code was adopted (Schwartz 1985).

For the WHO bureaucracy, the importance of having a code of pharmaceutical marketing did not justify the cost the organization would incur from the controversy. Mahler stated, "The strength of WHO derived from the willingness of Member States to try to focus on what enabled the Organization to get on with the job and not to dwell on *marginal, controversial* issues."[97] In a meeting of UNCTAD's Trade and Development Board, in which the spokesman of the G-77 "stressed that the drawing up of norms and standards on marketing, promotion, distribution, trade and technology in the pharmaceutical sector continued to be one of [the G-77] major preoccupations,"[98] a WHO representative responded:

---

93. WHO Document, 1984, WHA37/A/SR/10, pp. 139–140. WHO Library.
94. The board member from the United States warned, "The Board was in the position of being able to decide whether to promote or destroy the action programme—to bite the hand that fed would not provide a nutritious meal." WHO Document, 1984, EB73/SR/14, pp. 189–190. WHO Library.
95. WHO Document, 1982, EB69/SR/13. WHO Library.
96. WHO Document, 1984, EB73/SR/15. WHO Library.
97. Ibid. Emphasis added.
98. "Trade and Development Board, 28th Session," WHO Library.

The WHO secretariat was not lacking in courage, but it did try to exercise prudence, with the result that on occasion it might be considered somewhat overcautious. There was deep-rooted concern in WHO and its governing bodies that the preoccupation with an independent code of marketing practice for pharmaceutical products could divert attention away from the constructive progress that had been made by member states in developing national policies on essential drugs and by the pharmaceutical industry in accepting its responsibilities within the framework of the Drug Action Programme. Much more needed to be done in an atmosphere of collaboration rather than confrontation.[99]

The WHO secretariat resisted the code, but it did so strategically, by trying to convince developing countries that such a code was not in line with the NIEO spirit. In particular, the WHO staff made the case that a confrontation over pharmaceutical marketing would undermine the objective of equity. For Mahler, "the main objective was to get drugs to those who were in need of them, and that was why a dialogue should be kept up with the pharmaceutical industry."[100] Mahler made explicit his fear that the fight for a marketing code would come at the expense of "providing essential drugs for the masses," which, he urged, "was the least that could be achieved by those who believed in health for all and primary health care."[101] In expressing this position before the Executive Board, Mahler stated that

> in most developing countries, there were between 5% and 10% of drug "haves" and from 90% to 95% of drug "have-nots." While he had sympathy for the minority [of "haves"], who might be supplied with too many or the wrong kind of drugs and for whom WHO should take action with a view to improving drug-prescribing practices, the action programme was primarily concerned with the fact that so many people had no regular access to essential drugs. It was therefore of little value becoming involved in marginal, conflictual issues while there were governments which had no national policy for essential drugs or were not implementing such a policy. Consequently, WHO must concern itself first and foremost with the "have-nots" and focus its efforts on measures to ensure that they had access to essential drugs and that they were enabled to use them properly.[102]

---

99. Ibid.
100. WHO Document, 1982, EB69/SR/13. WHO Library.
101. Ibid.
102. WHO Document, 1984, EB73/SR/15. WHO Library.

Dr. Cohen of the Director-General Office similarly stated that the WHO member states should focus not on drugs sold to consumers but on "getting essential drugs to those 90% of people in developing countries who were non-consumers and wished to become consumers."[103]

Alluding to the NIEO principles of sovereign will and self-reliance, the WHO leadership also passionately argued against turning the WHO into a "supranational authority." A discussion paper by the director-general, just before the expert meeting, described what was within the WHO jurisdiction, including Health for All policies, and what was not:

> It can be seen that it is possible for WHO to support governments and people to take political action in support of policies for health for all and that it does so extensively. But while the Organization can firmly advocate compliance with health-for-all policy because that was agreed to collectively, it cannot enforce such compliance, nor can it enforce compliance with any other policy or with ethical or commercial codes of any kind.
>
> It is not possible for WHO to interfere in internal national political debates or struggles, no matter what their nature. . . . Nor can it interfere in internal national social unrest . . . even if the outcomes of such struggles are likely to affect health. What it can and does do is to advocate collectively adopted policy such as that enshrined in health for all by the year 2000. . . .
>
> It is not possible for WHO to enforce inter-country cooperation for health against the desires of the governments concerned since it is not a supranational organization but an international one.[104]

Following the World Health Assembly decision in favor of a meeting, the WHO staff organized a conference of experts on the rational use of drugs in November 1985, but it was criticized by supporters of the code for its reluctant efforts to make the conference successful. For example, the conference was held in Nairobi, Kenya, because it had an essential drugs program for delegates to visit, but allegedly also because the WHO staff was trying to lower the profile of the meeting by holding it outside Europe (Walt and Harnmeijer 1992: 37–38). The WHO secretariat was also criticized for keeping the list of invited participants secret and for asking them not to divulge the contents of the background papers in advance of the conference, apparently in an attempt to prevent controversies and lobbying before the conference took place (Hardon 1992: 53–54). Finally, critics

---

103. WHO Document, 1984, WHA37/A/SR/11. WHO Library.

104. WHO Document, 1985, "Global Strategy for Health for All by the Year 2000: Political Dimension," Discussion Paper by the Director-General, EB24, Annex 10, pp. 160–161. WHO Library.

complained about the decision not to have the conference reach resolutions or declarations, but that instead the director-general's summation at the meeting's close would provide an official conclusion that would also be reported to the World Health Assembly (Schwartz 1985). These accusations made Mahler particularly upset, as he described before the assembly in 1986:

> That decision [to arrange a meeting on the rational use of drugs] had given rise to a type of international social pathology the likes of which he has never experienced in his long career in WHO. It had threatened the very existence of the Organization, with passions running wild on all sides. Accusations had been made that the Secretariat was sabotaging the meeting. . . . Scandalously slanderous misinformation had been spread all over the world. Suspicions had been openly stated by one interest group that WHO was sold to the other and vice versa, and all seemed to be convinced that the meeting would only be a cover-up for predetermined conclusions—the opposite to the ones they wanted, of course![105]

In the end, the meeting had the results the WHO leadership was hoping for, as the experts decided against the possibility of an international code of conduct. The WHO leadership's desire to avoid confrontation was thereby satisfied (Schwartz 1985, Hardon 1992: 54). In summing up the conference before the assembly and justifying that decision, Mahler repeated the position that "there is no place for . . . regulation by WHO of drug promotion" and emphasized its opposition to assigning to the WHO a supranational role.[106] "There was a general understanding of WHO's international as opposed to supranational role. WHO is a cooperative of Member States and it is they who decide on its policy. . . . Policies can be defined in WHO but they cannot be imposed by WHO."[107]

The experts at the meeting also agreed on a "revised drug strategy," in which the possibility for international governance was replaced, in rhetoric and practice, with emphasis on national regulations. The experts agreed that prime responsibility for rational drug use—that is, for ensuring that drugs of acceptable quality, safety, and efficacy were available at affordable costs to all who needed them—rested with national governments, which should then be able to call on the support of the WHO in its international, rather than transnational, role (Fabricant and Hirschhorn 1987: 204). Mahler approvingly concluded that, "for the

---

105. WHO Document, 1986, WHA39/A/SR/11. WHO Library.
106. WHO, 1986, A39/12, "Director-General's Summing-Up, At the Conference of Experts, of the Issues, Proceedings, and Potential Implications for WHO's Programme," Annex 5. WHO Library.
107. Ibid.

first time in a decade of polemic, agreement had been reached to improve rationality in the use of drugs throughout the world by means of cooperation rather than confrontation—what the participants had called 'the spirit of Nairobi.'"[108]

In the previous clash, over the code on infant formula, the WHO staff was able to comply with developing countries while mediating a compromise. But this "passive" response, while successful in reaching a solution, still hurt the WHO's reputation and legitimacy. The debate over regulating the pharmaceutical sector, which was strongly supported by the G-77 and vehemently opposed by the United States and other developed countries, promised to lead to even more reputational damage. Moreover, given the gap in countries' positions, a compromise seemed unlikely. To protect the WHO's legitimacy, the secretariat was unwilling to support the position of developing countries. However, instead of "passively" resisting the demands of developing countries, they avoided the risk entailed in defying the wishes of the majority of countries by suggesting that the WHO's position was consistent with the NIEO principles and therefore acceptable.

Discussion

Developing countries' objective behind their call for a New International Economic Order was to change the uneven economic relations between North and South. It was also to change the related relations of exploitation between multinational corporations and governments of poor countries with limited regulative capacity. The UN and its agencies were asked to help governments to more effectively regulate the practices of multinational corporations in their countries, including through the development and implementation of international codes of conduct. The WHO was asked to help developing countries rationalize the purchasing of drugs by way of improved local manufacturing and by regulating the industry's marketing practices. Unlike the discussions over Health for All and primary health care, the subjects of appropriate technology and the inappropriate marketing of certain commodities led to heated debates between North and South. In such cases, the ideational position of the WHO bureaucracy had less impact on its response to the external pressures than its need to protect the legitimacy of the organization, which was severely undermined in the course of such clashes. Because conflicts among member states often did not involve direct negotiations but were rather manifested by parties attempting to influence the

---

108. WHO Document, 1986, WHA39/A/SR/11. WHO Library.

bureaucracy's position, outcomes were to a large extent shaped by the WHO secretariat's response to such attempts. Using adaptive strategies, the WHO secretariat was often able to protect the status of the organization even in the midst of particularly harsh debates.

The model list of essential drugs involved two analytically distinct phases of strategic adaptation. In the first stage, of strategic compliance, the WHO was able to incorporate the notion of essential drugs, which was an important aspect of primary health care, into the logic of the New International Economic Order by turning the "transfer of technology" into the transfer of *appropriate* technology. In the second stage, in order to appease the pharmaceutical industry, the WHO narrowed the scope of the list of essential drugs, limiting its applicability to poor people in poor countries. At this stage, it was not the NIEO principles that were compromised, as developing countries did not have a particular investment in the notion that primary health care should also apply to developed countries. Rather, in order to save the program, the WHO secretariat sacrificed the organization's own principles.

In the debates regarding both domestic production of drugs and codes of marketing practices, the WHO's reputation as a competent and responsible organization was at stake. In these cases, the WHO leadership responded to that threat by resisting at least some of the demands of developing countries. In the case of local production, the WHO, which was never at the center of the program, simply neglected to make it a priority. In the case of an international code of marketing of infant formula, the WHO generally supported the position of developing countries on the code but was also able to formulate a compromise that all countries, with the exception of the United States, could agree on. The WHO secretariat's support of the code, however, resulted in developed countries challenging its legitimacy by arguing it was going beyond its mandate. Consequently, when the possibility of a code of marketing of pharmaceutical products emerged, the WHO leadership opposed it. To avoid direct confrontation with developing countries, however, the WHO leadership resisted their demands strategically, by drawing on NIEO principles of equity and self-reliance to make the claim that its position was, in fact, compatible with the interests of developing countries.

These cases reveal that when compliance with G-77 demands had the potential for explicit confrontation with multinational companies and the rich countries that represented their interests, the WHO secretariat was more likely to resist, often employing strategic responses: the WHO secretariat steered clear of confrontations regarding nonessential drugs, it did not contribute much to the drive for local production, and while in principle supporting codes of conduct, it strategically resisted the call for regulating the pharmaceutical sector. In his last year as director-general, in 1988, Mahler reflected on the possibility of international codes of conduct, insinuating that the strategic resistance of the WHO was not driven by principles but by pragmatic realism in the face of a world that was not yet ready.

> The Constitution expected a great deal more from international cooperation than WHO had been able to provide so far: a much higher degree of concertation [*sic*] than had yet been achieved would be required to facilitate the development of binding international regulations. WHO was a very young organization and the world was not yet mature enough to permit [that] sort of international decision-making. . . . Although the optimal solution had not been found, important steps forward had been made, and WHO could be proud of the groundbreaking role it had played.[109]

Despite Mahler's optimism that the world might soon "mature" to the point of being able to accept large-scale international cooperation, the opposite was already beginning to happen. At the World Health Assembly in 1986, in which the Nairobi Conference was summarized and a strategy for the rational use of drugs formulated, U.S. representatives expressed their government's "strong position that the World Health Organization should not be involved in efforts to regulate or control the commercial practices of private industry, even when the products may relate to concerns about health" (quoted in Hardon 1992: 59). United States delegates lobbied, albeit unsuccessfully, for a resolution that decried the "alarming prospects of politicizing health" and the "attempts to regulate commercial projects" (Hardon 1992: 59). That year, the U.S. government failed to pay its assessed contribution to the WHO. Though no formal reason was given, the nonpayment was generally believed to be related to WHO's activities in the drugs field (Hardon 1992: 60). By then, conservative groups in the United States, with access to the Reagan administration, had been criticizing the WHO not only for the attempts to regulate infant food and pharmaceutical industries, but also for its Health for All strategy, which the Heritage Foundation described as a "blueprint that tilts far against private sector health care systems in favor of state run systems which, experience painfully teaches, fail to deliver medicines or care" (cited in Hardon 1992: 59–60). The New International Economic Order was dead. Neoliberal principles were to become the new dominant logic with which the WHO was expected to comply. The next chapter describes the rise of neoliberal thought and how it affected the World Health Organization.

---

109. WHO Document, 1988, EB81/SR/11. WHO Library.

THE WHO IN CRISIS

The missionary zeal that characterized Mahler turned into despair toward the end of his tenure. In an address in December 1987, Mahler mourned the failure of North-South talks.

> I have to say in all sadness that negotiations over any kind of new international economic order have reached beyond the state of even being frustrating; they have simply been shelved. And when they did take place, instead of dialogues they took the form of parallel monologues. . . . [It] is a matter of serious soul-searching. For not only has the gap between the "haves" and "have-nots" remained steadfast, it has grown even greater. Admittedly, some few "have-nots" have graduated to the ranks of the "haves," but the plight of the majority has become more sorry than ever.[1]

The demise of the New International Economic Order was reflected in the disintegration of NIEO-related programs, including Health for All and primary health care at the WHO. The crisis was not limited to specific programs, and it extended to the organization itself. Starting in the late-1980s, the WHO suffered from financial instability, its authority was undermined by competing institutions, and its stature as a legitimate institution was put into question.

---

1. "Health for All and Development," Address by Dr. H. Mahler, Director-General of the World Health Organization at the Conference on Italian Health Cooperation Activities in African Countries, Rome, Italy, 3–4 December 1987. WHO Library.

The financial, authority, and legitimacy predicaments at the WHO were caused by a radical transformation in the exogenous environment: starting under the leadership of President Ronald Reagan, and with pressure from an impatient Congress, the U.S. government made explicit its discontent with the dominance of Third World countries in UN agencies and vowed to fight back. Opposition to the NIEO, which advocated economic nationalism, intensified due to the rise of neoliberal thought spearheaded by the Reagan administration in the United States and elsewhere, which posited that economic growth could only be achieved through the self-efficiency of markets (Harvey 2005). Criticisms were aimed at UN-led initiatives and programs, but also at the alleged organizational malfunctioning of UN agencies, including irresponsible budget growth and managerial incompetence.

To generate the desired policy changes, the United States exploited the intensified economic vulnerability of developing countries in the context of the major debt crisis of the early 1980s. Taking advantage of developing countries' pressing need for renewed loans, the Reagan administration not only put an end to NIEO negotiations, but also introduced policies compatible with the neoliberal agenda into international organizations, especially the IMF and the World Bank. Under the new conditions, the United States and other industrial countries were also able to exploit, to a greater extent than in the 1970s, the resource dependence of international organizations. As a result of these pressures, the WHO experienced a crisis during the transition to the neoliberal logic. The WHO, which in the past had been highly regarded, was now resented for its NIEO-compatible policies, especially those affecting multinational companies. Starting in the early 1980s, and peaking during the tenure of Director-General Hiroshi Nakajima, who succeeded Mahler in 1988, the WHO experienced mounting exogenous pressures, which threatened the organization's finances and undermined its authority. The financial crisis was the result of a new budget policy, of zero growth, which developed countries forced on UN agencies. In addition, some countries, including the United States, did not pay their assessments in full. Rich countries also began contributing voluntary, rather than mandatory, donations to the WHO, which provided the donors, rather than the World Health Assembly as a whole, control over those funds. The authority crisis, in turn, occurred when other international organizations, including the World Bank and, in 1996, a newly established Joint United Nations Programme on HIV/AIDS (UNAIDS) developed global health policies and programs that directly competed with the WHO. In addition, the WHO suffered from a leadership crisis, as Hiroshi Nakajima, who was elected director-general against the position of the U.S. government, was blamed for weak leadership, poor management, and even cronyism and corruption. The mistrust in Nakajima likely contributed to the financial and authority crises, and it made the WHO secretariat unable to effectively respond to them.

The Neoliberal Turn at the International Level

Industrialized countries did not welcome the New International Economic Order. According to Rothstein (1979: 169), they found developing countries to be "occasionally irresponsible and narrowly self-interested," and they complained about the "politicization of even apparently technical issues" and about the resolutions that patched together everyone's demands, which were "masterpieces in the phraseology of ambiguity, and that result[ed] in uncertainty about what, if anything, [had] been decided."

In the United States, criticisms against the NIEO intensified under the Reagan administration. Doug Bandow, who served as special assistant to President Reagan and a deputy representative to the Third UN Conference on the Law of the Sea, complained against the "comprehensive and totalitarian system of global management" (Bandow 1985). The U.S. ambassador to the UN from 1981 until 1985, Jeane Kirkpatrick, called the New International Economic Order a philosophy of "global socialism" (cited in Bandow 1985). This was in line with the antimultilateralist, anti-Communist attitude of the Reagan administration, but it also reflected the triumph of neoliberal economic thought and the administration's opposition to the economic theories that informed import substitution industrialization (ISI) and other tenets of the New International Economic Order.

Criticisms in the United States were as often aimed at developing countries and supportive UN agencies as they were at the initiatives they promoted. A treasury department official exclaimed in the *National Journal:* "Ultimately, the [global] South wants our money. It's a scam. Our problem is that the whole mindset of the dialogue is objectionable. It's unreal" (cited in Livingston 1992). Vernon A. Walters, the U.S. ambassador to the UN who succeeded Kirkpatrick, and Daniel Mica, a Democrat from Delaware, referred to the nonaligned nations as "the lynching mob."[2] The conservative Heritage Foundation described the UN as being "dominated by a coalition of Third World developing countries and Soviet-bloc nations" (cited in Tickner 1990: 57). Referring to UN agencies as "union organizers for the Third World," Bandow (1985) complained that "the highly paid, professional staffs of the myriad UN agencies have discarded even the appearance of neutrality . . . and directly assisted countries in implementing indigenous policies reflecting the international collectivist ideology." Using harsher words, William S. Broomfield, a Republican congressman from Michigan, said that "the General Assembly . . . has largely degenerated into a forum for demagoguery practiced

---

2. "U.S. Policy in the United Nations," Hearings and Markup before the Committee on Foreign Affairs and its Subcommittee on Human Rights and International Organizations and the Subcommittee on International Operations, House of Representatives, Ninety-ninth Congress, First Session on H. Con. Res. 211, September 18, 1985.

by Third World dictatorships and Communist totalitarian regimes."[3] Benjamin Rosenthal, a Democrat from New York, referred to UN "hypocrisies," "biased resolutions," "incendiary rhetoric," and "anti-Semitism and racism."[4]

Although both in the General Assembly and in UN agencies the United States was, according to Kirkpatrick, "more often than not outvoted and outnumbered,"[5] the United States was financing these organizations.[6] Kirkpatrick complained that "countries that have the votes don't pay the bills, and the countries that pay the bills don't have the votes."[7] The blunt question that underlined congressional debates was why should the United States financially support an organization that does not do what the United States wants? Congressman Mica, for example, asked: "We pay $350 million a year, plus, to be there. It appears . . . that it is kind of an elite anti-U.S. debating society and we are paying for it. Now, why should we stay in the United Nations?"[8] In this way, the U.S. government's heads-on collision with the South over NIEO programs spilled over to a "crisis of multilateralism" (Ruggie 1985, Keohane and Nye 1985) and to conflict with the UN institutions themselves. In one heated moment, a deputy U.S. ambassador to the UN stated that if the United Nations wished to leave New York he would be on hand at the dock to bid a fond farewell. President Reagan seemed to endorse the idea by suggesting that most Americans agreed with those sentiments (Ruggie 1985).

Even while such rhetoric abounded, the Reagan administration never seriously considered leaving the UN. As Kirkpatrick admitted, "The price of withdrawal would be too high." She continued: "I think we are either confronted with improving the United Nations or leaving it. . . . But I took that to mean, therefore, that we simply had to do a lot better in that particular hardball game

---

3. "U.S. Participation in the United Nations," Hearings and Markup before the Committee on Foreign Affairs and its Subcommittees on international Operations on Europe and the Middle East and on Human Rights and International Organizations of the House of Representatives, Ninety-seventh Congress, Second Session on H. Con. Res. 322, April 22, 27; May 4, 1982.

4. Ibid.

5. Jeane Kirkpatrick, Hearings before a Subcommittee of the Committee of Appropriations, House of Representatives, Ninety-seventh Congress, First Session (part 5), May 12, 1981.

6. The waning of U.S. influence was supposedly reflected in the change in UN voting patterns. In the 1940s and 1950s, the United States voted with the winning side on roll-call votes in the General Assembly more than 60 percent of the time. By the 1980s this proportion fell to less than 20 percent. However, others reasoned that these calculations were distorted by the considerable amount of repetitive voting on resolutions relating to South Africa and Israel. See Harold K. Jacobson, professor of Political Science, University of Michigan, "U.S. Policy in the United Nations," Hearings and Markup before the Committee on Foreign Affairs and its Subcommittee on Human Rights and International Organizations and the Subcommittee on International Operations, House of Representatives, Ninety-ninth Congress, December 4, 1985.

7. "U.S. Policy in the United Nations," Hearings and Markup before the Committee on Foreign Affairs and its Subcommittee on Human Rights and International Organizations and the Subcommittee on International Operations. House of Representatives, Ninety-ninth Congress, First Session on H. Con. Res. 211, October 29, 1985.

8. Ibid.

of politics."[9] The debt crisis in 1982 made the game much easier to play. In subsequent years, the U.S. government successfully forced UN member states to abandon NIEO programs and initiatives and introduced neoliberal economic policies instead. The U.S. government also forced financial and managerial reforms on the UN.

Introducing the "Magic of the Marketplace"

Ronald Reagan's election in 1980 as the U.S. president was a turning point both in national and global economic history. The Keynesian economic theory that had informed economic policies in the United States since the New Deal in the 1930s was declared fallacious by the Republican Party, and replaced by a neoliberal economic program. In the United States, the new economic paradigm resulted in the deregulation "of everything from airlines and telecommunications to finance," tax cuts, budget cuts (albeit not in security spending), and attacks on trade union power (Harvey 2005: 26).

Neoliberalism was a global project and neoliberal economic policies eventually diffused from the United States, the United Kingdom, and Chile to other Latin American countries, Western European countries, South Africa, New Zealand, almost the entire Soviet bloc after the collapse of the Soviet Union, Sweden, India, and China (Harvey 2005). While the sources of this diffusion are contested (Fourcade and Babb 2002, Simmons, Dobbin, and Garrett 2006, Prasad 2006), scholars agree that the U.S. government had a major role in bringing the "magic of the marketplace," as President Reagan called it in many of his speeches, to developing countries. In the course of helping developing countries out of a major debt crisis, the U.S. government was able first to put an end to NIEO negotiations and programs and also to introduce new economic prescriptions informed by neoliberal principles.

THE DEBT CRISIS OF 1982

During the 1960s and 1970s, many developing countries embraced import substitution industrialization as their domestic economic policy (see chapter 3). One of the main objectives of ISI was to replace imports with locally manufactured commodities. Even as industrialization reduced imports of manufactured goods, however, it required the import of raw materials and machinery that were not available locally (Frieden 2006: 351). Imports required foreign currency that could be achieved only by way of exports, but while many ISI policies were designed to promote exports, most developing countries were unable to

---

9. Ibid.

export enough to buy the imports they needed. In the 1970s, the import-export gap worsened: inflation raised the price of the manufactured goods developing countries needed, stagnation in the West reduced the demand for the products of developing countries, and technological innovations, including new synthetic materials, pushed down prices of agricultural commodities and raw materials, which were developing countries' main types of exports (Castells and Laserna 1989). In addition, most developing nations were oil importers and, during the oil crisis that resulted from the embargo imposed by OPEC, they faced expensive oil import bills (Krasner 1987, Frieden 2006: 369; see also chapter 3).

The oil shocks also provided an unexpected source of loans. Frieden (2006: 370) succinctly explains: "The oil price explosion gave OPEC members far more money than they could spend, and they deposited much of it . . . into the world's financial markets. International bankers were eager to lend OPEC's 'petrodollars,' and among the principal users of these funds were the non-oil developing countries." By the early 1980s, the Third World as a whole owed $750 billion abroad, three-quarters to private financiers.

This "strange triangle" (Frieden 2006: 370) was ultimately put to an end by the U.S. Federal Reserve. To bring inflation down, the head of the Federal Reserve, Paul Volcker, who was appointed by President Carter in August 1979, pushed short-term interest rates up from about 10 percent to 20 percent and kept them at these high levels until late 1982. These interest rate hikes pushed the base lending rate to which Third World commercial debts were pegged from 10 to 20 percent in two years. Real interest rates on the debt of the least-developed countries, which barely kept up with inflation between 1974 and 1980, shot up to 6 percent in 1981, then to 8 percent in 1982 (Frieden 2006: 374). Poor countries were no longer able to pay their debts. In August 1982, Mexico announced that it had run out of money and that it could not even service its $62 billion debt to the United States. Shortly after, Brazil too suspended interest payments on foreign commercial bank loans. Within weeks, private lending to the developing world dried up. Countries that used to roll over their debt from one loan to another were cut off from the bank lending they had relied on for ten or fifteen years (Bradshaw and Huang 1991, Frieden 2006).

To protect American private banks from developing countries' defaults the U.S. government turned the IMF into a central coordinator of claims. The Reagan administration took advantage of the financial vulnerability of developing countries to also radically transform the international logic.

THE END OF THE NIEO

During the 1980s, the U.S. government intensified its opposition to any NIEO-informed demands or negotiations. The Reagan administration refused to sign the UN Law of the Sea Convention, which had been completed in the early 1980s after a decade of negotiations. In cases in which an agreement had been reached, as with the Common Fund for Commodities or the UNCTAD Liner Code, implementation was slow and the final outcome inconsequential (Krasner 1987: 179–181, Livingston 1992). The Reagan administration also took the extreme step of withdrawing from UN agencies. It threatened withdrawal from the Food and Agriculture Organization (FAO) and formally withdrew from UNESCO in 1983, accusing the organization of "politicization" (in regard to disarmament and human rights), "statist theories" (including pressures in UNESCO for a New World Information and Communication Order), and of exceeding "zero real growth" and having "extremely poor" management practices (Jacobson 1984).[10] The administration also considered withdrawal from UNCTAD and acted to weaken its influence. Citing "serious negative trends in the dialogue among the developed and developing countries," the State Department suggested overhauling UNCTAD, restricting its activities, and narrowing its agenda (cited in Livingston 1992). In addition, the U.S. government under Reagan began to bypass the UN system altogether, by negotiating issues through bilateral rather than multilateral channels (Tickner 1990, Sanders 1991: 310, Livingston 1992). Foreign aid, too, was increasingly distributed through bilateral aid programs rather than multilateral programs (Livingston 1992). This bilateralism helped weaken Third World solidarity, which had already been shaken by the financial crisis and geopolitical tensions. Finally, the U.S. government insisted on moving North-South negotiations to the "appropriate" international organizations, like the World Bank or the IMF, which it could control. As a Treasury Department official declared: "We will talk IMF issues—but in the IMF" (cited in Livingston 1992). The involvement of international financial institutions following the debt crisis allowed for this change in venue, and the new venues were then used to block NIEO initiatives and abandon the economic strategies that informed them.

THE PROMISE OF FREE MARKETS

The alternative to the economic nationalism of the NIEO was neoliberalism. The Reagan administration maintained that government involvement, inflated public sectors, and import substitution led to inefficiencies in the production process, and it sought to introduce neoliberal thinking, particularly the centrality of the market, into development programs (Tickner 1990, Livingston 1992, Adams 1993). According to the President's Task Force on International Private Enterprise, the new development model was based on the view that "greater reliance on private enterprise, individual initiative, and free competitive markets is

---

10. The United States returned to UNESCO in 2002, under President George W. Bush.

essential for sustained, equitable growth in the Third World" (cited in Tickner 1990: 56–57).

The debt crisis provided an opportunity to impose the neoliberal development model on developing countries. When the debt crisis broke out in 1982, the U.S. government persuaded private banks to agree to use the IMF as the central coordinator of their claims: developing countries could not negotiate with banks directly, but needed first to enter lending arrangements with the IMF (Cline 1995: 205–208). The "Baker Plan," a program of coordinated debt reduction conceived by U.S. Treasury Secretary James Baker in 1985, transformed the IMF into an active promoter of the neoliberal agenda. Under Baker's program, debt refinancing by the IMF would be made *conditional* on market-liberalizing policy reforms.[11] The Baker Plan gave rise to what has become known as the "Washington Consensus" (Williamson 1990): a set of ten market-liberalizing prescriptions, initially aimed at indebted Latin American countries, which were endorsed by a number of institutions located in Washington, DC, including the U.S. Treasury, the IMF, and the World Bank. The ten basic reforms that indebted countries were now obliged to follow if they were to receive IMF loans were: imposing fiscal discipline, reordering public expenditure priorities, instituting tax reform, liberalizing interest rates, creating a competitive exchange rate, liberalizing trade, removing obstacles to foreign direct investment, selling off public enterprises, deregulating businesses, and strengthening property rights (Williamson 1990, Adams 1993, Babb 2009: 126).

The World Bank also transformed itself in line with U.S. expectations (Babb 2009). The Reagan administration perceived the basic needs approach (see chapter 3) as having sacrificed growth and efficiency. According to the U.S. Department of State, basic needs policies "resulted from liberal impatience over the fact that economic growth is an uneven process. . . . But . . . this policy became divorced from the recognition that productivity—economic growth—is a *sine qua non* for development" (cited in Tickner 1990). A U.S. report, *United States Participation in the Multilateral Development Banks in the 1980s,* suggested that the United States reform the multilateral development banks "to encourage adherence to free and open markets, emphasis on the private sector as a vehicle for growth, minimal government involvement, and assistance to the needy who are willing to help themselves" (cited in Babb 2009: 88). The Baker Plan helped transform the World Bank in that direction by enhancing "coordinated lending" with

---

11. Even without conditionalities, the debt crisis would have probably led heavily indebted countries to abandon import substitution industrialization since, as Frieden (2006) explains, ISI was unsustainable without foreign loans, which paid "for the imported capital equipment and raw materials, subsidies, and public investments that governments needed to sustain industrial development."

the IMF: from that point forward, Bank and IMF lending were based on a common "policy framework paper," and the two organizations collaborated closely on plans for restructuring national economies (Chorev and Babb 2009: 469). The World Bank introduced structural adjustment lending programs, which instead of being "investment lending" and geared to concrete projects, as World Bank loans had been historically, were "policy lending," geared to the realization of policy changes and institutional reforms (Adams 1993). These programs focused on macroeconomic stabilization measures and were designed, according to the World Bank 1994 *Development Report,* to "unleash market forces so that competition can help improve the allocation of resources . . . getting price signals right and creating a climate that allows business to respond to those signals in ways that increase the returns to investment" (cited in Poku and Whiteside 2002: 192).

Developing countries transformed their economic policies following the new prescriptions, some enthusiastically and others more grudgingly. Livingston (1992) describes the shift from the call for a New International Economic Order to neoliberal policies in the following way: "Preoccupations with national sovereignty and controlling multinationals . . . have given way to efforts to attract foreign investment. Omnibus commodity programs have been superseded by dire compensatory financial needs. There has been a general move from trade regulation to export promotion." As Frieden (2006) shows, one developing country after another "liberalized trade, deregulated banks, sold off government enterprises, raised taxes and cut spending, and integrated its economy into world markets."[12]

UN: "Reform or Die"

Resentment among right-wing critics in the United States was not aimed only at developing countries and their NIEO initiatives, but also at UN agencies, where these initiatives had originated. A U.S. review of multilateral organizations from 1985 identified three systematic problems. Two were normative and were related to Third World dominance: the extraneous politicization in specialized technical agencies of the UN, and the UN's affinity with statist theory and concepts. The

---

12. Within a general trend toward liberalization, countries varied in their economic strategies. Amsden (2001) usefully differentiates between "integrationalists" and "independents." Most developing countries were "integrationists," which depended on technical licenses and economic collaboration with foreign firms for their long-run growth. A handful of "independent" countries, however, including China, India, Korea, and Taiwan, harbored ambitions to join the ranks of world-class innovators, and to base their expansion in high-tech sectors on national firms and investments in R&D. While "integrationist" countries opened the doors wider to foreign investment, "independent" countries used resistance mechanisms to promote science and technology and to buttress the market power of their national leaders. On divergence in the adoption of neoliberal reforms across states see also Evans and Sewell (forthcoming).

third related to the bureaucratic functioning of UN agencies and heavily criticized the budget management system.[13] In response to these concerns, the Reagan administration established a number of principles intended to improve the work of international organizations through financial and managerial reforms (Ghebali 1991: 28–29).

FINANCIAL REFORMS

Given the weakened influence of the United States in the international realm due to developing countries' procedural leverage, Congress thought it legitimate to reduce the relative contribution of the United States to the UN; given the alleged managerial incompetence and objectionable initiatives at the UN, Congress also thought it an imperative to reduce the overall growth in UN budget.[14] Already in 1972, Congress decided that U.S.-assessed contribution to UN bodies, including the WHO, would be reduced from more than 30 percent of the total contributions to 25 percent. An important issue of principle was involved, since contributions to the UN were determined by members' capacity to pay, as measured broadly by their gross domestic product and size of population, and on this basis of calculation a U.S. contribution of 25 percent was too low. In 1975, six members of Congress again called for the withdrawing of funds. Describing the United Nations as a "Third World dominated theater of the absurd," they wrote to President Gerald R. Ford, "It is one thing for the Third World, abetted by the Soviet Union, to lay claim to an organization which twists evil into goodness and darkness into light. It is another for our government to provide the financial wherewithal for such machinations."[15]

In 1983, budget-related tensions between the UN and the United States reached a new height, when criticisms were aimed not at the dominance of developing countries but the functioning of the UN organizations themselves. That year, Senator Nancy Kassebaum, a Republican from Kansas, introduced an amendment to Senate bill S.1342, to gradually reduce assessed payments of the U.S. government to the United Nations, UNESCO, the WHO, the FAO, and the

---

13. Gregory Newell, Assistant Secretary for International Organization Affairs, Department of State, Foreign Assistance and Related Programs Appropriations for 1986, Hearings before a Subcommittee of the Committee on Appropriations, House of Representatives, Ninety-ninth Congress, First Session (part 5), May 8, 1985.

14. The U.S.-assessed contributions to international organizations are controlled by Congress: a subcommittee in each of the House and Senate Appropriations Committees recommends appropriations for all such organizations, paid out of the annual budget of the Department of State. Voluntary contributions, in contrast, are run through the budget of the Department of State indirectly.

15. Letter to President Gerald Ford, December 4, 1974, WHCFSF, IT, Box 6. Ford Presidential Library.

ILO so that it would reach, by 1987, 70 percent of the 1980 level of U.S. contribution. The amendment provided that no contributions be made until the United Nations accepted the reduced amount as the full U.S. payment. In the hearings, Kassebaum justified her amendment by claiming that the UN organizations were "ineffective, top-heavy with high-paid officials, uncertain in their purposes, and unduly repetitious of other organizations."[16] The amendment, which the Reagan administration opposed because it found it too restrictive, was approved by the Senate but failed to pass the House (Ruggie 1985).

In 1985, Senator Kassebaum again tried to reduce U.S. relative contributions, but also to force change in the procedures by which the UN budget was decided. In an amendment to the Foreign Relations Act that Kassebaum cosponsored with Republican Congressman Gerald Solomon, U.S. contributions were limited to no more than 20 percent of the organizations' assessed budgets unless those organizations adopted voting rights on "matters of budgetary consequence" proportionate to the contributions of each member state (GAO 1986). According to the *State Bulletin*, "The law reflects dissatisfaction in the U.S. Congress over the fact that countries which contribute the great majority of the organization's money have little say in how it is spent."[17] The amendment was approved and from that year forward, the U.S. Congress refused to appropriate the full amount of the U.S. assessed contribution (Revzin 1988). By 1986, according to the UN Secretary General, "the United Nations [was facing] the most serious financial crisis in its history."[18]

At the UN General Assembly, member countries responded in 1986 by modifying the budget process to include consensus approval of the overall funding level before the detailed budget was prepared. This procedure gave each country a de facto veto power over UN spending, and since it satisfied the intent of the original Kassebaum-Solomon amendment, UN member countries hoped the United States would again pay its assessment in full.[19] In 1987, a crucial alteration to the Kassebaum-Solomon amendment, which permitted the adoption of consensus decision-making instead of the more restrictive original demand for weighted majority voting, was approved by Congress (Imber 1989: 132). Congress, however, continued to refuse to appropriate the full U.S. assessment, in spite of executive

---

16. "The U.S. Role in the United Nations," Hearings before the Subcommittee on Human Rights and International Organizations of the Committee on Foreign Affairs, House of Representatives, Ninety-eighth Congress, First Session, September 27 and October 3, 1983.

17. "UN Financial Crisis," October 1986, U.S. Department of State Bulletin.

18. Cited in Ibid.

19. Vernon Walters, Recent Developments in the United Nations System, Hearings before the Subcommittees on Human Rights and International Organizations and on International Operations of the Committee on Foreign Affairs, House of Representatives, One hundredth Congress, Second Session, February 25 and May 25, 1988.

officials pleading on behalf of the UN. Ambassador Walter urged members of Congress: "The initial shock of our withholding created the impetus for reform, but reforms are unlikely to take full effect in an organization paralyzed by financial instability."[20] In 1990, Gus Yatron, a Democrat from Pennsylvania, stated:

> The U.S. decision to start to withhold significant amounts of its assessed contributions to international organizations in the 1980s was part of an overall effort to spark much-needed management and political reforms within those organizations. The policy of using financial leverage within those organizations did in fact succeed. It also justifiably created the expectations that once UN reforms were realized, the US would pay its dues and arrearages. Unfortunately, this has not proven to be the case.[21]

Only during the George H.W. Bush administration was Congress persuaded to begin repaying the U.S. arrears, but not fully. Successive ambassadors to the UN continued to plead with Congress. Madeleine Albright maintained during her nomination hearings in 1993: "There is a fine line between the leverage gained by withholding funds in anticipation of reform, and losing credibility because you owe so much money."[22] Many members of Congress, however, maintained the position that the UN had failed to reform. Senator Jesse Helms from North Carolina still proclaimed in 1996:

> Withholding contributions has not worked. We have tried that. We have been there. Congress passage of the Kassebaum-Solomon bill, which sent a clear message if there ever was one to the United Nations either to reform or die, did not work either. The United Nations has neither reformed nor has it died. The time has come for it to do one or the other. You could flip a coin as far as I am concerned.[23]

FINANCIAL REFORMS: THE GENEVA GROUP

While the U.S. position on financial matters was generally more rigid than that of most other rich countries, the U.S. government was hardly alone in attempting to

---

20. Ibid.

21. "Recent Developments in the United Nations System," Hearing before the Subcommittees on Human Rights and International Organizations, and on International Operations of the Committee on Foreign Affairs, House of Representatives, One hundred first Congress, Second Session, April 25, 1990.

22. "Nomination of Madeleine K. Albright to be United States Ambassador to the United Nations," Hearing before the Committee on Foreign Relations, United States Senate, One hundred third Congress, First Session, January 21, 1993.

23. "United Nations Reform," Hearing before the Subcommittee on International Operations of the Committee on Foreign Relations, United States Senate, One hundred fourth Congress, Second Session, September 11, 1996.

reduce its contribution to the UN agencies. Already in 1964, the UK and the U.S. governments invited other governments contributing more than 1 percent to the budgets of the UN Specialized Agencies to join a forum, the Geneva Group, which would meet once a year, in which the "principal contributors" for the Specialized Agencies would be able to discuss a common agenda.[24] It was the same year UNCTAD was founded and the developed countries became concerned with what they regarded as a developing countries attempt to "gang up" on them in various institutions within the UN System (Williams 1987: 86). Participants of the Geneva Group were invited "to discuss the problems posed by . . . rapid growth in the activities and budgets of the main Specialized Agencies and the accompanying decline in our influence in the Agencies as their membership has expanded."[25] According to a confidential memorandum, "The main object of the Geneva Group has been to re-establish the proper influence of the principal contributors in the process of programmes and budget preparation in the Specialized Agencies."[26] Australia, Belgium, Canada, France, Germany, Italy, Japan, and the Netherlands accepted the invitation. Sweden and Switzerland chose to maintain observer status.[27]

Developing countries and UN secretariats did not welcome the new cooperation among the major contributors and the Geneva Group soon gained the unflattering reputation of "budget bashers." The Swiss delegate to the Geneva Group meeting reported of "a fairly strong current of resentment" directed against the Group. According to a British official, "To at least some of the Secretariats and non-members, it appeared to be a pressure group under Anglo-American, or NATO, control, which aimed at undermining the authority of the Organizations (and thus of the United Nations) and at concentrating control in the hands of a minority of members."[28] At the WHO, Director-General Candau did not allow senior officials to meet with Geneva Group representatives. Candau alluded privately to the Geneva Group as the "source of all evil."[29]

Until the 1980s, however, the Geneva Group had only little influence. Many of the initial obstacles in pushing the Geneva Group agenda was not due to the opposition of developing countries or secretariats, but stemmed from internal tensions among its members. It was often difficult to reach an agreement between the hard-

24. "UN Specialized Agencies," Note by the Foreign Office, October 2, 1964, OD 29/61. UK National Archives.

25. Ibid.

26. "Anglo-American Talks on the United Nations to be Held in the Foreign Office on 3 and 4 March," March 1966, FO 371/189918. UK National Archives.

27. "UN Specialized Agencies," Note by the Foreign Office, October 2, 1964, OD 29/61. UK National Archives.

28. Note, British Embassy in Berne, Germany, 11 February 1966, FO 371/189917. UK National Archives.

29. Geneva Group, Fifth Consultation on Specialized Agencies, May 21–22, 1968, FCO 61/78. UK National Archives.

liners and the other countries;[30] and even when an agreement had been reached, it was difficult for members to keep it when it was time to vote. A British official complained that "it has been very irksome at recent [world health] assemblies to have people like the French and the Australians purporting to be very tough about budget increases and then speaking with such still, small voices that they are hardly noticed. They are very bellicose in the Geneva Group."[31] The Geneva Group also had difficult time agreeing on appropriate tactics. The Americans, in particular, were criticized for their pettiness, insisting on small and controversial issues instead of focusing on the most important ones, and refusing compromises that other Geneva Group members would have been willing to accept. Many members agreed that, "American tactics . . . may, on future occasions, seriously reduce the effectiveness of the Group in the pursuit of our common objective."[32] By the early 1980s, as the U.S. position hardened, the criticism also intensified. A UK report following an Executive Board meeting held in 1983 complained:

> The Americans' . . . obsession with reducing spending has led them to challenge all, even the most minor, increases, with the result that the effectiveness of their arguments was impaired and many members were alienated by their negative approach. Overall the USA has ceased to play a constructive and respected part in the work of the Board.[33]

But the Geneva Group survived the initial difficulties and in subsequent years it adopted an increasingly more ambitious agenda. Originally, the Geneva Group's main focus was "to try to ensure acceptable rates of budget expansion" in the various Specialized Agencies.[34] In the late 1970s, the Geneva Group insisted on substantially lowering budget growth. Following the demands of the Reagan administration, by the 1980s the Geneva Group called for "zero real growth and maximum absorption of nondiscretionary cost increases occasioned by inflation and unfavorable rates of exchange."[35] Again echoing the U.S. government, the Geneva Group combined these budget demands with calls for managerial reforms.

---

30. "Steering Committee on International Organizations," Note by the Foreign and Commonwealth Office, 3 March 1970, FCO 61/634. UK National Archives; "Steering Committee on International Organizations," Note by Foreign Office, 18 March 1966, FO 371/189918. UK National Archives.

31. Letter, From Department of Health and Social Security to Peter Hayman, Foreign and Commonwealth Office, 7 February 1969, FCO 61/487. UK National Archives.

32. "Report on Anglo-American Talks on UN Matters," London, 11/12 July 1968, FCO 61/79. UK National Archives.

33. Memo from Department of Health and Social Security to Foreign and Commonwealth Office, 17 March 1983, MH 148/1047. UK National Archives.

34. Letter, UK Mission to Geneva to UN (Economics and Social Department) Foreign Office, 10 January 1966, FO 371/189917. UK National Archives.

35. Gregory Newell, Assistant Secretary for International Organization Affairs, Department of State, Departments of Commerce, Justice, and State, The Judiciary, and Related Agencies Appropriations for 1986, Hearings before a Subcommittee of the Committee on Appropriations, House of Representatives, Ninety-ninth Congress, First Session, Part 6. May 8, 1985.

MANAGERIAL REFORMS

Already in the early 1970s, the Geneva Group sought to better justify its demands by refocusing the discussion from the size of budgets, which developing countries deeply resented, to the effective use of those budgets. A note to the UK Foreign and Commonwealth Office explained:

> Major non-Communist contributors have not wished to appear concerned solely to limit the size of their contributions without regard to the need for the resources of the UN system to be efficiently used. They have therefore been interested in reforms designed to promote such efficient use.[36]

Hence, the Geneva Group tried to change its "former image as simply a 'budget-basher'" and to create the impression that it was "genuinely concerned to help improve efficiency and cost-effectiveness."[37] Issues requiring reform included: budgetary excesses (partly due to lack of financial accountability), a bloated bureaucracy characterized by administrative mismanagement, duplication of effort (due to insufficient coordination), an unnecessary plethora of meetings and documentation, and an uneven record on program effectiveness (Rothstein 1979: 169, Ruggie 1985, Lee and Walt 1992). As we saw, these complaints were reiterated in the concentrated attack of the U.S. government against the UN in the 1980s. As Nicholas Platt, acting assistant secretary of state for international organization affairs, told Congress: "We believe it is particularly important that [international] organizations regularly evaluate their programs, reduce and phase out low-priority and obsolete activities, operate with lean staffs, and minimize support and overhead costs."[38] These concerns were arguably linked to the issues of politicization and waning influence: according to industrial countries, the agencies had so politicized their technical tasks and deliberations that the United Nations as a whole accomplished too little of what it had been designed to accomplish, and at great expense (Ruggie 1985).

What's New in the Neoliberal Era?

With the debt crisis in the early 1980s, the United States and other Western countries rediscovered their ability to impose their will by using others' dependence

---

36. Note, "Geneva Group—Future Role and 'Extraordinary Measures,'" 2 March 1971, FCO 61/781. UK National Archives.

37. Note, "Geneva Group: Performance and Prospect," From UK Mission in Geneva to the UN (Economic & Social) Department, Foreign Office, 15 February 1972, FCO 61/919. UK National Archives.

38. Departments of Commerce, Justice, and State, the Judiciary and Related Agencies Appropriations for 1983, Hearings before a Subcommittee on Appropriations, House of Representatives, Ninety-seventh Congress, Second Session, March 16, 1982.

on their funds. The Reagan administration, often with the support of other rich countries, used this influence to radically transform North-South relations at the international level. The U.S. government was able to break up the Third World coalition and roll back NIEO programs. In addition, the U.S. government used its control over needed resources to transform the IMF, the World Bank, and other international organizations into adopters and promoters of neoliberal economic policies. These policies, as we have seen, were governed by a number of fundamental economic maxims, including the reliance on the efficiency of the market and suspicion of most governmental interventions (Harvey 2005). More broadly, neoliberal thinking brought to international organizations a tendency for conceptual reductionism of social well-being into economic development (Somers 2008). This allowed the spread of neoliberal maxims also into noneconomic realms of governance, including health, through the imposition of economic logic onto issues that had previously been relatively autonomous from it. Such neoliberal orientation led to policies that, for example, favored market-driven solutions over governmental interventions, or that defined goals, listed priorities, and measured success in purely economic terms.

The neoliberal-compatible principles that were introduced to the international level differed from the guiding principles of the New International Economic Order in a number of ways. The one central tenet the NIEO and the neoliberal logics shared was emphasis on economic growth. However, the NIEO concern, even if secondary, with social development was completely lost under neoliberalism, and the NIEO interest in economic growth as a tool for achieving the goal of sovereign equity between North and South also disappeared. Most important, the means to achieve economic growth in developing countries were distinctly different. Neoliberal economic theory disputed economic nationalist strategies such as ISI and saw the only course for economic growth to be participation in the global market through trade liberalization and other measures that would open domestic markets to international competition (McMichael 2000). The new emphasis on exports was perhaps unavoidable given the need for foreign currency to pay old and new debts but, unlike the export-led industrialization of South Korea and other newly industrializing countries, IMF conditionalities discouraged export subsidies or other such protectionist measures that allowed governments to participate in national economic planning. Rather, the Washington Consensus supported the weakening of all forms of state intervention. Furthermore, economic recovery was to be achieved not by nurturing domestic companies but with the involvement of foreign capital. Multinational companies were to be lured rather than regulated, thereby reversing the NIEO notion of economic sovereignty. Given the Third World struggles during the 1960s and 1970s against the presence and intervention of multinational corporations in their domestic affairs, this was indeed a radical shift. Participation in the global economy did not allow for the delinking of North and South or even for more moderate versions of collective self-reliance. In addition, there was no longer room for developing countries' argument that former colonizers and other rich countries were obligated to support the poor; instead, rich countries' foreign aid had become a matter of charity. Finally, nonuniversal international organizations such as the World Bank and IMF were preferred over international organizations where developing countries had a majority vote.

The new era of international politics that started in the mid-1980s should not, however, be reduced to the adoption of neoliberal economic policies as it was combined, especially in the United States, with conservative foreign policy that included deep mistrust in international bureaucracies. In a lecture before The Heritage Foundation, titled *Defining a Conservative Foreign Policy,* Ambassador Kirkpatrick suggested: "It is accurate, I believe, to say that a conservative would not have designed and worked to realize the United Nations" (Kirkpatrick 1993). Indeed, in the 1980s, U.S. hostility to the UN reached a new height and, as we saw, the attempt to weaken the political influence of the G-77 turned into a crisis of multilateralism in which international bureaucracies were also targeted. In the same lecture, Kirkpatrick (1993) defined a "conservative foreign policy" as "above all, worry[ing] about growth in the size and powers of government and about the problems of holding government responsible." Such sentiment was partly a façade to justify anti–Third World policies but partly a genuine concern with the effective functioning of governments and international organizations.

Crisis of Transition at the WHO

By the late 1980s, the international arena looked very different than it had a mere ten years earlier. Developing countries were economically crushed, their solidarity shaken, and with urgently needed loans conditioned on policy reforms, the number of their votes no longer mattered. For the WHO, like other international organizations, the exogenous environment had been radically transformed, with pressures now coming from industrial countries with new demands, expectations, and considerably more political leverage. A transition period ensued in which the WHO suffered an authority crisis as other international organizations became involved in global health issues, a severe financial crisis as contributions were sharply reduced, and a leadership crisis following the retirement of Mahler.

Financial Crisis

The WHO's financial crisis was the result of two developments: zero nominal growth and countries' failure to pay their full assessments on time. Rich countries' voluntary contributions helped prevent financial disarray, but it deepened the dependence of the WHO secretariat on rich countries' resources and weakened the procedural influence of poor member states.

ZERO NOMINAL GROWTH

When the Geneva Group was established in the 1960s to discuss "rapid growth in the activities and budgets of the main Specialized Agencies"[39] and influence the way budgets were developed, the WHO was not an obvious target for its efforts. At the time, Belgium's opinion, for example, was that "WHO had an unusually low proportion of administrative costs."[40] Similarly, Sweden stated that "considering the needs of the developing world, [WHO's] expansion had not been excessive" and that "it was difficult to see where savings might be made without damaging effects."[41] But by the late 1970s, there was no longer a budgetary consensus regarding the WHO.[42] A U.S. report, laconically titled "US Participation in the World Health Organization Still Needs Improvement," harshly criticized "the continuous and excessive increases in the budgets of the UN specialized agencies," including the WHO (GAO 1977).

In addition to internal disagreements among Geneva Group members (see also above), the procedures governing the determination of budgets at the WHO made it difficult for rich countries, at least until the 1980s, to impose their wishes on the institution. The WHO budget was prepared by the director-general, examined by the Executive Board, and voted by the World Health Assembly (see chapter 1). The Geneva Group respected the notion that for the director-general, who holds "the philosophy of the medical man," "the 'acceptable' rate of expansion must be the maximum possible, and this in practice means the maximum that the Assembly will be likely to accept."[43] The Geneva Group also tolerated the fact that members of the Executive Board, who functioned as experts rather than

---

39. "UN Specialized Agencies," Note by the Foreign Office, October 2, 1964, OD 29/61. UK National Archives.

40. Geneva Group, Fifth Consultation on Specialized Agencies, May 21–22, 1968, FCO 61/78. UK National Archives.

41. Ibid.

42. Letter from S. Paul Ehrlich, Acting Surgeon General, Director, Office of International Health, HEW, May 25, 1977, Staff Offices, Peter Bourne, Box 34. Carter Presidential Library.

43. Aide Memoire on the WHO, Meeting of UN Ad Hoc Committee on UN Finances at Geneva on 20–21 April 1966, FO 371/189916. UK National Archives.

representatives of their governments, were often in alliance with the director-general: "It is companies of people who, on the one hand, are doctors, and proud of it, and on the other hand are independent, and proud of it."[44] It was at the assembly, therefore, that the Geneva Group tried to use the WHO's resource dependence on its members in order to counterbalance the procedural dependence on developing countries, which had the majority of votes.[45]

During the era dominated by the call for a New International Economic Order, the impact of the Geneva Group on the WHO budget was modest, and it failed to reduce the budget, which increased at more than 10 percent a year. Given "the ever-greater disparity that is developing in health programmes between the developed and the newly independent countries,"[46] developing countries called for greater international assistance, although without increasing the previous rate of budget growth. In an emotional speech given before member states in 1968, the representative of Senegal reminded the states that had been members of the WHO during its first decade that "the resolutions and the guiding principles for WHO's work had been laid down before the entry of the newly independent countries" and that "there was a saying that what was done without you was against you." He quickly added that that was not true of the present situation: "If the countries of the newly independent countries had believed that, they would not have applied to be, and become, Member States." Nonetheless, "the fact remained that those countries had not been present at the beginning. They had not been able to express their point of view at the outset. Consequently, the principles followed by WHO, especially those regarding assistance to Member States, did not always meet present realities." Those present realities, according to the Senegalese delegate, required increasing material assistance to the programs of developing countries.[47] Other delegates assured rich countries, however, that "there was no intention to increase the budget; what was in mind was to readjust or redistribute the budget."[48]

Also in later years, developing countries kept their demands within the limits of the previous rates of budget growth. In 1975, Resolution WHA28.76, sponsored by African, Arab, and some Asian delegations recalled in its preamble the

---

44. Note, UK Mission to Geneva to UN (Economic & Social) Department, Foreign Office, 4 April 1966, FO 371/189916. UK National Archives.

45. To reduce the budget, the Geneva Group also tried its hand at institutional changes, which often required constitutional amendments. Some initiatives, such as changing the status of Executive Board members so they functioned as state representatives rather than in their individual capacity or having a World Health Assembly only once every two years, failed; other initiatives, such as having biannual instead of annual budgets, passed.

46. WHO Document, 1968, A21/P&B/SR/20. WHO Library.

47. Ibid.

48. Ibid.

NIEO resolutions, and called on the assembly to decide "that the regular programme budget shall ensure a substantial increase, in real terms, of technical assistance and services for developing countries."[49] The UK Mission in Geneva reported:

> A Geneva Group meeting, hastily convened . . . revealed strong reservations on the part of several members of the Group (FRG, Italy, Canada and Japan) regarding a sweeping commitment to increase the overall size of the regular programme budget to provide for an expansion in technical assistance, which they agreed should normally be financed from extra budgetary sources. And, while some (Netherlands, Sweden) were happy to support an increase in the overall budget to accommodate expanded technical assistance, most could only accept its expansion within an unchanged total.[50]

The resolution passed with half of the Geneva Group abstaining.

The following year, the G-77 sought to define more precisely the resolution's reference to "substantial increase . . . of technical assistance and services." Accordingly, Resolution WHA29.49 called for 60 percent of the WHO's regular resources to be devoted to technical cooperation (WHO 2008: 29). Mahler declared this "unforgettable" resolution to be, "one of the most important political decisions in the history of the organization" (cited in WHO 2008: 29). For Mahler, the resolution "was a striking symbol of a new balance of power in the world of health in which the health representatives of the countries of the world came to realize their mutual dependence."[51] According to the "Technical Discussions on the Contribution of Health to the New International Economic Order," the "re distribution of resources in the health sector, as exemplified by trends in WHO's budget policy," was "fully consistent with the NIEO" (WHO 1980a).

Although several representatives who were not members of the G-77 found the request for fixing a percentage for technical assistance "undesirable," "premature," "arbitrary," and one that might "produce rigidity in programmes" (cited in WHO 2008: 29), the Geneva Group was ultimately pleased with the resolution. According to the Americans, "For the developing countries this action means a more significant proportion of the Organization's resources devoted to the pressing health needs they perceive. For ourselves, and other developed countries, this signals a major *management* effort to utilize resources more effectively,

---

49. WHO Document, 1975, WHA28.76, A28/VR/13. PAHO Library.

50. Note, "28th WHA: Administrative and Financial Questions," from UK Mission in Geneva to Foreign Office, 26 June 1975, FCO 61/1351. UK National Archives.

51. "Action for Health," Address by Dr. H. Mahler, Director-General of the WHO to the Thirty-Second World Health Assembly, 8 May 1979. WHO Library.

eliminate unnecessary overhead costs, and discontinue programs which are no longer found to be productive."[52]

However, budget bashing, now tightly intertwined with reform issues, came back with a vengeance, when in 1979 the Geneva Group successfully demanded annual growth of no more than "real increase of up to 2 percent per annum, in addition to reasonable estimated cost increases."[53] From then on, major donors continued to press for even lower budget increases. In the early 1980s, for example, they introduced a policy, which applied to all UN organizations, of zero real growth of regular budget funds (Godlee 1994a). In 1993, the WHO introduced a policy of zero nominal growth, which unlike real growth, no longer allowed for adjustment for inflation and exchange rate movements. Due to the zero nominal growth budgets, during the 1990s contributions to the WHO declined by 20 percent in real terms (People's Health Movement et al. 2008).

ARREARS

The financial difficulties of the WHO worsened due to unpaid contributions, including from Russia, but also from the United States which, following the 1985 Kassebaum-Solomon amendment, withheld its contributions and paid only 20 percent of the organization's assessed budget. At the WHO, the withholding of funds was considered a protest against the list of essential drugs that was opposed by U.S.-based pharmaceutical companies (Godlee 1994b, Brown, Cueto, and Fee 2006) and, more broadly, against turning the WHO into a "sort of super international regulatory body," as Alan Keyes, a former U.S. assistant secretary of state in charge of international organizations, called it in 1988 (Revzin 1988). A year before retirement, Mahler did not conceal his frustrations.

> For more than a year now your Organization [has been] held financial hostage due to the uncertainty of payments of assessed contributions.... What crime has WHO committed against those who are withholding mandatory contribution? Surely it cannot be the influence of commercial lobbies who falsely believe that WHO is blocking their expansion, whereas in fact adding resources for the health of underprivileged as part of WHO's value system could open up new markets in the most ethical of ways. What crimes then has WHO committed? That it has stimulated Member States to adopt health policies in line with the WHO health culture? That it has saved them more than they have ever contributed to

---

52. Letter from S. Paul Ehrlich, Acting Surgeon General, Director, Office of International Health, HEW, 25 May 1977, Staff Offices, Peter Bourne, Box 34. Carter Presidential Library.
53. Memo, "Tentative Budgetary Projections for 1982–83," May 7–25, 1979, RG25, vol. 14979, file 46–4-WHO-12–1979. Canada National Archives.

WHO by eradicating smallpox? That WHO has taken the international lead in the battle against AIDS . . . and that it has done so with very meager means, scraped from the bottom of the barrel. . . . Or that your Organization has displayed outstanding fiscal responsibility?[54]

Mahler's rage was of little effect. In 1986, the rate of collection of mandatory assessments was 72.18 percent. In 1989, it was 70.22 percent (Beigbeder et al. 1998: 163). In the following years, the rate of collection improved somewhat but in the end of 1996, the rate of collection for that year still amounted to only 77.72 percent. Only 102 Member States had paid their current-year contributions to the budget in full that year, and 63 Members had made no payment toward their contributions. The total unpaid arrears of contributions exceeded $169 million (Beigbeder et al. 1998: 163).

EXTRABUDGETARY FUNDS

In addition to mandatory assessments, from the very beginning the WHO had relied on voluntary contributions, called extrabudgetary funds (EBFs), especially for major initiatives, such as the malaria and smallpox eradication programs. However, EBFs were not a central component of the WHO budget, and most funds were drawn from member states' mandatory assessments. In the early 1970s, for example, the extrabudgetary funds for programs such as the Onchocerciasis Control Programme, Tropical Diseases Research Programme and Human Reproduction Programme accounted for only about 20 percent of the total WHO expenditure and over half of these funds came from other UN agencies, not directly from member states (Vaughan et al. 1996).

In the mid-1970s, however, at the same time that rich countries began to aggressively challenge their contribution to the regular budget, the share of voluntary contributions coming from donations by multilateral agencies or "donor" nations increased significantly, and has since continued to grow steadily over the past several decades. EBFs increased to almost 30 percent of WHO total expenditures in 1974–1975, and then to 53 percent in 1980–1981. During the 1980s, EBFs remained around 50 percent but increased to closer to 60 percent during the 1990s. By 2004 it was 70 percent (Lee 2009). There was also a significant shift in the source of the EBFs, with a clear increase in the contribution of countries. Vaughan et al. (1996) calculate that since WHO started to receive EBFs for assisted activities, UN funds and the World Bank have donated only about 6 percent of the total to date and donor governments have contributed directly nearly 80 percent of all EBFs.

---

54. "World Health for All: To Be," Address by Dr. H. Mahler, Director-General of the WHO, in Presenting his Report for 1986 to the Fortieth World Health Assembly, 5 May 1987. WHO Library.

Extrabudgetary funds saved the WHO from the need to rely solely on assessed contributions which, given the zero growth and arrears, helped the WHO avoid an absolute financial disarray. EBFs also intensified the WHO's resource dependence on rich countries and weakened its procedural dependence on poor countries. Extrabudgetary funds, which are granted unilaterally, allowed a small number of rich countries—the United States, Japan, and a number of Western European countries—to bypass the World Health Assembly where mandatory budgets and organizational priorities are decided (Godlee 1995, Vaughan et al. 1996). Godlee of the *British Medical Journal* cites a spokesman for a European aid organization, who said: "We invest in these programmes because we have control over what we invest in. If we don't like what happens we can vote with our check book" (Godlee 1995). Ambassador Kirkpatrick, who found a selective approach to U.S. contributions more effective than the Kassebaum initiative, made a similar argument already in the 1980s. Speaking before Congress, Kirkpatrick supported the practice "of earmarking our funds to specific agencies and for specific projects," which would allow the United States to "reward the specialized agencies which do work of which we approve and discontinue or reduce our funding of agencies which engage in practices we do not endorse."[55] Godlee concluded that "the shift to extrabudgetary funding restore[d] to donor countries much of the influence they lost during the 1970s" (Godlee 1995).

Bypassing the assembly and relying solely on donors' preferences had substantive implications for the WHO (Frenk et al. 1997, Yamey 2002b). There were concerns that EBFs would turn the WHO into a top-heavy bureaucracy, unfocused in its mission (NIC 2000). Others warned of a potential bias in the type of programs that would be prioritized, as donors tended to invest in short-term, technically driven programs and to judge them by short-term outputs, such as the number of immunizations given, rather than long-term outcomes, such as improved quality of life, which are more difficult to quantify (Godlee 1995). Indeed, the move from mandatory to voluntary contributions soon contributed to a new focus on disease-specific vertical programs (see chapters 6 and 7).

In short, over the course of the 1980s, the WHO financial situation had significantly worsened with fewer contributions of mandatory funds and with the funds that were available often provided voluntarily. Fewer funds had a negative impact on the ability of the WHO secretariat to function effectively. In addition, it changed the balance in the relations of the secretariat with rich and poor countries. The emerging financial needs made the WHO particularly dependent

---

55. "The U.S. Role in the United Nations," Hearings before the Subcommittee on Human Rights and International Organizations of the Committee on Foreign Affairs, House of Representatives, Ninety-eighth Congress, First Session, September 27 and October 3, 1983.

on the countries providing the funds. In turn, the shift from mandatory to voluntary contributions intensified this dependence by bypassing the capacity of poor countries to effect rich countries' decisions through votes on the budget and program in the World Health Assembly.

Authority Crisis

In addition to a severe financial crisis, the WHO also suffered from an authority crisis as the World Bank became involved in public health programs beginning in 1987 and advocated policies that directly competed with, and—given their neoliberal orientation—often contradicted, the WHO's own policies. In addition, in 1996 donor governments decided to establish the Joint United Nations Programme on HIV/AIDS (UNAIDS), which took the issue of AIDS away from the WHO and put it under the authority of an independent organization.

WORLD BANK'S LENDING FOR HEALTH

The World Bank's interest in health started during its "basic needs" phase, under President Robert McNamara (see chapter 3). In the mid-1970s, the Bank began to include components for health-related activities in its loans, which reflected "an attempt . . . to broaden lending in ways which directly attack[ed] problems of poverty."[56] The number of health–related projects supported by the Bank increased from four in 1969 to twenty-two in 1973 (Buse 1994). The World Bank, however, did not grant direct loans for health. A full policy review of lending for health in the World Bank, conducted in 1973, made the World Bank board conclude, "with full US support," that "investment in agriculture, water and sewerage, education, nutrition and population was a surer means of improving health than directly lending to the sector, but that health should be included as a component in other lending."[57]

The Carter administration, however, pushed for greater World Bank involvement. In 1977, "the Treasury Department requested that the World Bank reassess its effectiveness in health, and examine the possibilities for future lending either as an expanded component of other lending or a discrete and separate sector."[58] A White House review of international health policy reported that "the World Bank has responded positively to the US request."[59] In 1979, the World Bank created

---

56. "World Health Strategy," Preliminary Draft, Report of Working Group III: Multilateral Agencies, 14 July 1978, Staff Offices, Peter Bourne, Box 35. Carter President Library.

57. Ibid.

58. Ibid.

59. White House Review of International Health Policy, Working Group III: Multilateral Health Organizations, Prospectus, 15 May 1978. Carter Presidential Library.

the Population, Health and Nutrition Department and allowed, for the first time, stand-alone health loans. Between 1981 and 1990, annual loan disbursements for health (excluding population and nutrition) rose from about $33 million to $263 million (Lee et al. 1996). In 1990 the World Bank sharply increased the amount of loans to an amount surpassing the entire WHO budget. In 1996, the World Bank again sharply increased the amount of loans, while the WHO budget remained almost the same (Buse and Gwin 1998, Yamey 2002d).[60]

Following the general shift at the World Bank from "investment lending" to "policy lending," the World Bank's funds devoted to health were not aimed at financing infrastructure but focused instead on structural reform components considered crucial for the performance of the health sector. The World Bank was now providing loans not for building hospitals and clinics or for financing equipment but for "chang[ing] the incentive framework that would allow these . . . new investments to be fully effective" by way of financial incentives, insurance schemes, regulations and so on.[61]

The World Bank's policy recommendations were informed by the neoliberal paradigm, which assigned to the private market the ability to best allocate and use resources, also in the field of public health (Armada, Muntaner, and Navarro 2001). The World Bank's position on health policies was formulated in three seminal publications: *Financing Health Services in Developing Countries: An Agenda for Reform* (Akin, Birdsall, and Ferranti 1987); *Strengthening Health Services in Developing Countries through the Private Sector* (Griffin 1989); and *World Development Report: Investing in Health* (World Bank 1993), which was the first *World Development Report* (WDR) devoted entirely to health.

The three reports considered the major problems with international health care systems to be the misallocation of funds to less cost-effective interventions, inefficient use of funds, inequity in access to basic health care, and the explosion of healthcare costs outpacing the growth of income (Abbasi 1999). These reports then called for a number of policies that would transform the provision and financing of health care in low- and middle-income countries. Some of the bank's recommendations were compatible with the primary health care approach, such as shifting the focus of government investment away from tertiary health care toward public health (Abbasi 1999). The most central recommendations, however, contradicted existing WHO recommendations. First, the World Bank maintained that public health systems were often wasteful, inefficient, and ineffective, and it

---

60. The increased spending on health in the 1990s was part of a broader attempt to mitigate the social costs of the World Bank's structural adjustment programs, in response to critics who called attention to the frequently negative consequences of these programs (Einhorn 2001, Parker 2002).

61. Interview by the author with Cristian Baeza, Lead Health Policy Specialist in the Latin America and the Caribbean Region of the World Bank, 28 May 2009.

argued in favor of reducing public funds for health services delivery. As part of the World Bank's structural adjustment programs, many lower-income countries were therefore encouraged to reduce public expenditure on health throughout the 1980s and 1990s (Lee and Dodgson 2000, Brown, Cueto, and Fee 2006). Second, World Bank reports announced that the "faith that health care should be totally paid for and administered by governments needs to be vigorously challenged" and recommended the partial "cost-recovery" of public health services by charging user-fees (de Ferranti 1985, Akin, Birdsall, and de Ferranti 1987; see also Gilson, Russell, and Buse 1995). Third, the World Bank insisted on an increased reliance on the market to finance and deliver health care. In *Financing Health Services in Developing Countries,* the authors suggested that some privatization of health care in developing countries held out the promise of increasing both efficiency (i.e., greater improvement in health indicators at lower cost) and equity (i.e., greater health gains for the poor) (Akin, Birdsall, and Ferranti 1987, Birdsall and James 1993); *Strengthening Health Services in Developing Countries through the Private Sector* (Griffin 1989) called for a mixture of private and public health services; and the *World Development Report* (World Bank 1993) recommended the introduction of private or social insurance schemes to foster competition in the delivery of health services (Ugalde and Jackson 1995, Abbasi 1999).

In addition to policy recommendations, an equally consequential contribution of the World Bank to the transformation in global health perspectives was the development of a new way for calculating health priorities. The *World Development Report* (World Bank 1993) introduced the unit of Disability-Adjusted Life Year (DALY) for measuring both the global burden of disease and the effectiveness of health interventions (Lerer and Matzopoulos 2001, Yamey 2002b). The innovation of DALY was in measuring the burden of a disease not only by number of years lost due to premature death but also number of years of productive life lost to disability, and in that way directly linking diseases to the issue of economic productivity (Specter 2005: 66). The WDR ranked existing health interventions by calculating the cost required for every "DALY saved." Using DALYs, the WDR concluded that the most cost-effective health services included promotion of breast-feeding, immunizations, salt iodization (to prevent iodine deficiency) and vitamin A supplementation, anthelmintics (drugs that expel parasitic worms), smoking prevention, use of condoms, and cataract removal. The least cost-effective interventions included surgical and medical treatment of chronic diseases and cancers.

Using DALYs, the World Bank inaugurated cost-effectiveness as the new paradigm to guide global health programs in poor countries, which replaced its previous focus on strengthening health systems (Buse 1994, Yamey 2002b). A cost-effectiveness approach to health, which is compatible with the neoliberal focus on economic reductionism and population-level outcomes, explicitly challenged the WHO's emphasis during the 1970s and early 1980s on equity, where priority in resource allocation was to be afforded to those most in need. The WHO was always mindful of costs, and the secretariat objected, as previously described, to the purchase of expensive medical interventions that poor countries could not afford. But the World Bank introduced economic reasoning that marginalized all other considerations, including equity. Some health interventions needed by the poor, such as immunizations, were found to be cost-effective, but this was a matter of chance, not of methodological design: while an equitable approach to resource allocation would have attached weight to the illnesses of more disadvantaged people, DALY calculations considered only age, sex, disability status, and time period and did not take into account individuals' socioeconomic circumstances (Segall 2003, Yamey 2002b).

The WHO's contribution to the *World Development Report: Investing in Health* reflected the marginalization of the organization with the World Bank's growing interest in public health, even though the WHO secretariat was actively involved throughout the process. The report was the long-term outcome of a meeting between Mahler and McNamara (Kickbusch 2000) and dozens of WHO staff were involved in the background work for the report. At the same time, it was "unmistakably a World Bank product" (Lancet 1993) while the WHO secretariat's role as technical adviser prevented it from criticizing the report's conclusions (Godlee 1994b). The WHO's cooperation possibly helped the World Bank to gain status as the new, and unchallenged, authority on health (Buse and Gwin 1998, Muraskin 1998: 140). More significant was the enormous fiscal and policy leverage that the World Bank exercised over lending governments, which the WHO lacked (Simms 2007). The WHO was "the gentlemen's club for the health people": it could only act through member states, advising their governments on technical matters; in contrast, the World Bank could impose its preferences on governments (cited in Abbasi 1999). In addition, the WHO's access point was through health ministries, while the World Bank had influence on finance ministries, which have greater influence over governmental policies than health ministries do (Abbasi 1999). Consequently, countries obliged. Following World Bank recommendations, "there has been [in the health sector in many countries] liberalization, increased use of non-government sources of finance and greater emphasis upon market mechanisms and incentives to help to structure health sector operations" (WHO 1993b). The *Lancet* editorial announced that "*Investing for Health* marks a shift in leadership on international health from the World Health Organization to the World Bank" (Lancet 1993) and a study by the U.S. Institute of Medicine claimed that the most significant change in the global health arena had been the growth in both financial and intellectual influence of the World Bank (cited in NIC 2000).

By the late 1990s, then, the World Bank established itself as a dominant authority in the global health field. The threat to the WHO was twofold: not only did an organization with much greater resources and influence now develop its own policies on health, but these policies reflected a rigid application of neoliberal economic theories and were in conflict with the WHO's policies of the 1970s and 1980s.

LOSING LEADERSHIP ON AIDS: FROM GPA TO UNAIDS

While World Bank policies challenged the authority of the WHO, the World Bank did not explicitly try to undermine it. In another case, donor countries publicly embarrassed the WHO by deciding to close an existing WHO program on AIDS and establish a joint UN program independent of the WHO.

The WHO, like the rest of the world, was very slow to recognize the catastrophic consequences of AIDS in Africa and elsewhere (Slutkin 2000). In the mid-1980s, the WHO staff still regarded AIDS as an ailment of the promiscuous few (Gellman 2000a). It was not until 1985, four years after the first recognition of the disease, that the WHO became actively involved (Booth 1995: 144). Two men were responsible for the beginning of the WHO's more serious engagement with AIDS: Fakhry Assad, head of the Division for Communicable Diseases, and Jonathan Mann, who was at the Harvard School of Public Health and later became known for being "a bold visionary, idealist, and fighter for human rights and equity" (Slutkin 2000: S24). In a 1985 meeting organized by Assad, Mann convinced Mahler that AIDS was a problem that would seriously affect the developing world and that it was time for the WHO to respond to it (Slutkin 2000, Gellman 2000a).

In July 1986, the WHO formally established the Control Program on AIDS under Assad's division. In February 1987, the Control Program was renamed the Special Program on AIDS (SPA) and was made independent. Mann was appointed the SPA's first director. In January 1988, SPA became GPA, or the Global Programme on AIDS. From 1987 to 1990, GPA quickly grew into the largest single program at the WHO. The staff grew from three to more than two hundred at headquarters alone, and the budget grew from $30 million to $82 million; 91 percent of the funding came from voluntary contributions of donor countries' bilateral assistance agencies (Parker 2000, Booth 1995: 198–199).

For a short time, the AIDS program put WHO "on the map" again (Gibbons 1990). When in October 1987, the UN General Assembly received a special briefing on AIDS—debating on a disease for the first time in its history—it designated WHO as the "lead agency" in the global response to AIDS (UNAIDS 2008: 15) and confirmed WHO's "essential global directing and coordinating role" (cited in Mann and Kay 1991).

Under Mann's directorship, the GPA held a then-unconventional rights-based approach, rather than a classic public health quarantine approach (Tarantola et al. 2006). The GPA opposed policies such as bans on immigration and on employment of people with AIDS, or on mandatory HIV tests for foreigners. Under Mann, the program emphasized the language of empowerment and participation of nongovernmental organizations and networks of people living with HIV, and the GPA engaged with sex workers, men who have sex with men, and drug users (Tarantola et al. 1997, Poku 2002, UNAIDS 2008).

In spite of these novel developments, the GPA under Mann still developed a vertical orientation: the GPA was centrally organized, adopted a top-down style of intervention, and focused on technical support (Booth 1995: 196). Concretely, the GPA adopted a series of short- and medium-term policy "packages," which were developed in Geneva and exported to Africa, Asia, and Latin America (UNAIDS 2008: 18). By the end of Mann's tenure, in 1990, "the AIDS program . . . established itself in miniature in the governments of more than one hundred countries" (Booth 1995: 143). The short-term plans emphasized public education and information on how HIV is, and is not, transmitted, and encouraged persons to avoid unprotected sex. The programs also emphasized HIV surveillance to monitor trends and estimate effectiveness at the national level. Other elements included blood screening and guidance on care and counseling (Slutkin 2000, UNAIDS 2008). Critics claimed that such a standardized, one-size-fits-all approach did not meet the need for culturally sensitive plans and programs, and African countries, in particular, found it culturally inappropriate.[62] In 1992, GPA started to work with a number of countries in preparing their second medium-term plans, which were more country specific (UNAIDS 2008: 18). By then, however, Mann had already resigned from the WHO.

Given its unprecedented growth, the GPA had come to be seen by other WHO staff as competing with the WHO's established hierarchy for funding, authority, and influence, and with Mahler's retirement, power struggles between the GPA and the WHO leadership became intolerable (Gibbons 1990, Parker 2000: 42, Gellman 2000a). The new director-general, Hiroshi Nakajima, was displeased with Mann's privileged status and unorthodox style. In addition, Nakajima did not share the position that favored AIDS over other diseases, such as malaria, which, at the time, had killed many more people than AIDS. He also seemed reluctant to draw attention to a problem that few nations wished to acknowledge (Gellman 2000a). Consequently, Nakajima set out to "normalize" the program's

---

62. Interview by the author with Peter Piot, Executive-Director of UNAIDS, Geneva, Switzerland, 20 May 2008.

status, by cutting resources and subjecting it to layers of unsympathetic management. Mann was excluded from meetings, was blocked from spending his program's budget, and his travel requests were denied (Gellman 2000a). In March 1990, Mann and many of his staff resigned in protest (Booth 1995: 201).

Following Mann's resignation, Nakajima selected Dr. Michael Merson, previously head of the WHO's Diarrheal Disease Programme, to serve as director of GPA and charged him with the task of bringing the program into conformity with standard WHO procedures (Parker 2000: 42). Merson was, by all accounts, a very different person from Mann: he was pragmatic and was thought of not as an innovator but as a manager (Gibbons 1990). A UNAIDS official reflected on the transition from Mann to Merson:

> [As in any organization,] first you have an entrepreneur. But Jonathan [Mann] was unable to deliver the goods. And here you have Mike [Merson], a systematic manager. Not charismatic. Absolutely not . . . he was seen as someone to put order and bring the troops in the WHO. Order. And that was part of it. In hindsight, 20 years later, it was necessary to have a Merson type there. If Jonathan continued, it would have been a mess.[63]

With Mann's resignation, a fundamental shift began to take place, with the perceived "activist excesses" of the earlier institutional response to the epidemic gradually being replaced by an orderly, professional, and coordinated response—aimed less at stimulating action from the top down than at "coordinating" efforts and providing support for the initiatives taking place nationally (Gibbons 1990, Parker 2000). The GPA under Merson faced close involvement and scrutiny by donors. While aid from official development assistance agencies steadily increased through 1990, in 1991 it fell for the first time from its peak of $255.5 million to $236.8 million (Booth 1995: 212). The two-year budget for 1992–1993 (nearly $190.5 million) reflected a 15 percent decrease in real terms. The budget for 1994–1995 was less than $150 million (GAO 1998). Donors also began to demand the identification of priorities, the development of evaluation indicators to measure the GPA's achievement, and financial accountability (UN Chronicle 1994, Booth 1995: 215–219, Slutkin 2000). Under the donors' gaze, AIDS was now considered, first and foremost, a problem of management (Booth 1995: 204).

Under Merson, the WHO effort was focused more on the medical and public health aspects of the disease and less on the social, economic, or developmental

---

63. Interview by the author. UNAIDS, Geneva, Switzerland.

issues affecting the spread of HIV/AIDS, leading to critics' accusations that WHO's technical base was too narrow for effectively dealing with AIDS prevention and control (Godlee 1994b, GAO 1998, UNAIDS 2008: 18). When other UN specialized agencies "discovered" AIDS—including donors' willingness to spend money to fight the disease—they used the medical focus of the WHO to challenge its competence, and a turf war ensued (Gellman 2000a). The United Nations Development Program (UNDP), the United Nations Children's Fund (UNICEF), the World Bank, and others complained that AIDS was hamstrung by its place within the WHO and that the GPA was unable to work effectively with other UN agencies (Poku 2002). These interagency rivalries raised a genuine concern regarding the quality of international AIDS programs. An external review of GPA's work criticized the "inefficiency of coordination between different UN agencies," noting that, at the country level, "duplication of effort and territorial rivalries threaten to weaken the global response to AIDS" (cited in UNAIDS 2008: 20). In addition, donors wanted more control over their funding and some hoped that a new program could be created that was cheaper, more flexible, more rooted at country level, and more accountable to donors (UNAIDS 2008: 24). Susan Holck, who joined GPA when Merson took over as its director, reflected: "The push for [an independent AIDS agency] certainly did not come from the UN agencies. The push came from the donors, who were fed up with having to individually respond to requests for funding from each of these different agencies, fed up with the lack of coordination, and fed up with WHO's inability to really be operational at country level" (cited in UNAIDS 2008: 23).

While most of the relevant agencies did not want a new international body that would coordinate and potentially control their activities, they had little choice as donors threatened that if the agencies did not work through an independent agency, they would stop funding multilateral AIDS programs and start funding bilateral programs instead (UNAIDS 2008). In 1995, the Joint United Nations Programme on HIV/AIDS was created by the UN General Assembly and designated as the key site for establishing a global response to the epidemic. It became fully operational in January 1996. The six original cosponsors were the WHO, UNICEF, UNDP, the United Nations Population Fund, the United Nations Educational, Scientific and Cultural Organization, and the World Bank. Later, four other agencies joined: the Office of the United Nations High Commissioner for Refugees, the World Food Programme, the United Nations Office on Drugs and Crime, and the International Labor Organization. The cosponsoring agencies wanted the power to select board members, but the board was eventually made of states: five each from Africa and Asia, two from Eastern Europe, three from Latin America and the Caribbean, and seven from Western Europe and other states. Five NGOs and the cosponsoring agencies participate as non-voting members (UNAIDS 2008: 34).

In the negotiations preceding the establishment of the independent AIDS agency, UNICEF, UNDP, and the World Bank successfully rejected the suggestion that the new program would be a funding agency (UNAIDS 2008: 22). In its first year, UNAIDS was given a budget that was 15 percent lower than GPA had had in its last year.[64] It also had significantly reduced staff: GPA's roughly 275 professional employees were cut to less than half that number (Poku 2002). With a small annual budget that restricted its role to one of a coordinator of action rather than an implementing agency, UNAIDS could only offer the promise of "a thin layer at the top which can take innovative steps to reach the grassroots" (Awuonda 1995, Piot 2000: 2177). The UNAIDS secretariat was expected to advocate political and financial support for HIV/AIDS activities, coordinate the work of the various agencies in each country and bring their diverse activities under a single strategic plan, provide technical support and information to facilitate development and implementation of national HIV/AIDS strategies, and develop a framework for measuring the objectives and performance of HIV/AIDS activities (GAO 1998: 3–4). UNAIDS also worked to keep the epidemic at the forefront of international political attention through, for example, the collection and compilation of data on HIV prevalence, and by consistently monitoring and publicizing the status of the global response to the crisis (Piot 2000: 2177). The complexity of this mandate—getting six UN agencies whose priorities range from UNICEF's concern for the welfare of children to the World Bank's preoccupation with development issues to work in concert—was described by Jonathan Mann as comparable to "walking six cats on a leash" (cited in Poku 2002: 288). Nonetheless, public health experts concurred that UNAIDS was an effective advocate, one that helped promote a strong global response to HIV/AIDS and eventually increased spending for the disease (Das and Samarasekera 2008, Poku 2002).

The establishment of UNAIDS threatened the WHO's authority in a different way than the World Bank's. The policies the World Bank recommended often contradicted the WHO's principles, which was not the case with UNAIDS. Also, the World Bank had greater resources than the WHO while UNAIDS remained a small organization. However, the World Bank could justify its input by referring to its economic expertise as complementing the WHO's public health expertise. There was no similar reason to justify moving away the authority over AIDS from

---

64. In addition, when UNAIDS was established, its cosponsoring agencies cut back sharply on the resources and personnel they devoted to AIDS. World Bank loans dropped from $50 million to less than $10 million, WHO spending dropped from $130 million to $20 million, and UNICEF from $45 million to $10 million (Gellman 2000a, GAO 1998).

the WHO and the decision to establish an independent AIDS organization was widely perceived as "clear evidence of the . . . lack of confidence in WHO's abilities to tackle the broader health issues" (Godlee 1994b).

Leadership Crisis

During the transition from the logic of a New International Economic Order to neoliberalism, in which the WHO saw its funds shrink and authority undermined, the WHO was under leadership that was ill-suited to respond effectively to the new environment. Director-General Mahler, who was highly respected by both developing and developed countries for his response to the New International Economic Order, was not willing, or capable, to change course when the political environment around him no longer fit with the programs and policies he had fought hard to implement. His overt rage at member states not paying their dues, quoted above, suggests his disinterest of transforming the organization in a way that would fit better with the new demands. In the end of his third term, in 1988, Mahler decided to retire, partly in response to the disintegration of his ideas and programs.

The World Health Assembly elected as director-general Dr. Hiroshi Nakajima, a Japanese researcher, who had been director of the WHO Western Pacific Regional Office in Manila. Nakajima's candidacy was supported by developing countries, but not by the United States and a number of European and Latin American countries, which preferred another candidate, Dr. Guerra de Macedo (Chetley 1988, Brown, Cueto, and Fee 2006). This original conflict was followed by continuous tension between the director-general and many donor countries. During Nakajima's tenure, from 1988 until 1998, WHO's reputation as "the most efficient and capably managed of the Agencies"[65] was severely damaged. The accusations made against Nakajima were often personal. Donors, but also WHO staff, found him too reserved and a poor communicator (Godlee 1994a). Nakajima himself complained, "Many countries are not in favor of me, for political or personal reasons. Most criticism was of my management style. Maybe mine is too Asian for some people, and not European or American enough" (cited in Walgate 1997). But there were also serious concerns regarding poor management, combined with an autocratic style (Brown, Cueto, and Fee 2006). A report prepared by a Danish overseas development organization, Danida, suggested that the WHO's budget in individual countries was used for "ad hoc financing

---

65. Aide Memoire on the WHO, Meeting of UN Ad Hoc Committee on UN Finances at Geneva on 20–21 April 1966, FO 371/189916. UK National Archives.

of fellowships, study tours, workshops, local cost subsidies and miscellaneous supplies and equipment" rather than being allocated according to a strategic plan (cited in Godlee 1994a). Worse, there were charges of mismanagement and improper staffing, including complaints that three-quarters of the budget went on salaries and overheads, that under Nakajima the number of directors at the WHO had almost doubled, and that new directors were named at Nakajima's discretion without approval by the organization's senior selection committee (Lerer and Matzopoulos 2001: 421, Brown, Cueto, and Fee 2006).

When Nakajima's first five-year term ended, Western governments took the unprecedented step of asking Japan to withdraw his candidacy for reelection. His renomination by the Executive Board led to allegations that Japan had exerted undue pressure on developing countries, including threats to withdraw trade and aid agreements, if they did not vote for Nakajima. Opponents also alleged that the WHO's funds had been misused to influence the election (Godlee 1994a). An external audit to examine the allegations found no evidence of corruption, but criticized the WHO for shortcomings in management and found that the number of contracts to members of the Executive Board had doubled in the six months leading up to the election (Godlee 1994a). In 1994, Sweden, normally a supporter and second in its donations only to the United States, announced it was halving its grant in protest at what it saw as a lack of coherence and rationale in the organization and because management reforms Sweden had called for had not taken place (*The Guardian* 1994, Pilkington 1995). Six months later, in May 1995, Britain's National Audit Office announced that, after sixteen years as the WHO's external auditor, it no longer wished to continue. The clash was prompted by a report on the WHO's operations in Africa, which concluded that the bookkeeping was so sloppy there was a risk of "fraudulent transactions remaining undetected over long periods" (Pilkington 1995).

Rich countries' mistrust in Nakajima exacerbated the WHO's vulnerability and contributed to its financial crisis, as donor countries were pushed in the direction of earmarked funding, and to its authority crisis, with the successful usurpation of the international health agenda by other agencies (Walgate 1997). The leadership crisis also prevented a suitable response by the WHO to those difficulties.

Discussion

The Reagan administration strongly opposed programs drawing on the call for a New International Economic Order and showed little respect for UN agencies. In such a hostile environment, many of the WHO initiatives of the 1970s and early 1980s were abandoned, either formally or informally. The strategy developed to achieve Health for All, primary health care, was questioned early on (see chapter 3). While Health for All survived as the organization's objective, the passion died. By 1993, a WHO working group had found that

> the Organization and Member States had perhaps not been entirely successful in defining and implementing the goals and programmes set, and . . . the Organization now faced the dilemma of whether to concentrate greater resources on achieving those targets or to revise them.[66]

In the discussion that followed this verdict by the working group, Executive Board members declared Health for All to be a "quasi-philosophical ideal, the dignity of which suffered from the imposition of a target date," while endorsing the view that "health for all without a target date should remain WHO's mission." The chairman of the board concluded that there was "a consensus that the present situation was untenable and that some rethinking of the goal of health for all by the year 2000 was necessary."[67]

The rise of neoliberalism did not only threaten NIEO-related programs. Reduced funds and earmarked contributions also undercut the WHO's autonomy and its ability to maintain a coherent agenda. The increased intervention of the World Bank in national health policies and the creation of UNAIDS indicated a beginning of a structural transformation in which the WHO could no longer assume it was the agency responsible for global health issues. The World Bank involvement was doubly provocative, as the bank supported neoliberal policies that often contradicted the WHO position.

In the mid-1990s, analyses in leading medical journals described in alarming terms the dire condition of the WHO. Typical titles included "What Role for WHO in the 1990s?" (Lee and Walt 1992), "WHO in Crisis" (Godlee 1994a), and "WHO in Retreat" (Godlee 1994b). Godlee (1994b) of the *British Medical Journal* saw "signs that, instead of leading the way on health policy, WHO is becoming simply the agency that advises other agencies . . . on medical matters." An editorial at the *Lancet* warned in its title, "Where There Is no Vision, the People Perish" (Lancet 1997). According to Lerer and Matzopoulos (2001: 421), "The WHO was increasingly thought of as fairly unimportant by other groups competing for limited health funding, sometimes even in projects that the WHO had helped establish. . . . After ten years of poor performance, the WHO was no longer setting the international public health agenda" (Lerer and Matzopoulos 2001: 421). Others similarly concluded that "WHO has become a follower rather

---

66. WHO Document, January 1993, EB91/SR/16. WHO Library.
67. WHO Document, January 1993, EB91/SR/17. WHO Library.

than a leader while other agencies have promoted their respective agendas" (Gillies, von Schoen-Angerer, and 't Hoen 2006).

In considering the future of the WHO just before the election of a successor to Nakajima in 1997, a more hopeful piece in the *Lancet,* titled "A Vital Opportunity for Global Health: Supporting the World Health Organization at a Critical Juncture," agreed that "Despite its mandate and achievements, WHO has not been able to respond as effectively as necessary to the world's new complexities." However, the editorial also thought that "the need to improve that response . . . has created a broad constituency for a changed and strengthened WHO" (Al-Mazrou and Bloom 1997). The complexities were organizational: a new director-general had to deal with the financial and the authority crises, but they were also substantive. Vincent Navarro (2009) describes the "new policy environment" that was created by the neoliberal reforms in the health sector.

> The need to reduce public responsibility for the health of populations; the need to increase choice and markets; the need to transform national health services into insurance-based health care systems; the need to privatize medical care; a discourse in which patients are referred to as clients and planning is replaced by markets; individuals' personal responsibility for health improvements; an understanding of health promotion as behavioral change; and the need for individuals to increase their personal responsibility by adding social capital to their endowment.

The following two chapters describe how the WHO under the leadership of Dr. Gro Harlem Brundtland, who was elected to succeed Nakajima, strategically adapted to this new policy environment.

HEALTH IN ECONOMIC TERMS

Once again, the world turns its attention to . . . the World Health Assembly. You are the health leaders of the world, and your World Health Organization is the lead agency in health. Ours are the crucial issues of the time: health, survival, development, equity, and opportunity. Global public opinion is starting to realize where health belongs: at the core of every child's opportunity to reach his or her full potential; at the core of every parent's opportunity to work, to care and to innovate. It is at the core of every community's opportunity to secure sustainable economic development for its citizens; and at the core of our efforts to combat poverty, and foster development for all.

"Challenges and Opportunities for the Health Leaders of Today," Address by Gro Harlem Brundtland, director-general of the WHO to the Fifty-Third World Health Assembly, 15 May 2000

When Dr. Gro Harlem Brundtland was elected director-general, in 1998, the political environment of the WHO was markedly different from the environment that had confronted Mahler when he was elected back in 1974: in the new balance of influence, rich countries were now able to exploit the WHO's dependence on their resources to a much greater extent than poor countries could utilize the organization's dependence on their votes. This was largely due to the WHO's severe financial crisis, itself the outcome of rich countries' institutional manipulation. As described in chapter 5, rich countries enhanced the WHO's vulnerability and its dependence on their resources by imposing limits on mandatory contributions on the one hand and, on the other hand, increasing voluntary contributions that allowed the WHO to survive financially but under conditions determined by the donors. Rich countries' ability to achieve these institutional victories was partly due to the Geneva Group, which coordinated their positions and strategies. The WHO's resource dependence also increased with the competition for limited funds with new organizations that had overlapping mandates, such as UNAIDS. Some of the same institutional transformations also led to the decline in poor countries' procedural leverage over the organization. Developing countries could still influence the WHO's regular budgetary funds in the assembly, but by the 2000s these funds accounted for only 30 percent of the total budget (Lee 2009, WHO 2009). Moreover, following the debt crisis and the demise of the NIEO, the coalition of developing countries was much less unified and, importantly, the great structural dependence of poor countries on rich countries with the rise of a global economy made developing countries reluctant to vote against the position of rich countries or multinational companies.[1]

In short, the balance between procedural dependence on developing countries and resource dependence on rich countries was now tilted in favor of rich countries, which were using it to press for new policies and reforms, compatible with neoliberal rather than NIEO principles. Initially unable to respond to the new expectations, the WHO transformed from a leading organization to a potentially redundant one. But in the late 1990s, under the leadership of Brundtland, the WHO underwent programmatic and organizational changes in a conscious attempt to pacify the exogenous forces. Similar to the WHO secretariat's response to the call for a New International Economic Order in the 1970s, the WHO leadership of the late 1990s strategically adapted to the neoliberal logic by fitting its programs to reinterpreted demands, so to protect the WHO's principles and, this time, also to increase the organization's legitimacy, regain its authority, and let it benefit from old and new sources of funds.

The central component of the WHO leadership's strategic adaptation to the new environment was the replacement of a social logic, which dominated WHO's programs during the NIEO era, with economic logic as the foundation for the organization's decisions and policies. The economic replaced the

---

1. Import substitution industrialization, dominant in the 1970s, was based on the assumption that economic development could be achieved without the support of foreign capital, which allowed developing countries, in their call for a New International Economic Order, to challenge multinational companies. The neoliberal turn, which led to the opening up of developing countries' markets to international competition, made the support of multinational capital a principal condition for growth. First of all, developing countries now heavily relied on foreign direct investment (see Kentor and Boswell 2003, Beer and Boswell 2002, Amsden 2001, Amsden 2003, Frieden 2006). Second, the globalization of production also changed developing countries' relations with foreign capital. In the "new international division of labor," developing countries no longer merely served as the source of raw materials but became the preferred location of low-cost production (Fröbel, Heinrichs, and Kreye 1980). This global shift in the locus of manufacturing was combined with the fragmentation of production across a large number of sites, so that "production of a single good commonly [came to span] several countries" (Gereffi 1989). Global commodity chains did not allow production to be isolated within national boundaries, as exporting firms were enmeshed in subcontracting relationships with multinational corporations (Gereffi 1989). The need for foreign direct investment and the fragmented nature of global production meant that economic growth was no longer conditioned on the rise of domestic industrialists independent of foreign capital but, on the contrary, on the ability to integrate domestic industries into the global system, and accordingly, multinational corporations were no longer viewed as a threat but as a promise.

social in informing the WHO leadership's position in regard to two funda-mental questions. First, how could the WHO regain international interest in national health policies and programs? Following a neoliberal reasoning, WHO officials now justified investment in health by referring to the impor-tance of health for economic growth rather than as a fundamental part of a nation's social development. Second, which health programs should the WHO prioritize? In line with contemporary economic perceptions, the WHO staff now allowed cost-effective programs rather than considerations of equity to determine priorities.

Neoliberal reasoning made the transformed WHO policies and programs agreeable to donor countries. However, a strict reading of economic reduction-ism would have maintained the organization's financial and authority crises—because it was the very same neoliberal perceptions which informed the World Bank's call for reducing health budgets and for restricting the public provision and finance of health services. However, the WHO secretariat was able to use the same economic maxims, by contrast, to defend positions and promote programs that called for enhancing investment in health and that allowed for international intervention in the control of a number of diseases, including those of greatest impact on the poor.

Under Brundtland's leadership the WHO's central aim and one of its successes was to broaden the "development agenda" so that it would prioritize health is-sues rather than marginalize them. The first part of this chapter describes how the WHO secretariat was able to advance the seemingly indefensible position of "investment in health" by recruiting economists who provided evidence that im-provements in health were one of the most effective ways to bring about economic development and growth. The second part of the chapter describes the strategies used in selecting the WHO's flagship programs. Following World Bank prescrip-tions, the WHO leadership ranked priorities based on their cost-effectiveness. Such ranking led to two important divergences from the practices of the 1970s: cost-effective reasoning led to the reemergence of disease-specific interventions, which replaced the previous concern with health systems and other structural issues; and when selecting among competing interventions, cost-effectiveness calculations prioritized the cost of intervention over the need of the popula-tion in question. Methodologically, therefore, equity was no longer a dominant concern and the category of "those most in need" lost its relevance. Yet the WHO leadership was able to use the donors' concern with economic growth and cost-effectiveness to advance a competing value of the WHO, that of universal access. Thus the WHO leadership promoted the concept of "new universalism"—the delivery of high-quality essential care to all—as a viable alternative not only to primary health care but also to the neoliberal-informed market-oriented approach to health care delivery.

The WHO: Effective, Accountable, and Receptive to a Changing World

Already during Nakajima's tenure, delegates to the WHO discussed solutions to the organization's increasing financial constraints and its ongoing crisis of authority. In 1992, the Executive Board, "concerned with the need to respond to . . . profound [global political, economic, social and health] changes," appointed a working group to "undertake a review of the extent to which WHO could make a more effective contribution to global health work" (WHO 1993a; see also Godlee 1997, Brown, Cueto, and Fee 2006). The report that was prepared by the Working Group conceded that

> WHO's recent attempts to attract resources from other sectors into health and its broader ventures into the general field of development have not been fully successful. Moreover, other United Nations agencies or international bodies have increased their efforts to assume direction of specific health and environmental initiatives (WHO 1993a).[2]

The realization that the WHO was at a crossroads and that reforms were necessary came not only from the Working Group report, but also from external voices, ranging from the *British Medical Journal* (Godlee 1994a, 1994b) to the Rockefeller Foundation, which organized a series of meetings of health experts, in 1996 and 1997, to explore how international institutions concerned with health could do better (Frenk et al. 1997, Lancet 2002b). Two reports commissioned by the Swedish government also pushed for WHO reform (Godlee 1997).

When Nakajima announced, giving in to U.S. demands, that he would not seek a third five-year term, the Executive Board was under pressure to nominate a person who could lead such reform (Lerer and Matzopoulos 2001: 420–421). A *Lancet* editorial, for example, published an open letter with a set of ten questions to the candidates, including: "WHO used to have a reputation as being a preeminent technical organization in health. During the previous decade, its position has been eroded. What would you do to reestablish its credibility and

---

2. The working group's final report recommended that the WHO—if it were to maintain leadership of the health sector—must overhaul its fragmented management, diminish competition between regular and extrabudgetary initiatives, and above all, increase the emphasis within the WHO on global health issues and WHO's coordinating role in that domain (Stenson and Sterky 1994).

role in this area?" (Al-Mazrou and Bloom 1997). The forerunners for taking on this challenging task were: Nafis Sadik, the executive director of the United Nations Population Fund since 1987; Ebrahim Malick, the WHO's regional director for Africa since 1995 who had the backing of the nations of sub-Saharan Africa; George Alleyne, director of PAHO, the WHO regional office for the Americas; and Gro Harlem Brundtland, the former prime minister of Norway who was known as "an energetic campaigner on environmental and economic development issues" (Balter 1998).

Brundtland had a number of advantages over the other candidates. She was a doctor (albeit with little public health experience), she was a woman in an era where there were finally some pressures for having more women in leadership roles, and as Japan and others desired, she had no links with the United States (Godlee 1997, Balter 1998). Also, it was understood that the "WHO needs someone from the outside" (Godlee 1997) and Brundtland, while still having experience working for the UN, was an outsider. In Norway, she had first been minister for environmental affairs (1974–1979) and then prime minister (1981, 1986–1989, 1990–1996). She gained international prominence when she chaired the UN World Commission on Environment and Development ("The Brundtland Report"), which produced in 1987 a report, *Our Common Future*, that eventually led to the Earth Summit of 1992. The Brundtland Report developed the concept of "sustainable development," which championed the possibility of environmental protection in the context of economic growth (Rich 1994: 196–197). In addition to other qualities, then, her record promised that she would be able to position health in the larger context of development, as she had done with the environment (Brown, Cueto, and Fee 2006). Indeed, in an interview with *Science*, given before she was elected, Brundtland stressed the relation between health and development issues, noting that "not only does poverty breed ill health, but ill health breeds poverty. Investing in health increases productivity and economic output" (cited in Balter 1998). Members of the Executive Board could therefore expect an emphasis on such issues if she were to become the director-general. In January 1998, the Executive Board nominated Dr. Brundtland and in May that year, the World Health Assembly elected her to the post. At the Fifty-first World Health Assembly, as a director-general elect, Brundtland promised: "WHO can and must change. It must become more effective, more accountable, more transparent and more receptive to a changing world."[3]

In the five years in which Brundtland served as director-general—she chose not to serve a second term—she engaged in a "systematic attempt to return

---

3. WHO document, May 1998, A51/VR/6, p. 102. PAHO Library.

WHO to its leadership role" (Kickbusch 2000). Against unlikely odds, analysts agree that she achieved that goal. Brown, Cueto, and Fee (2006) concluded that "Brundtland succeeded in . . . reposition[ing] WHO as a credible and highly visible contributor to the rapidly changing field of global health," and Yamey (2002b) stated in the *British Medical Journal* that, with Brundtland, the "WHO made a comeback to the global political stage." Horton (2002) reported: "Corrupt, bureaucratic, inefficient, unresponsive, unaccountable, overly medical, and far too male. These are some of the more unkind accusations thrown at WHO during the past decade. Brundtland successfully restored WHO's international credibility. WHO has become an agency to be reckoned with." Given the difficulty of the task, how was Brundtland able to save the WHO?

In part, success was due to an internal reform intended to recover the WHO as a competent bureaucracy. According to a report by the U.S. National Intelligence Council, which summarized approvingly some of Brundtland's organizational changes, the reform included expanded internal oversight and transparency, closer scrutiny over programs and budgets, improved management accountability, and strengthened and potentially more responsive regional offices (NIC 2000). More than organizational reforms, however, the WHO's revival was the outcome of a complete makeover of its legitimating strategies and a corresponding transformation of its policies and programs.

"Anchoring Health on the Development Agenda"

Similarly to Mahler's support of the call for a new international order, Brundtland perceived neoliberalism, and the global economy it helped create, an opportunity rather than a threat. As she told the World Health Assembly:

> The landscape reflects our increasingly interdependent world. Yes, globalization frightens some people and causes uncertainty to many more. But it also presents us all with genuine opportunities. We live at an important moment in history. . . . It is our responsibility to shape events in line with our values—of equity and fairness. As health workers, we are increasingly well placed to make sure that greater economic integration brings benefits to those who need them.[4]

Brundtland was forthright and unsentimental in her conviction that the only way to revive the WHO's deteriorating finances, legitimacy, and authority was by

---

4. "Challenges and Opportunities for the Health Leaders of Today," Address by Dr. Gro Harlem Brundtland, the Director-General of the WHO to the Fifty-Third World Health Assembly, 15 May 2000. PAHO Library.

actively incorporating the organization into the new environment in which it was expected to function, and that, to do so successfully, the WHO had to broaden the range of its allies to include the relevant audiences and to develop a revised message that the new audiences would find appealing.

Traditionally, the WHO secretariat had regarded health ministers as its main audience. With a somewhat brutal frankness, Brundtland assessed that they were not a useful audience. Health ministers were already convinced of the importance of health so that the WHO did not need to readdress them and, given the subordinate position of health ministers in most executives, they were of little use in delivering the message that health was a paramount objective. Indeed, because of the organizational transformation of many governments under neoliberalism, by the late 1990s health ministers had even less influence over national budgets than they had had in the past (Cox 1986). Instead, Brundtland was convinced that the WHO leadership should communicate directly with policymakers who had influence over the distribution of budgets. As Brundtland wrote in an editorial in *Science,* not long before taking office, "Health ministers need little convincing, but WHO will remind presidents, prime ministers, finance ministers, and science ministers that they are health ministers themselves" (Brundtland 1998).

Drawing on her experience as the chair of the World Commission on Environment and Development, Brundtland was convinced that the only effective way to persuade finance ministers to care about health and earn their support was not to talk about health but to talk about finance. To satisfy its new audience, therefore, the WHO staff abandoned its position that health was an aspect of social development that should be pursued independently of economic concerns and, accepting the reduction of social development to economic development, adopted instead the premise that health was good for economic growth (Horton 2002).[5] As Brundtland put it in the *Science* editorial: "Our message will be that healthy people help build healthy economies" (Brundtland 1998). Speaking before the World Health Assembly in 1999, Brundtland stated that, "WHO needs to remind prime ministers and finance ministers that . . . investments in the health of the poor can enhance growth and reduce poverty" (Brundtland 1999b). In another early speech as director-general, Brundtland asserted before the Executive Board, "We . . . know that sound investments in health can be one of the most cost-effective ways of promoting development and progress. Improving health

---

5. Note that both NIEO and neoliberalism involved economic reductionism. While in the 1970s the WHO had responded by diverting attention from economic to social development, the WHO in the 1990s responded by reversing the causal link between economic development and health.

in poor countries leads to increased GDP per capita" (Brundtland 1999a). In the same speech she emphasized the importance of making such knowledge public and utilizing it for the sake of promoting the WHO agenda.

> I believe the international health community, including WHO, has undersold this fact. In a time . . . where nations are searching for ways to make ends meet, we have been sitting on a secret. We haven't fully seen that this is a powerful message we should take to the political decision-makers and to the private sector. . . . My own experience tells me that this strategy was instrumental in taking the environment from being a cause just for the already convinced, to becoming a real issue of political importance to major players. (Brundtland 1999a)

In short, Brundtland was formulating a message, relating health to development, which would be palatable to those with decision-making powers.

The objective for linking development and health was financial, an explicit attempt to resolve the WHO's financial crisis. Given the dire financial conditions of poor countries and recent cuts in public health services throughout the developing world, this focus had a reason beyond the WHO revival. Brundtland wanted to help "[increase] investments in the health of the poor," by convincing donor countries to channel their contributions to poor countries into health-related projects (Brundtland 1999b).

This was a difficult task as neoliberal economists conceived of the health sector as an "unproductive consumer of public budgets," while Brundtland wanted to argue that wise investment in health was "key to productivity itself" (quoted in Birmingham 1999). The promise of development could be a legitimate justification for such investment. Brundtland recognized that for the message to be effective, the reasoning, too, had to appeal to finance ministers. As she said in an interview: "Anchoring health on the development agenda . . . involves not just reaching the minds of people who have decision-making power in the broader fields of economics and politics, but also increasing the evidence base so that you have convincing arguments" (cited in Yamey 2002e). To make her arguments convincing, Brundtland wanted "to stress the importance of health in economic terms" (cited in Birmingham 1999). Here, as in other cases, Brundtland relied on her past experience:

> The environment moved on from being a cause for the marginal few to becoming a key issue once . . . the economic implications of environmental degradation were properly understood. The same approach now needs to be applied to analyze the role of sound health policies and interventions. (Brundtland 1999c)

To provide the economic evidence needed to claim that investment in health was good for development, in January 2000 Brundtland established the Commission on Macroeconomics and Health (CMH).

Investing in Health for Economic Development (CMH Report)

The setting up of the Commission on Macroeconomics and Health marked a watershed in the involvement of economists in health (Banerji 2002). It also marked their co-optation into the World Health Organization. The commission was chaired by the economist Jeffrey Sachs, then of Harvard University, described by the *New York Times* as "probably the most important economist in the world" (cited in Banerji 2002). At the time, Sachs was known for implementing economic "shock therapy"—the sudden release of price and currency controls, withdrawal of state subsidies, privatization of public-owned assets and immediate trade liberalization within a country—in developing and transitional countries such as Bolivia, Poland, and Russia (Waitzkin 2003). But Sachs was also advising the United Nations on various global issues, and a UN Commission he headed in 1999 had called for the creation of a fund for AIDS (Cannon 2005).[6] In addition to Sachs and other world-leading economists, the commission also included former ministers of finance and officers from the World Bank, the IMF, the WTO, the UNDP, and the Economic Commission on Africa, as well as public health leaders (Ashraf 2001, Brown, Cueto, and Fee 2006). Most of the CMH economists, including those from the poorer countries, had been educated in prestigious universities in the West, such as Harvard, MIT, Berkeley, Princeton, Oxford, and Cambridge. Many of them were involved in the World Bank's *Investing in Health* report (Banerji 2002, Waitzkin 2003). In short, Brundtland clearly decided to co-opt leading economists by giving them the task of presenting the WHO's position. By contrast, the commission did not include representatives of NGOs, trade unions, professional organizations in medicine and public health, organizations of indigenous or ethnic minorities, or activists in occupational and environmental health (Waitzkin 2003). The commission's activities were funded by contributions from the UK Department for International Development, the Grand Duchy of Luxembourg, the governments of Ireland, Norway, and Sweden, the Rockefeller Foundation, Ted Turner's United Nations Foundation, and—not

---

6. Sachs continued to be an influential figure at the international level following his work with the WHO. From 2002 to 2006, Sachs was Director of the UN Millennium Project and Special Advisor to UN Secretary-General Kofi Annan on the Millennium Development Goals, a set of internationally agreed goals to reduce extreme poverty, disease, and hunger by the year 2015.

normally an enthusiastic contributor for WHO initiatives—the Bill and Melinda Gates Foundation (Banerji 2002).

Brundtland made explicit the conclusions she expected the commission to reach. In an early CMH meeting, she announced: "Placing health at the heart of the development agenda. This is the purpose of the Commission" (Brundtland 2000c). In the same meeting, Brundtland explained the reason behind her turn to economists:

> Some people may think that addressing the health needs of poor people and poor communities is a task for technical experts and public health physicians. In part that is true. But one thing I have learnt over the years is that to reach the minds of those who hold sway over real financial and political power, we—and I speak now as a health professional—have to communicate in a language that these decision makers understand. Good health is intrinsically important in its own right. But we cannot ignore the fact that governments will take more notice when faced with robust evidence showing the true economic impact of avoidable illness. This information also has to be presented in such a way that it stands out amongst all the other information and choices that governments face every day. (Brundtland 2000c)

Brundtland continued: "I am convinced that the full economic cost of communicable diseases has been under-estimated," and then summarized her expectations for the commission report: "That poverty causes ill health is well known. But good health can fuel the engine of development. Healthy people add significant momentum to the forces of economic development and poverty reduction. This is the case we have to make" (Brundtland 2000c).

The commission issued its report, *Macroeconomics and Health: Investing in Health for Economic Development,* in December 2001 (CMH 2001). As instructed, the report presented evidence showing that improving the health of the poor was not only an outcome of economic development but also a means for achieving economic growth. According to the commission's analysis, good health contributed to economic development by lowering the fertility rate, improving educational performance, increasing labor productivity, and improving macroeconomic stability. The commission also established that for low- and middle-income countries, investing in health was one of the most effective means to achieve development. As Sachs maintained before the World Health Assembly:

> Accomplishing this investment in the life-saving technologies for your countries is the *sine qua non* of ending the poverty trap which afflicts so

many of the poorest countries in the world and is the *sine qua non* of the economic progress that you so ardently desire and deserve.[7]

The policy implications that followed were obvious: the way to achieve economic growth was a massive injection of financial resources into health services (Lancet 2002a). Indeed, one of the main proposals of the commission's report was "an expanded aid effort to the world's poorest countries" (CMH 2001: 9). At the same time, the authors of the report were able to assure rich countries that to generate enormous health benefits in the developing world would only require minimal resources. The report estimated that $25 billion per year—or only 1 cent out of every $10 of the gross national product in rich countries—was needed to control HIV/AIDS, malaria, and tuberculosis in poor countries (Banta 2002).

The Executive Board welcomed the CMH report and the central role it gave to health in the fight against poverty.[8] At the World Health Assembly, member states expressed similar support of the link made between health and development. France, for example, "congratulated WHO and the Commission on their . . . attempt to change the basic paradigm according to which health was a secondary effect of development."[9] Member states also supported the recommendation to increase aid. Finland was alone in criticizing the heavy reliance on economic thinking:

> Although it was important for macroeconomic decision-makers to understand health issues, WHO must ensure that the health and health policy implications of macroeconomic and trade policies continued to be assessed and that health priorities were not compromised by other interests. . . . The Organization's health policy directions should come from its governing bodies. Discussions on essential policy issues must take place in the governing bodies before positions were promoted outside the Organization.[10]

Other member states accepted the reliance on economists, whose opinion was considered legitimate among international financial institutions and rich countries, because it was an effective way to bring attention to health. Sachs himself referred to his economic expertise as a unique source of legitimacy when presenting the report to the World Health Assembly: "I am asking you to take on . . . the challenge of ending absolute poverty in our generation. Why do I think it can be done? Because, if I have any talent at all to justify my being here, I have my

---

7. WHO Document, 2002, A55/VR/5, p. 109. PAHO Library.
8. WHO Document, 2002, WHA55/A/SR/5, pp. 17–18. PAHO library.
9. Ibid.
10. Ibid.

doubts, but if I do, it is because I can add up the dollars, because I am trained to put a price tag on what it would cost to meet this challenge."[11] Unlike most WHO reports, the commission report received adequate media attention, partly thanks to Sachs himself who was "a campaigner and an advocate in addition to being a macroeconomist."[12]

With the CMH report, the WHO secretariat relied on the legitimacy of expert economists to grant the field of public health what was then the only justification for intervention and "investment" (rather than aid) in the developing world: the possibility of economic growth. By relying on such justification, the WHO secretariat reversed two principles central to its agenda during the 1970s (see chapter 3). First, in justifying investment in health by referring to its potential contribution to economic growth, the WHO accepted a perception of development that reduced it to its economic dimension and no longer defended the notion of social development that allowed concern with individuals' quality of life independently of the economic realm.[13] Second, the WHO now focused on the question of overall growth at the national level at the expense of its previous prioritization of equitable distribution within a country (Kickbusch 2002, Banta 2002).

However, the CMH report was not a passive capitulation to the economic reasoning of exogenous forces, but rather a strategic modification of that very reasoning. The World Bank emphasized the causal link between poverty and disease to prioritize economic development and to downplay the need for direct attention to the health sector. The CMH report emphasized instead the opposite vector, which went from disease to poverty, postulating that improved health leads to economic development.[14] By insisting that improvement in health was necessary for achieving the goal of economic growth, the report turned the World Bank's reasoning on its head. Instead of agreeing with the World Bank's call for budget cuts in the public health sector, the WHO secretariat used the goal of economic growth, on the contrary, to call for greater investment in public health.

Through this strategic compliance—manipulating the link between economy and health to gain economists' attention to health matters—the WHO secretariat was able to incorporate the organization into the neoliberal environment.

---

11. WHO Document, 2002, A55/VR/5, p. 109. PAHO Library.
12. Interview by the author with Dr. Steven Phillips, Medical Director, Global Issues and Projects, Exxon Mobil Corporation, Washington, DC, 12 January 2009.
13. In the UN, the notion of social development has been maintained in the Human Development Report, which has been published by the UNDP since 1990. Its first publication stated, "Even in the absence of satisfactory economic growth ... countries can achieve significant improvements in human development through well-structured public expenditures" (UNDP 1990: 3); see also Parker 2000: 45.
14. Interview by the author with Dr. Steven Phillips, Medical Director, Global Issues and Projects, Exxon Mobil Corporation, Washington, DC, 11 January 2009.

In other international settings as well, the economic reasoning used in the CMH report was utilized to transform the position of international organizations and of rich donors regarding the primacy of health matters. The Millennium Development Goals, which provided UN member states benchmarks for tackling extreme poverty, include three (out of eight) health-related goals: reducing child mortality; improving maternal health; and combating HIV/AIDS, malaria, and other diseases. In 2001, UN member states established the Global Fund to Fight AIDS, Tuberculosis, and Malaria (see chapter 7), which received, since its founding, donations of almost $22 billion.

Objecting to User Fees

With the help of the Commission on Macroeconomics and Health, the WHO bureaucracy was able to turn the exclusive focus by donor countries on economic growth into an advantage: by elevating investment in health to a fundamental strategy for economic development in poor countries, the WHO inverted the World Bank recommendation for budget cuts in health. In response to the World Bank recommendation for user fees, the WHO staff employed strategic resistance rather than strategic compliance, in which it opposed the recommendation but, by relying on economic considerations of growth, was able to justify its opposition and avoid direct confrontation with the exogenous environment.

As we saw in chapter 5, the World Bank questioned governmental provision of health care services and recommended partial cost-recovery of public health services by charging patients. Drawing on moral hazard arguments, *Financing Health Services in Developing Countries* (Akin, Birdsall, and de Ferranti 1987) argued that free services were used also by those who did not truly need the service, and that to permit an efficient allocation of scarce medical resources, patients needed to be willing to pay for those services. In later years, user fees have become a condition for World Bank's loans and donor support. UNICEF launched its own program, the Bamako Initiative, which experimented with community-based "revolving" drug funds (Gilson et al. 2001). At the regional meeting of the WHO in Africa, in 1987, UNICEF proposed to provide essential drugs for use in maternal and child health clinics on condition that charges be made for drugs or services, with the resulting income being spent on health workers' salaries or other aspects of building up primary health services (Walt and Harnmeijer 1992: 41). By 1993, a WHO report identified the increasing use of user fees for government services as one of the most significant recent changes in the financing of health services (WHO 1993b).

The WHO secretariat did not follow UNICEF's example. Relying on economic reasoning and economic methods of evaluation, the WHO report, *Evaluation of*

Recent Changes in the Financing of Health Services (WHO 1993b), made a number of critical claims regarding the increased use of fees: that the development of a private sector would not necessarily generate further resources for health, that fees would not necessarily improve allocative efficiency, and that it would negatively effect equity as poor people would drop their use of health services (WHO 1993b: 21–25). A decade later, WHO publications and reports more explicitly criticized user fees as harmful and discriminatory. For example, a World Health Report on maternal and child health asserted that "financial barriers to access have to be eliminated and users [have to be] given predictable financial protection against the costs of seeking care, and particularly against the catastrophic payments that can push households into poverty" (WHO 2005a). The report asserted that "to attain the financial protection that has to go with universal access, countries throughout the world have to move away from user charges" (WHO 2005a). The report also criticized existing efforts "to mitigate the exclusion that goes with the introduction of user fees" as "disappointing," since "exemption schemes for the poor rarely work" (WHO 2005a). In other reports, the WHO called for a phaseout of user fees for disease-specific interventions, including tuberculosis (WHO 2003) and HIV/AIDS (WHO 2005b). The report on HIV/AIDS was unequivocal: "It is apparent that user charges at the point of service delivery institutionalize exclusion and undermine efforts towards universal access to health services." Therefore, "even with sliding fee scales, cost recovery at the point of service delivery is likely to depress uptake of antiretroviral treatment and decrease adherence by those already receiving it." The report advised countries "to adopt a policy of free access at the point of service delivery to HIV care and treatment, including antiretroviral therapy." Nonetheless, the report emphasized that, "this recommendation is . . . warranted as an element of the *exceptional* response needed to turn back the AIDS epidemic" (WHO 2005b, emphasis added).

In regard to user fees, then, the WHO staff positioned itself in opposition to the neoliberal perception held by the World Bank, and emphasized instead the responsibility of governments for universal access to health services, particularly access by the poor (on universal access see more below). However, consciously avoiding passive resistance, the most explicit declarations did not criticize user fees in general but merely referred to particular health issues (maternal health, tuberculosis, and HIV/AIDS) and, somewhat defensively, emphasized exceptional circumstances. Additionally, while emphasizing the principle of universal access, the WHO staff specifically used economic reasoning to justify its concern for access. Regarding maternal health, the WHO reports warned of catastrophic payments that could push households into poverty. The report on HIV/AIDS shifted focus from the individual household to the entire economy: "For AIDS treatment and care services to have any impact, HIV-infected people must actually be able to access them. When fees are an insurmountable barrier to end users, the economy may experience a large net loss due to ill health, as people are pushed into poverty or prevented from moving out of it" (WHO 2005b). In other words, user fees should be avoided, first and foremost, because they have detrimental effects on economic growth.

As with the call for investment in health, therefore, the WHO secretariat chose not to question the dominant focus on economic growth. Instead, it criticized the practice of user fees by arguing that those fees prevented universal access, and WHO reports then defended the principle of universal access not on normative grounds but economic ones: the "institutional exclusion" (WHO 2005b) of the poor had a detrimental impact on economic development, and it is for that reason that universal access should be protected and fees be avoided.

A Cost-Effective "New Universalism"

Establishing the Commission on Macroeconomics and Health exemplified the WHO secretariat's position in response to neoliberal pressures: instead of asserting the WHO's leadership by offering an alternative vision—for example, one that would rely on public health knowledge—the WHO bureaucracy circumvented the neoliberal challenge by using neoliberalism's own tools. Just as the WHO secretariat incorporated into its programs developing countries' concern with equity and justice during the NIEO era, it accepted economic formulations and strategies as a way to fit into the neoliberal logic. To justify its programs, the WHO leadership adopted the World Bank's economic reasoning as well as its programmatic priorities, shifting its focus from serving those most in need to seeking cost-effective interventions. While signifying a move away from equity considerations, the WHO leadership used this shift to protect another significant principle, that of universal access.

In an early indication of this transformation, Brundtland chose the World Bank's *World Development Report: Investing in Health* (World Bank 1993) as her roadmap for guiding her position on various WHO policies, and the strategies that Brundtland's transition team proposed for the WHO were strongly based on that report (Lerer and Matzopoulos 2001, Yamey 2002b). Brundtland's reading of the *World Development Report* ignored the argument that governments should focus on economic growth, which would then enable households to care for health using their private means; this, as we have seen, contradicted her mission to convince governments to invest, on the contrary, in public health as a strategy to improve growth (Lerer and Matzopoulos 2001). But Brundtland did embrace the report's highly rational, evidence-based, and programmatic approach to health policy. In particular, under Brundtland, the WHO secretariat adopted the World Bank's ranking of health interventions based on cost-effectiveness calculations, that is, based on the relative "reduction in disease burden from a health intervention *in relation to the cost*" (World Bank 1993, emphasis added). The 2000 World Health Report, *Health Systems: Improving Performance* (WHO 2000a), formally endorsed cost-effectiveness as a tool for priority setting and the World Bank's suggested unit of measures, Disability-Adjusted Life Years (DALYs, see chapter 5), for calculating cost-effectiveness.

World Health Report 2000

In addition to recruiting economists to write reports on behalf of the WHO, Brundtland also hired them, including many of the authors of the World Bank's *World Development Report* (World Bank 1993), to staff a new WHO unit, Evidence and Information for Policy. As many of these economists came from Harvard, cynics said that the WHO had become "a branch of Harvard and the World Bank" (Yamey 2002b). Soon after it was established, the Evidence and Information for Policy Unit was asked to produce a World Health Report that evaluated countries' health systems (Yamey 2002b, Ollila and Koivusalo 2002).

Paradoxically, the decision to have a WHO report on health systems was originally conceived as a critical counter to positions held by the World Bank. The initial interest in the issue derived from concerns shared by some member states that international financial organizations and aid agencies were promoting health care and public sector reforms copied from developed countries—reforms such as user fees, privatization, and market mechanisms—with no evidence for their benefits to health systems in countries with scarce administrative resources and capacities. The report's focus on health systems was also intended to be a response to concerns over a recent emphasis on disease-focused approaches (Ollila and Koivusalo 2002). Ultimately, the report had little to offer toward addressing the concerns that had brought it into being, as it closely reproduced the World Bank's assumptions and logic (Ollila and Koivusalo 2002), but by utilizing the methods and considerations deemed acceptable by donors, it was able to provide a robust and ambitious new agenda for the WHO. Indeed, Brundtland hoped that the report would become "a landmark publication," and for that purpose the WHO launched the report as close as possible to 19 June 2000, to commemorate the opening of the International Health Conference in New York in 1946.[15]

One part of the report evaluated the health systems of 191 countries, and ranked them based on their "effectiveness," "responsiveness," and "fairness."

---

15. WHO Document, 2000, A53/4. PAHO Library.

These three components were also aggregated into a single overall indicator of the performance of health care systems, in which France was ranked first and Sierra Leone last (Navarro 2002). At the WHO, the report generated, as one member state put it, "a widespread and frequently hostile reaction."[16] Many WHO member states objected to their ranking, and with the help of experts, fiercely criticized the report's methods (Williams 2001, Braveman, Starfield, and Geiger 2001, Yamey 2002b). Brazil, for example, "believed that the use of a single overall health system attainment index was excessively reductionist . . . [and] its validity as a measure of the effectiveness of health systems was doubtful."[17] Discussions therefore focused on the improvements needed in collecting the data and in fine-tuning the methodologies. Critics outside the WHO, in turn, also pointed at the report's neoliberal bias in supporting minimal state intervention and showing faith in market efficiency. For example, the report seemed to endorse the World Bank's call for privatization of public health services by considering the private U.S. health care system to have the most responsive system in the world, and considering the health system of Colombia, which had undergone in-depth reform that favored participation of the private sector in provision and financing, first in fairness of financial contributions (Armada, Muntaner, and Navarro 2001, Navarro 2002). In contrast, the report referred to national health care systems that relied on public funding as examples of "heavy handed state intervention . . . the type of intervention discredited everywhere"; considered them "highly impersonal and inhuman (as in the pre-1990 Soviet Union)"; and criticized them as "monolithic" (cited in Navarro 2001). The report also called for strengthening the role of governments in supervising private provision of health services as a way to facilitate the role of the private sector in health care (Armada, Muntaner, and Navarro 2001).

The overall message of the report, however, has utilized neoliberal sensibilities to offer a new articulation of WHO values, which could also fit the organization's public health perceptions (Ollila and Koivusalo 2002, Yamey 2002b). This was made most explicit in the part of the report that advised on the most appropriate means for "choosing priorities" in health interventions (WHO 2000a). Relying heavily on the approach adopted in the *World Development Report* (World Bank 1993), the *World Health Report* stated that emphasis should be put on those interventions that would give most value for money (WHO 2000a: 52, Ollila and Koivusalo 2002, Segall 2003). The main concern, as a title of one section of the report suggested, was "getting the most health from resources" (WHO 2000a: 52). The prioritization of cost-effectiveness was explicitly presented as an improved

---

16. WHO Document, 2001, EB107/SR/4. WHO Library.
17. Ibid.

alternative to the WHO's previous focus on those most in need. An algorithm in the report, which offered a list of questions that should guide governments' process of decision making, recommended interventions that benefited the poor *only* if they were cost-effective (see figure 6.1).

Cost-effectiveness, however, was utilized in the report not to restrict health programs but to introduce a new, potentially broader, scope for health intervention. On the one hand, the report unequivocally rejected what it termed "primitive" health care, that is, "basic" or simple interventions only to the poor—namely, primary health care. The reference to "primitive" rather than "primary" health care was part of the report's harsh evaluation of primary health care programs:

> Despite . . . efforts, many such programmes were eventually considered at least partial failures. Funding was inadequate; the workers had little time to spend on prevention and community outreach; their training and equipment were insufficient for the problems they confronted; and quality of care was often so poor as to be characterized as "primitive" rather than "primary," particularly when primary care was limited to

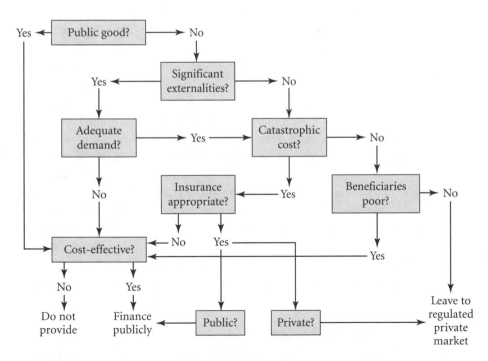

FIGURE 6.1 *World Health Report* (WHO 2000a) on how governments should decide what interventions to finance

the poor and to only the simplest services. Referral systems, which are unique to health services and necessary to their proper performance, have proved particularly difficult to operate adequately. Lower level services were often poorly utilized, and patients who could do so commonly bypassed the lower levels of the system to go directly to hospitals. Partly in consequence, countries continued to invest in tertiary, urban-based centers. (WHO 2000a: 14–15)

On the other hand, the report called for replacing primary health care with a "new universalism," which, like selective primary health care, promised cost-effective interventions, but *for everyone.*

Rather than all possible care for everyone, or only the simplest and most basic care for the poor, ["new universalism"] means delivery to all of high-quality essential care, defined by criteria of effectiveness, cost and social acceptability. It implies explicit choice of priorities among interventions, representing the ethical principle that it may be necessary and efficient to ration services, but that it is inadmissible to exclude whole groups of the population.[18]

Hence, while abandoning helping the poor *first,* the WHO staff utilized neoliberal logic to offer, instead, cost-effective remedies for a larger population, *including* the poor (see figure 6.2).[19]

The notion of "new universalism" had already been presented by Brundtland to the World Health Assembly a year earlier. In her discussion of the *World Health Report 1999,* Brundtland rhetorically asked, "Where . . . do the values of WHO lead when combined with the available evidence?" (Brundtland 1999b). Brundtland argued that "they cannot lead to a form of public intervention that has governments attempting to provide and finance everything for everybody (i.e., 'classical' universalism)," an approach that failed to recognize both resource limits and the limits of government. However, Brundtland also explicitly rejected a neoliberal solution that would rely entirely on the market. In the same speech, Brundtland forcefully asserted that "WHO's values cannot support market-oriented approaches that ration health services to those with the ability to pay," since such approaches lead to intolerable inequity with respect to a fundamental human right, and further, because "growing bodies of theory and

---

18. WHO Document, 2000, A53/4. PAHO Library.
19. Rejecting primary health care while replacing it with new universalism may explain why the report was criticized both from the left and from the right. While critics from the left thought the World Health Report 2000 to be the mouthpiece of "US financial and political circles" (Navarro 2000), critics from the right could describe its policy message in the pages of the *Wall Street Journal,* as "healthcare à la Karl Marx" (Helms 2000).

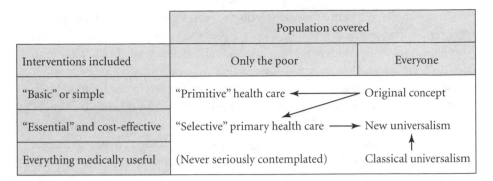

Interventions included	Population covered	
	Only the poor	Everyone
"Basic" or simple	"Primitive" health care ←	Original concept
"Essential" and cost-effective	"Selective" primary health care →	New universalism
Everything medically useful	(Never seriously contemplated)	Classical universalism

FIGURE 6.2   *World Health Report* (WHO 2000a) on "new universalism"

evidence indicate that markets in health are . . . inefficient as well." A year later, in presenting the *World Health Report 2000,* Brundtland explicitly presented the new approach as an adaptive strategy to the new environment. Brundtland explained that the new strategy "has been due in part to the profound political and economic changes of the last 20 years or so, including the transformation from centrally planned to market-oriented economies, reduced State intervention in national economies, fewer government controls, and more decentralization. Ideologically, this has meant greater emphasis on individual choice and responsibility. Politically, it has meant limiting promises and expectations about what governments should do." Brundtland offered the report as guidance for governments in the context of those new limits. "Clearly, limits exist on what governments can finance and on what services they can deliver. The report intends to stimulate public policies that acknowledge these limits—recognizing that if services are to be provided at all, then not all services can be provided."[20] And, once the need to make priorities was established, Brundtland insisted that "the most cost-effective services should be provided first" (Brundtland 1999b).

Disease-Specific, Cost-Effective Interventions

Cost-effectiveness calculations were most often used to identify risk factors and recommend particular interventions in specific diseases. Using DALYs, the *World Health Report* offered a table with "examples of interventions that, if implemented well, can substantially reduce the burden of disease, especially among the poor, and do so at a reasonable cost relative to results" (WHO 2000a: 53).

---

20. WHO Document, 2000, A53/4. PAHO Library.

These included direct observation treatment, short-course (DOTS) treatment of tuberculosis,[21] maternal health and safe motherhood interventions, family planning, school health interventions, integrated management of childhood illness, HIV/AIDS prevention (targeted information for sex workers, mass education awareness, counseling, screening, mass treatment for sexually transmitted diseases, safe blood supply), immunization, treatment of malaria (early assessment and prompt treatment and selective preventive measures such as impregnated bed nets), tobacco control (tobacco tax, information, nicotine replacement, legal action), and treatment of noncommunicable diseases and injuries (selected early screening and secondary prevention) (WHR 2000: table 3.1).

Cost-effectiveness was also a central recommendation of the Commission on Macroeconomics and Health report, which was published a year after the *World Health Report* (Ashraf 2000, Lerer and Matzopoulos 2001). In some respects, the CMH report offered a more limited public health agenda than the *World Health Report,* as it suggested that "poverty could be considerably reduced by addressing a *few* health conditions responsible for a high proportion of avoidable deaths and disabilities"[22] and focused largely on malaria, tuberculosis, and HIV/AIDS (the report also supported intervention regarding childhood infectious diseases, maternal and perinatal conditions, micronutrient deficiencies, and tobacco-related illnesses, all compatible with the *World Health Report*). In other respects, however, the CMH report brought attention back to those "most in need," albeit for economic reasons rather than considerations of equity: a concern with economic growth led the commission to focus significantly on "diseases of poverty." The CMH report also broadened the global health agenda: while the *World Health Report* relied on *existing* cost-effective interventions, the CMH report urged donor countries to invest in funding research that would lead to cost-effective solutions, where those did not yet exist.

Most comprehensively, the 2002 World Health Report, *Reducing Risks: Promoting Healthy Life,* was a large-scale study of the cost-effectiveness of 170 interventions. The report calculated how much of the burden of disease, disability, and death that could be attributed to twenty-five of the world's major risk factors

---

21. DOTS, which the WHO had adopted as a new approach to tuberculosis control in the 1990s, included short-course chemotherapy (taking anti-TB drugs for six months instead of the previous standard twelve-month treatment) and direct observation of drug intake (where someone watches each patient take the medicines daily, rather than relying on unsupervised self-administered treatments). The new strategy also comprised of case finding through examinations of patients with respiratory symptoms attending primary health care units (Okie 1999, Raviglione and Pio 2002). Thanks to DOTS, the World Bank and WHO reports crowned tuberculosis control as one of the most cost-effective health interventions available.

22. WHO Document, The representative of the Executive Board at the Fifty-fifth World Health Assembly, 2002, WHA55/A/SR/1, p. 16. WHO Library. Emphasis added.

could be avoided if the risk factors were reduced using existing cost-effective interventions. The report identified five risk factors that were responsible for at least 30 percent of all disease burden in high-mortality developing countries—underweight, unsafe sex, micronutrient deficiencies, unsafe water, and indoor smoke—and identified cost-effective interventions for reducing these risks (WHO 2002, Brundtland 2002).

This new emphasis on cost-effective interventions was generally welcomed by WHO member states.[23] The Canadian delegate, for example, "agreed with the commission's suggestion that the emphasis should be placed on the delivery of select interventions known to meet priority needs in a cost-effective manner."[24] Other members, however, saw the focus on particular diseases as the reintroduction of the vertical approach, which had been rejected in the 1970s, and criticized the reliance on cost-effectiveness calculations. The delegate from Finland stated:

> The Commission's report acknowledged the need to develop the health sector as a whole but ended up recommending increased funding for certain vertical outcome-oriented approaches focused on communicable diseases and maternal and child health. Finland was concerned about some of its recommendations from a public health point of view. . . . [The] Commission appeared to have overlooked many recent lessons regarding the development of health systems in poor countries, which had shown that vertical interventions to tackle specific diseases did not work as expected but simply diverted human and financial resources from the building of comprehensive and universal health services.[25]

Similarly, the delegate from Mozambique, who "welcomed the long-overdue initiative to emphasize health as a key element in development," nevertheless suggested, in a way that also subtly criticized the composition of the commission, that "input from public health specialists from developing countries would have avoided proposals for a vertical approach and furthered integrated development by dealing with other crucial determinants of health, such as safe water, roads and education, particularly for women."[26] Such concerns notwithstanding, cost-effectiveness calculations reinforced the WHO's move away from a comprehensive approach to primary health care toward a selective approach that concentrated on specific health interventions.

---

23. WHO Document, 2002, WHA55/A/SR/1, p. 16. WHO Library.
24. WHO Document, 2002, WHA55/A/SR/5. WHO Library.
25. WHO Document, 2002, WHA55/A/SR/1. WHO Library.
26. Ibid., p. 21; for other criticisms of the report see, for example, Katz 2004, 2005, Motchane 2003.

In addition to the prioritization on the basis of cost-effectiveness, other considerations further pushed the WHO in the direction of vertical programs. A particularly important one was the increasing reliance on earmarked extrabudgetary funds at the WHO, a source of funding that relied on the goodwill of rich countries' development agencies (see chapter 5). The United States in particular had a tendency to prefer disease-specific contributions more than beneficiary countries, so the shift in decision-making authority from the World Health Assembly to individual donor governments led to a shift in the WHO programs.[27] This tendency increased with the greater involvement in global health matters of private foundations and health activists, both of which, for different reasons, favored a focus on particular diseases. Another factor contributing to the rise of vertical programs was the WHO's new commitment to forming partnerships, which often had a targeted, disease-specific mission (see chapter 7).

Starting in the late 1990s, then, the WHO's priorities focused on health problems that had a major socioeconomic impact on development, partly by having an effect on the lives of the poor, and for which cost-effective interventions were available (McCarthy 2002, Yamey 2002b). In that way, the WHO replaced its comprehensive approach of the 1970s with a selective approach, which concentrated on specific health interventions to which medico-technical solutions were available (Lerer and Matzopoulos 2001, Katz 2004). At the top of the WHO's priorities were the three major communicable diseases, malaria, tuberculosis, and albeit somewhat later, HIV/AIDS.[28] All three initiatives were presented as contributing to development. All three initiatives were structured as WHO-led partnerships (see chapter 7): Roll Back Malaria, Stop TB Partnership, and 3-by-5, respectively. For all three diseases, cost-effectiveness was to be achieved by preferring cheap solutions (for example, preventive) over expensive ones (for example, medication). As a more detailed description of the malaria strategy shows, the outcome was a combination of "appropriate technologies"—as they might have been called in the 1970s—with some market-driven innovations, following the WHO's new "new universalism" perception (Brundtland 1999b).

---

27. According to Andrew Natsios, Administrator of USAID: "We take a disease-directed approach. In other words, we will target malaria or tuberculosis or HIV/AIDS. [The Europeans] take a health systems approach. We do that too, but if you looked relative to the amount of money we spend, Congress has preferred—and [US]AID agrees with this approach—that a disease-focused approach is a better one." See Halting the Spread of HIV/AIDS: Future Efforts in the U.S. Bilateral and Multilateral Response," Hearings before the Committee on Foreign Relations, U.S. Senate, One hundred and seventh Congress, Second session, February 13 and 14, 2002.

28. The attention to these three diseases also moved beyond the WHO, in large part thanks to the report of the Commission on Macroeconomics and Health and the personal influence of Jeffrey Sachs. As we saw, one of the eight Millennium Development Goals was to combat HIV/AIDS, malaria, and other diseases. The Global Fund to Fight AIDS, Tuberculosis, and Malaria was established in 2002.

Roll Back Malaria

Following the failure of the malaria eradication program in the 1960s, the WHO secretariat was reluctant to get caught up in another unachievable attempt to fight malaria. Brundtland's decision to nonetheless focus on malaria again partly stemmed from political considerations. By the late 1990s, according to WHO estimates, malaria killed more than 1 million people a year, especially young children, and there were an estimated 300–500 million acute cases annually, pre-dominantly in Africa.[29] For decades, malaria accounted for the highest morbidity and mortality rates in sub-Saharan Africa, although by the 1990s it was overtaken by HIV/AIDS.[30] The African political leadership, demanding action, made a re-newed malaria control campaign a pivotal condition during the election of the WHO director-general in 1998.[31]

These political considerations were also given an economic reasoning. One slogan for the initiative was, "Roll Back Malaria, Roll in Development," and the first executive director for the Roll Back Malaria initiative, Dr. David Nabarro, stated, "Malaria is taking costly bites out of Africa. . . . It is feasting on the health and development of African children and it is draining the life out of African economies" (cited in Packard 2009). The WHO leadership relied on an economic report prepared by Jeffrey Sachs and colleagues at the Harvard University Center for International Development and the London School of Hygiene and Tropical Medicine that pointed to the negative economic impact of malaria. The report calculated not only the short-term costs of malaria, such as loss of labor and the cost of treatment and prevention, but also longer-term costs such as tourists and foreign investors avoiding malaria-prone countries, large numbers of sick children missing school, and the increase in population and impoverishment that typically ensues when parents decide to have more children because they know some will quite likely die.[32] By including these long-term costs, the report concluded that malaria was taking a far greater toll of the economy of many developing countries than had been previously estimated. As with the CMH re-port, the inevitable conclusion was that malaria was not just a health matter but

---

29. In 2008, using improved statistical techniques, the WHO modified these numbers and sug-gested that there were 250 million cases of malaria in the world each year, and about 880,000 deaths. Virtually the entire drop in this estimation was accounted for by revisions of the figures for India, Indonesia, Pakistan, and other Asian countries. The number of cases in Africa has not changed (McNeil 2008).

30. WHO Document, 1999, WHA52/A/SR/5. PAHO Library.

31. Interview by the author with Allen Schapira, formerly at the WHO Roll Back Malaria Depart-ment, Geneva, Switzerland, 31 May 2008; see also Crossette 1998.

32. The report appeared as an appendix to a WHO review of the African Summit on Roll Back Malaria in Abuja, in April 2000 (WHO 2000b). For an insightful critic of the economic rationale, see Packard 2009.

a development issue, and therefore something rich countries should care about (McNeil 2000, Boseley 2000).

In October 1998, the WHO, together with the World Bank, UNICEF, and UNDP, established a multiagency campaign, with the WHO as a lead agency, called Roll Back Malaria (RBM) (Goshko 1998). The WHO Executive Board "approved the innovative concept of the Roll Back Malaria project, welcoming in particular its ability to generate new working methods in WHO and to act as a development strategy for the health sector."[33] Over time, RBM became an alliance of more than five hundred partners, including malaria-endemic countries, bilateral and multilateral development agencies, the private sector, nongovernmental and community-based organizations, foundations, and research and academic institutions.

Learning from the experience of past malaria projects, which had fallen short of their aims, Roll Back Malaria was not an attempt to eradicate the disease. Instead, the formal goal was to halve malaria-associated mortality by 2010 and again by 2015 (Nabarro and Tayler 1998). Without a "magic bullet," even this was considered an ambitious goal. According to Dr. Steven Phillips, the medical director of Global Issues and Projects at Exxon Mobil Corporation,

> Most global health interventions are single point-of-service interventions, so a child getting an immunization, or a child getting anti-worming medication, or a child getting vitamin A.... And you can do dramatically good things because you have magic bullets. But because the need for human organization and human cooperation . . . is limited . . . it's not a huge challenge on the system. Malaria . . . is a huge challenge on the system. . . . For malaria interventions you need to figure out, on a broad population basis, how to spray households, how to distribute medicines, not just one time but for any fever. You need to figure out how to distribute that medicine in a way that people will actually use them and value them. You need to figure out how to deliver health services at maternal antenatal clinics. And you need to figure out how to do this systematically everywhere all the time, not just in some places some of the time.[34]

In choosing strategies to "roll back" malaria, the WHO focused on cost-effective interventions. Indeed, evidence of the availability of cost-effective solutions played a role in Brundtland's decision to focus on malaria. According to Allan Schapira, of the Roll Back Malaria Department:

33. WHO Document, 1999, WHA52/A/SR/5. PAHO Library.
34. Interview by the author with Dr. Steven Phillips, Medical Director, Global Issues and Projects, Exxon Mobil Corporation, Washington, DC, 12 January 2009.

Research in the 1980s had started to show good results of insecticides-treated mosquito nets, and building on that, TDR [WHO Special Programme for Research and Training in Tropical Disease] conducted multi-center studies on insecticide-treated nets during the 1990s, and it was somewhere around 1997 . . . that it was possible to publish that in four different sites in Africa with different transmission intensities there had been a quite marked reduction in overall childhood mortality. That provided a background for really going out into the world and [saying] what to do about malaria and what to do especially about malaria in Africa. So it was not just the worsening situation, but it was also that there was an evidence base for identifying at least one highly effective intervention.[35]

In addition to bed nets treated with insecticide, RBM partners decided to support the spraying of insecticide to kill larvae.[36] Emphasizing measures geared for small communities, the program also planned to train people at the local level to institute preventive measures, recognize new malaria cases, and treat them quickly with cheap and effective remedies (Goshko 1998, McNeil 2000).

Although focused on one disease, some of the cost-effective measures adopted by RBM were compatible with certain principles of the primary health care approach, including the reliance on auxiliary personnel and on "appropriate technologies." Other aspects of the program, however, reflected the dominance of a new logic, including market-driven solutions—that is, solutions that were based on imitating competitive market conditions or solutions that could transfer responsibility from the public realm to the private sector by creating the possibility for profit. This was the case, for example, with the provision of bed nets. As part of RBM, the WHO announced, in October 1999, a five-year program to increase thirtyfold the use of insecticide-impregnated mosquito nets in Africa. Normally, such a program would rely on public funds. This time, the WHO attempted to promote the spread of bed nets by using market forces. The WHO reasoned that, unlike residual spraying or vaccination, bed nets were something people could

---

35. Interview by the author with Allen Schapira, formerly at the WHO Roll Back Malaria Department, Geneva, Switzerland, 31 May 2008.

36. Insecticide spraying, which was a prominent aspect of the malaria eradication program in the 1950s, became controversial when reports in the 1960s, including that by the environmentalist Rachel Carson in her book *Silent Spring*, showed that DDT was killing off bald eagles, in part by thinning their eggshells, and seeping into the food chain. Environmental protests led the Environmental Protection Agency in the United States to ban the use of DDT in 1972. Soon thereafter, the WHO also stopped using DDT as an antimalaria measure. However, restrictions on the use of the DDT to combat malaria have been attacked by campaigners who said the limitations cost lives in the developing world (Boseley 1999). Subsequently, the WHO reversed its policy and supported the indoor spraying of pesticides generally, and DDT specifically, to control mosquitoes in countries with high rates of malaria.

do for themselves, and the WHO's advice to governments was therefore to build sustainable private for-profit markets for insecticide-treated bed nets or to create a not-for-profit commercial sector (Noor et al. 2007).[37]

The WHO also thought to rely on market forces for the distribution of expensive drugs. Initially, RBM supported as the first line treatment for malaria the use of drugs that were cheaper but less effective than newer drugs, particularly artemisinin-based combination therapies (ACT).[38] In 2004, a number of malaria researchers published a letter in the *Lancet,* saying that, because of the WHO recommendations, international funds were being wasted on useless malaria drugs (Attaran et al. 2004). In response to this public pressure, the WHO bureaucracy changed its policy and began urging countries affected by drug-resistant malaria to switch to the more effective ACTs. The new policy raised new difficulties. More than half of malaria patients in Africa got their drugs from private outlets rather than public health systems. Most drugstores in Africa, moreover, did not carry ACTs, and if they did, they were much more expensive than older drugs, like Chloroquine. There were also concerns over counterfeit drugs and over cheap artemisinin monothrerapies, which increased resistance to artemisinin (Enserink 2008).

In 2004, a report published by the U.S. Institute of Medicine (IOM), entitled *Saving Lives, Buying Time,* and prepared by a group chaired by the Nobel laureate Kenneth Arrow, proposed a solution for the affordability of ACTs (Arrow, Panosian, and Gelband 2004). The report proposed a "high-level subsidy" backed by a centralized procurement mechanism to increase production volumes and drive down prices of ACTs to the level of cheaper drugs. In other words, rather than paying the governments that would buy the drugs and then provide them for free or cheaply to its poor population, donors should pay manufacturers of ACTs so they would be able to sell their drugs as cheaply as competing alternatives in the private market. According to one health economist who sat on the IOM panel, "For years, we've been saying in public health: If only we knew how Coca-Cola gets its cans into the most remote African villages, we could do the same for drugs. Well, this is how they do it—by relying on the market" (cited in Enserink 2008). Others voiced concern that, even with the subsidy, the price would remain unaffordable for many consumers, who might start treatment and then drop it, triggering greater drug resistance and an increase in the number of victims of malaria. There was also the worry that instead of passing the benefit

---

37. The strategy has arguably failed, however, as it increased the coverage of bed nets only from 1 percent to 3 percent over three years. Interview by the author with Allen Schapira, formerly at the WHO Roll Back Malaria Department, Geneva, Switzerland, 31 May 2008.

38. Artemisinin is refined from the qinghaosu plant, which is available mostly in China and Vietnam. In the early 1990s, Chinese scientists developed a combination therapy that put together an artemisinin-based drug called artemether and lumefantrine, an older antimalarial drug.

on to patients, intermediaries would pocket most of the subsidy (Enserink 2008). But in 2007, RBM threw its weight behind the idea and launched with the Global Fund to Fight AIDS, Tuberculosis, and Malaria the Affordable Medicines Facility for malaria (AMFm).[39]

Roll Back Malaria, then, adopted elements that mirrored a neoliberal, market-oriented program, which, where possible, favored solutions that attempted to bypass governmental interventions by relying on the forces of the market. These and other examples illustrate the sharp transition of the WHO bureaucracy and its adherence to the exogenous expectations of those who financially supported the malaria programs—more than 90 percent of the funds for RBM came from voluntary contributions. While incorporating exogenous norms and strategies, however, the WHO's adaptation enabled the protection of the organization's material as well as ideational goals, by assuring sustainable attention to the diseases of the poor, including malaria, tuberculosis, and HIV/AIDS.

Discussion

Like Mahler, who had been elected at the height of the mobilization for a New International Economic Order, Brundtland was elected at a time when the WHO was in turmoil due to exogenous circumstances, and when both the staff and member states were eager for an adequate response. Both the election of Mahler in 1974 and Brundtland in 1998 reflected disillusionments with the past. In the 1970s, the past was represented by Director-General Candau and his support for vertical programs; in the 1990s, this past was represented by Mahler and his call for health for all and support of primary health care. Both Mahler and Brundtland were suitably embedded in the respective environment and were able to successfully integrate the WHO into it—deferring to the procedural dependence on the G-77 and the resource dependence on rich countries, respectively.

Facing a broken organization with a discredited agenda and desperate need for new financial resources, Brundtland was determined to revitalize the global health agenda, relying on strategies that she had used to integrate environmental concerns into the development agenda. Under Brundtland's leadership, the WHO embraced neoliberal principles and used economic formulations to rethink its programs and priorities. As this chapter shows, a neoliberal transformation was evident in every layer of operation. The WHO considered health through the lens of economic growth, prioritized cost-effective programs, and as the malaria

---

39. Interview by the author with Renia Coghlan, Medicines for Malaria Venture, Geneva, Switzerland, 27 May 2008; see also Enserink 2008.

program illustrates, accepted market-driven solutions and business-friendly arrangements. While accepting the exogenous logic, however, the WHO bureaucracy was also able to manipulate existing economic maxims to defend its own preferences and values. In the 1970s, the WHO secretariat relied not on public health expertise but on reworking NIEO principles to justify its policies; similarly, in the late 1990s, the WHO secretariat relied not on public health or medical logic but on neoliberal principles and economic reasoning. For that purpose, Brundtland invited established economists to help the WHO frame its central agenda and used their reports, which showed that health was fundamental for economic growth, to reverse the neoliberal neglect of noneconomic spheres and to successfully reclaim the centrality of health. This enabled the WHO secretariat to then declare the organization's "central task" to be "the reduction of poverty through improving health."[40] In addition, the WHO secretariat relied on cost-effectiveness calculations to introduce the concept of the "new universalism," which promised "'essential' and cost-effective" interventions for everyone (WHO 2000a). New universalism rejected primary health care, but it also rejected rigid market-oriented approaches and thereby maintained the WHO's responsibility to the poor. Finally, the formal rejection of interventions "only to the poor" did not negate attention to diseases "which affected the poorest and weakest and impoverished those [they] afflicted."[41] Although limiting the importance of health interventions only to their potential contribution to economic development ostensibly neglected issues of inequity, in practice concerns with economic growth led to programs that prioritized the poor by favoring interventions in "diseases of poverty" such as malaria, tuberculosis, and HIV/AIDS. Similarly, while cost-effectiveness and the "new universalism" did not methodologically favor the poor, in practice, the reliance on DALYs—which took into consideration the global burden of disease and the cost required for every "DALY saved"—focused on relatively cheap preventive and curative measures for conditions mostly affecting the poor.

Using economic considerations, then, the WHO was able to emphasize the value of universal access as part of its "new universalism" and to broaden the cause of universal access so it was concerned "not just . . . with improving people's health, but also with protecting them against the financial costs of illness."[42] The next chapter, which examines the WHO's relations with multinational corporations, describes additional cases of strategic compliance and resistance, in which, while adapting to the exogenous environment, the WHO was able to protect universal access and other ideational goals.

---

40. WHO Document, 2001, Report by the Director-General, EB107/SR/1. PAHO Library.
41. Ibid.
42. WHO Document, 2000, A53/4. PAHO Library.

HOW TO WIN FRIENDS AND INFLUENCE ENEMIES

Although describing the WHO as the "lead agency in health,"[1] Director-General Brundtland engaged in a strategy of co-opting other agencies and actors rather than competing with them. In her first speech before the World Health Assembly after her election, Brundtland declared that the WHO must "reach out to others" (cited in Yamey 2002c). As we have seen, the WHO secretariat chose to work with, rather than challenge, more influential international organizations, such as the World Bank. The WHO staff also transformed its relations with the private sector, including both charitable foundations, such as the Bill and Melinda Gates Foundation, and for-profit companies and their associations. Brundtland and subsequent directors-general invited business to participate in WHO-led partnerships, in which companies were asked to contribute money and to share knowledge. The WHO also welcomed companies' in-kind donations and staff on loan (secondments).

This welcoming attitude to external contributions was mostly due to the budget freeze imposed on the WHO by the U.S. government and other Geneva Group members, which forced the organization to look for funds from alternative sources (see chapter 5). Companies became a legitimate source for donations because the shift from the New International Economic Order to neoliberal principles brought with it a radical change in the appreciation of business' potential contribution to governance: President Reagan's call to engage with the private sector outlived his administration, and subsequent U.S. administrations pressed

---

1. "Challenges and Opportunities for the Health Leaders of Today," Address by Dr. Gro Harlem Brundtland, Director-General of the WHO to the Fifty-Third World Health Assembly, 15 May 2000.

UN agencies for private sector involvement as part of a broader agenda of adopting market-friendly strategies. Private foundations also began to condition their contributions on private sector involvement.

Although they accepted business as legitimate partners in programs for improving global health, the WHO secretariat chose certain instances to strategically resist the new truism that "business was part of the solution" and continued to treat business as the source of the problem. Paradoxically, during the New International Economic Order the WHO leadership had avoided explicit confrontations with multinational companies, but in the era of neoliberalism the WHO leadership positioned itself against a number of influential industries, including tobacco and pharmaceuticals. The WHO launched a global campaign against the tobacco industry as part of its antismoking mission, and the WHO staff took a position against the pharmaceutical industry in the dispute over intellectual property protection and access to AIDS drugs. In both cases the WHO secretariat attempted to minimize the risk of sanctions, which donor countries would have been likely to impose in response to its resistance, by redefining the exogenous pressures it was expected to follow. The WHO bureaucracy justified its attack on the right of tobacco companies to sell their products to informed consumers not by criticizing market principles but emphasizing a list of characteristics that made the tobacco sector a legitimate exception to the general rule. The WHO staff challenged the right of pharmaceutical companies to protect their patents on AIDS drugs not by questioning the principle of intellectual property protection but providing a legal interpretation to the disputed text that suggested that the international agreement protecting patents was entirely reconcilable with exceptions for particular cases such as AIDS. In short, when opposing exogenous prescriptions, the WHO secretariat was careful not to tarnish its new business-friendly reputation and refrained from explicitly criticizing probusiness principles and relying, instead, on those very principles to justify its deviant position.

The first part of the chapter analyzes the new era in WHO-business relations. The second part describes the strategies of resistance used by the WHO to oppose the tobacco and pharmaceutical companies.

Business Is Part of the Solution

In an address before the World Health Assembly in 1999, entitled "Looking Ahead for WHO after a Year of Change," Brundtland announced that "WHO needs to be more innovative in creating influential partnerships" (Brundtland 1999b). In that speech, Brundtland praised UNAIDS, which was still regarded with suspicion by most WHO staff. She also promised—and, as we have seen, later delivered—a closer working relationship with the World Bank, including "deeper dialogue on policy issues," and with the International Monetary Fund and the World Trade Organization. As this address reveals, Brundtland considered that the most "influential partnerships" the WHO should be interested in were not with its more traditional allies, such as UNICEF or UNDP, but rather with the international financial institutions. In the same address, Brundtland also spoke favorably of the fact that "WHO [was] making progress in building partnerships with nongovernmental organizations and the private sector" (Brundtland 1999b). In this and subsequent speeches, Brundtland downplayed the fact that seeking cooperation with the private sector constituted a substantial departure from the WHO's past position on the issue. Relations between the WHO bureaucracy and business had historically been founded on mutual suspicion. Hostility was exacerbated during the 1970s, when some WHO member states called for international codes of conduct to regulate the marketing of infant formula and medicines. During that period, conversations between the WHO leadership and pharmaceutical associations in attempt to promote discounts of essential drugs intensified rather than lessened the lack of trust between the parties (see chapter 4).[2] With the dominance of neoliberal thinking, new constraints and incentives led the WHO bureaucracy to reconsider its rejection of cooperation with business. In particular, the WHO was in a dire financial situation as a result of a zero budget growth (see chapter 5) at the same time that both donor governments and private foundations pressed UN agencies, including the WHO, to improve their relations with business.

Cooperation with the private sector was one solution the U.S. government pushed for in its attempt to fix the alleged UN inefficiency. Echoing neoliberal sentiments, the Reagan administration promulgated the perception that bureaucracies were inherently less efficient than companies competing in the private market (Lee and Walt 1992, Utting and Zammit 2006). In addition to internal reforms, therefore, the Reagan administration encouraged "private sector involvement in problem-solving on the development issues in the United Nations

---

2. There were some precedents in which the WHO got involved, albeit reluctantly, in partnerships with the private sector. In one case, Merck offered the WHO a donation of Mectizan against onchocerciasis (river blindness). The WHO initially refused to collaborate with Merck. Stefanie Meredith, who was involved in the negotiation from Merck's side, recounted: "[Merck] first went to WHO and said they had this really good drug . . . but people at [the WHO] headquarters wouldn't touch it. . . . This was back in 1983. . . . [WHO] said no, we don't need it, we wouldn't know how to work with you, we can't work with a pharma company directly." Eventually, a partnership of Merck with the WHO and the World Bank, among others, was established in 1995 (interview by the author with Stefanie Meredith, Director of Public Health Partnerships, IFPMA, Geneva, Switzerland, 23 May 2008). Another partnership established during that period was between the WHO and Rotary International, which helped to eradicate polio in the Americas by 1991 (Seytre and Shaffer 2005).

system."[3] Testifying before the House Committee on Appropriations, in May 1982, Jeane Kirkpatrick, the U.S. ambassador to the UN, stated that "our basic approach toward the rest of the world in development programs" moved "toward more emphasis on the private sector." Kirkpatrick assured the committee that "we have undertaken a genuine offensive," that "we do a lot of talking about private sector and market systems," and finally, that "there is more interest today in the United Nations in the private sector role in economic development than there has been in human memory there."[4]

Support of private sector involvement included calls for shifting prerogatives to business, by means of privatization, contracting-out, and so on—but it also included calls for bringing the private sector *into* the public realm. The U.S. government actively pressed international organizations, including the WHO, to engage the private sector in their programs. Scholarly reviews similarly equated private-sector participation with efficiency, including arguments that a UN engagement with the private sector would "provide access to . . . skills and management talents" (Buse and Walt 2000b) and "enable UN agencies to be more effective and efficient" (Richter 2004).

Support for a meaningful private-sector participation in global health initiatives also came from private foundations, which began to play an increasingly influential role in shaping WHO policies and its institutional arrangements. In the late 1990s, private foundations involved in global health programs developed a new perception of how global health should be run and began to condition their donations on particular managerial reforms, including greater involvement of business. In a report by the director-general to the Executive Board, in 1999, Brundtland announced two new private sources of funds: the UN Foundation, a charity established by CNN founder Ted Turner—which committed $100 million annually over ten years to organizations of the UN system in the fields of children's health, population, and women—and the Bill and Melinda Gates Foundation, which pledged two grants of more than $10 million each for the WHO programs on human reproduction and children's vaccines. Brundtland then informed the Executive Board: "Significantly, both these two foundations have made partnerships and collaboration with the private sector a key feature of their grant giving" (WHO 1999a). Older foundations, including the Rockefeller Foundations, introduced similar conditions.

---

3. Gregory Newell, Assistant Secretary for International Organization Affairs, Department of State, "Foreign Assistance and Related Programs Appropriations for 1986," Hearings before a Subcommittee of the Committee on Appropriations, House of Representatives, Ninety-ninth Congress, First Session (part 5), May 8, 1985.
4. "Foreign Assistance and Related Programs Appropriations for 1983," Hearings before a Subcommittee of the Committee on Appropriations, House of Representatives, Ninety-Seventh Congress, Second Session, May 14, 1982, pp. 131–132.

The WHO leadership responded favorably to these demands, as it saw in the participation of the private sector a potential solution for the ongoing financial crisis the organization had been suffering (Buse and Walt 2000a, Motchane 2003). The WHO leadership was encouraged by the impressive growth in the overall number of corporate foundations and the value of their grants during that period (Utting and Zammit 2006). Dr. David Nabarro, the executive director at the Director-General Office, stated: "We certainly need private financing. For the past decade governments' financial contributions have dwindled. The main sources of funding are the private sector and the financial markets" (cited in Motchane 2003). Brundtland personally perceived the integration of business not as a threatening necessity but as an opportunity. Chris Hentschel, CEO of Medicines for Malaria Venture, noted that at the time "many of the people in Geneva were anti-the private sector. [Brundtland] was not. She thought they were part of the solution, not the problem."[5] He attributes her view to the fact that, unlike previous directors-general, Brundtland "had come from politics."[6] During the run-up to the 1992 UN Conference on Environment and Development, Brundtland was centrally involved in the initial moves by the UN to work more closely with the commercial sector (Motchane 2003). Already in 1990, Brundtland had declared her strong support for building constructive relations between the UN and the private sector:

> Partnership is what is needed in today's world, partnership between government and industry, between producers and consumers, between the present and the future . . . We need to build new coalitions. . . . We must agree on a global agenda for the management of change. . . . We must continue to move from confrontation, through dialogue to cooperation. . . . Collective management of the global interdependence is . . . the only acceptable formula in the world of the 1990s. (cited in Richter 2004)

In short, pressures from donor governments and private foundations, combined with a WHO leadership desperate for new sources of funds while accepting the potential utility of working with the private sector, led the WHO bureaucracy to reform its relations with business and to integrate companies into its global health projects. The WHO invited the private sector to participate as "partners" in new initiatives, including Roll Back Malaria (RBM), Stop TB Partnership, and, in 2003, the "3 by 5" initiative. The WHO also encouraged in-kind donations, secondment

---

5. Interview by the author with Chris Hentschel, CEO of Medicines for Malaria Venture, Geneva, Switzerland, 19 May 2008.

6. Ibid.

of personnel, and other forms of business contributions. At least initially, there was little attention to the reputation of potential partners, and Brundtland commended the WHO cooperation with companies that had questionable operations in the global South, such as diamond and mining companies (WHO 1999a). The WHO staff also worked to improve its relations with old adversaries, including Nestlé, the company most associated with the unethical marketing of infant formula in poor countries in the early 1980s, and the pharmaceutical sector.

Member states generally supported in-house partnerships, both with other international organizations and with the private sector. Given the general neoliberal turn of many developing countries, their position in regard to multinational companies has radically changed since their call for a New International Order in the 1970s: they no longer cultivated antagonistic relations with business, and they had no principled objection to working with them. Representatives from developing countries were also genuinely concerned about WHO's declining authority and "abdication of its responsibilities to others," and hoped that partnerships could help WHO regain "the vanguard on health."[7] The representative from Uganda saw collaboration as providing the potential for the WHO to reclaim leadership:

> In the not-so-distance past, other UN specialized agencies had regrettably assumed responsibility for implementing certain country programmes which clearly fell within WHO's remit. Inter-sector collaboration was to be welcomed, provided the Organization did not relinquish its turf to other agencies.[8]

Other member states agreed that the WHO had no choice but to support the trend toward public-private partnerships and to involve the private sector.[9] The representative from Canada, like others, "fully supported the WHO partnership policy, since clearly WHO alone could not achieve what it wished or was expected of it."[10]

In contrast, other WHO member states and some of the WHO's staff feared that bringing new actors into the organization would lead to an institutional capture and weaken the autonomy of the WHO. They also feared that reliance on corporate cash would skew the WHO policies toward vested interests.[11] In the same meetings in which some countries congratulated the WHO's revival by way of partnerships, others warned that collaboration with the private sector would lead to conflicts of interest and to the WHO's loss of impartiality. The Executive

---

7. WHO Document, 1999, WHA52/A/SR/5. WHO Library.
8. Ibid.
9. WHO Document, 2000, EB105/SR/2. WHO Library.
10. Ibid., p. 42.
11. See also Boseley 2002, Ollila 2003, Utting and Zammit 2006.

Board member from France cautioned that the WHO "should not be naïve, for the interests of the Organization and industry were not the same. WHO should not be market-controlled."[12] In a different meeting, France again warned that "the credibility of the Organization was at stake. It was essential that there should be no suspicion that the Organization had been influenced in any way by its private partners."[13] The board member from Venezuela "stressed that the principal objectives of partnerships should be consistent with the strategic directions of WHO,"[14] and the member from Chad said that "the relations between WHO and the private sector should be fully transparent in order to avoid any conflict of interest and to protect the independence of the Organization."[15] The board member from Belgium warned that "[donations] would need to be scrutinized . . . since it was known that providing something free of charge often had a perverse effect, interfering with the way in which normal systems operated."[16] The member from India urged that "in mobilizing resources . . . no compromise in the credibility and moral standing of WHO should be allowed."[17] Some WHO staff, in turn, made accusations that the secretariat was self-censoring itself so as not to alienate existing and potential partners. One member of the policy group concerned with essential drugs and medicines, Daphne Fresle, who subsequently resigned in protest in 2001, accused the WHO of playing safe in its public statements and of silencing criticism made of the pharmaceutical industry (Horton 2002: 1605). Staff also accused the WHO leadership of manipulating discussions to avoid confrontation with infant formula manufacturers (Ferriman 2000, Boseley 2001).

In response to such concerns, Brundtland conceded that there were some risks involved and that "there is a need to ensure that health systems are not distorted by donations; that costs remain under control; and that advice is independent. There is potential for real or perceived conflicts of interest" (WHO 2001). Dr. Lyagoubi-Ouahchi, the executive director for External Relations and Governing Bodies, assured member states that "in extending its partnership with the private sector, the Organization's main concern must always be to preserve its integrity and independence. It thus consistently refused to work with companies where actual or potential conflict of interest might be involved."[18] Brundtland also supported the formulation of guidelines that would put "safeguards in place to prevent conflicts of interest or infringement of WHO's impartiality."[19] Still, in

---

12. WHO Document, 2000, EB105/SR/2, p. 43. WHO Library.
13. WHO Document, 2001, EB107/SR/12, p. 157. WHO Library.
14. WHO Document, 2001, EB107/SR/11, p. 154. WHO Library.
15. WHO Document, 2001, EB107/SR/12, p. 157. WHO Library.
16. WHO Document, 2002, EB109/SR/2, p. 42. WHO Library.
17. WHO Document, 2001, EB107/SR/11, p. 154. WHO Library.
18. WHO Document, 1999, WHA52/A/SR/5. WHO Library.
19. Ibid.

this debate, supporters of improved relations with the private sector generally had the upper hand (Bruno 2000). At least in one case, when facing the prospect of alienating a powerful industry, the WHO secretariat chose to pacify it instead, as I describe below.

"Food Is not Tobacco"

The WHO started focusing on the problem of obesity in the 2000s, citing a rise in the number of obese adults from an estimated 200 million in 1995 to more than 300 million in 2000, many of them in the developing world (Brody 2005). In 2003, a joint WHO/FAO scientific report, *Diet, Nutrition, and the Prevention of Chronic Diseases,* analyzed the increasing rates of obesity, heart disease, strokes, and diabetes in poorer countries, and made a number of policy recommendations (WHO/FAO 2003). The report, which was prepared by a group of independent scientists, identified sugar in soft drinks and television advertising aimed at children among the primary reasons for the dangerous global rise in these conditions. The report recommended that sugar should account for no more than 10 percent of a person's energy consumption (Boseley 2003a, Naik 2003). This recommendation infuriated the sugar industry, which claimed that a 25 percent sugar intake was acceptable (Boseley 2003b).

The WHO secretariat planned to publish global guidelines on healthy eating based on the WHO/FAO report, including the recommendation that sugar should account for no more than 10 percent of a healthy diet. Before these guidelines were published, however, the American Sugar Association sent a letter to Brundtland, in which it warned that it would "exercise every avenue available to expose the dubious nature" of the report, and threatened to challenge U.S. funding of the WHO (Boseley 2003b). In an attempt to avoid a full-scale confrontation with the sugar industry, the WHO secretariat immediately asserted that the recommendations on sugar consumption were guidelines rather than standards requiring regulation (Barber and Sevastopulos 2003). In another conciliatory step, Brundtland invited top food industry executives from big multinational companies—including Unilever, Coca-Cola, Pepsico, Nestlé, and McDonald's—to discuss the WHO's future strategies and share *the companies'* ideas on how to encourage consumers to eat a healthier diet and exercise more (Williams 2003). The WHO, somewhat defensively, justified it relations with the food industry by declaring that

> Food is not tobacco. The food and beverage industries are part of the
> solution. They have an important role to play in achieving the best pos-

sible global strategy. We have been arranging a series of transparent discussions where all parties can discuss practical solutions for better diet, which do not in any way compromise the interests of public health.[20]

In the meeting with the executives, an accommodating Brundtland stated, "We believe that companies such as yours can make a major contribution towards . . . promoting healthier diets and lifestyles" (Kapp 2003). Brundtland insisted that the report would form "the critical science-based foundation" of the WHO's strategy and that the WHO would safeguard the integrity of its policymaking process (Kapp 2003). However, the Global Strategy on Diet, Physical Activity and Health, which was endorsed by the World Health Assembly in resolution WHA57.17 in 2004, did not set specific limits on consumption, but instead emphasized that dietary recommendations were a matter for national governments (Williams 2004). The cultivation of better relations with the food sector continued into the implementation stage of the Global Strategy. The food industry was not involved in determining standards or guidelines, and the WHO put limits on the type of programs food and sugar companies could endorse—for example, the WHO objected to food companies financially supporting physical activity programs—but the WHO secretariat attempted to incorporate the food and sugar sectors in other ways.[21] According to Tim Armstrong, from the WHO Department of Chronic Diseases and Health Promotion,

> When I started working on this project in 2002 . . . [food companies] were very suspicious of us. They didn't want to talk with the WHO at all. They were terrified that there's going to be some sort of [regulatory] action on "junk food." . . . But at least since 2004 we established a private sector dialogue group to address some of the recommendations that were made in the Global Strategy document. And we had a very different relationship with the industry. We worked particularly hard to allow them to discuss their issues, look to see how they can address the issues and recommendations that emerged in the strategy. . . . We recognize that they don't have public health at heart . . . no matter what they may say, but WHO recognizes that—although it's a cliché—industry is part of the solution not part of the problem, that food is not tobacco and it's very clearly a different set of issues around

---

20. WHO statement, 9 January 2003, available at http://www.who.int/mediacentre/news/statements/2003/statement1/en/index.html.

21. Interview by the author with Tim Armstrong, Department of Chronic Diseases and Health Promotion, WHO, Geneva, Switzerland, 28 May 2008.

food. And there are opportunities to harness the private sector expertise. If we want product reformulation . . . the only people that can do it is in the industry . . . industry has to be part of that discussion.[22]

In this case, then, even as the sugar and food companies tried to undermine the WHO's legitimacy and expertise, the WHO secretariat insisted on cultivating working relations with them.

In practice, however, the WHO's attempts to lure industry did not lead to a large volume of corporate donations or other forms of participation. One explanation for the limited engagement by business in global health initiatives is that the WHO staff was still regarded with suspicion by many companies. In response to a question regarding the WHO's relations with the private sector, Seth Berkley, the CEO of International AIDS Vaccine Initiative suggested:

> They [the WHO staff] are better than they were. [For years] there's been this very negative feeling about industry. In those days . . . industry wasn't allowed in the building. And if one industry came everybody had to come . . . otherwise you're giving special preference. There were all these kinds of rules. . . . And so [compared to the past] it's gotten better. And certainly today people [at the WHO] understand the importance of industry, but it's still hard to work with [the WHO] and there's a lot of discomfort about it.[23]

Indeed, the number of companies working with the WHO has been quite limited and their donations unimpressive. As of 2000, business contributions represented less than 1 percent of the WHO budget.[24] By 2006, the WHO had entered into approximately ninety partnerships, compared to UNICEF, which reported approximately a thousand partnerships or alliances (Utting and Zammit 2006). While in principle the new attitude deviated greatly from that of the past, in practice the WHO did not have great success in incorporating business into its partnerships.

When Business Is Part of the Problem: The Tobacco Industry

While enthusiastically seeking partnerships with business, the WHO also embraced a number of policies and programs that contradicted its new probusiness orientation. Most prominent was the WHO's crusade against the tobacco sector.

---

22. Ibid.
23. Interview by the author with Seth Berkley, CEO and founder of IAVI, New York, 19 February 2009.
24. WHO Document, 2000, EB105/SR/2, p. 43. WHO Library.

Discussions at the WHO on the health hazards of smoking had begun in the 1970s. At the time, WHO activities around smoking were mostly educational, involving conferences, reports, and information kits, with little attention given to the actual activities of the tobacco industry. Part of the reluctance was the negative effect that a campaign against smoking would have had on tobacco growers, who mostly resided in the global South, while most smokers were in the global North.[25] In the 1980s, however, the WHO noted a shift in tobacco consumption from developed to developing countries and began to criticize the tobacco industry for actively contributing to this shift. Director-General Mahler stated before the Executive Board that smoking in developing countries was on the increase due mainly to "intensive and ruthless promotional campaigns on the part of the tobacco industry."[26] During most of the 1990s, such criticisms were no longer heard and observers complained that "there is nothing bold . . . in WHO's approach to the tobacco industry" (Godlee 1994b), but toward the end of Nakajima's term smoking turned into a major WHO campaign. In May 1996, the World Health Assembly adopted resolution WHA49.17 for the development of a WHO framework "convention" on tobacco control. For the first time in the WHO's history, member states agreed to make the policies binding.[27] When Brundtland was elected director-general, she declared tobacco control as one of her priorities and the implementation of the 1996 tobacco resolution began in earnest (Roemer, Taylor, and Lariviere 2005). Given Brundtland's attempt to change the antibusiness reputation

---

25. In an Executive Board meeting, in 1989, the representative from Malawi stated that

[Malawi] had never disputed or belittled the health hazards of tobacco. . . . However, there was another side to the story, where the realities and problems were equally genuine, and remained unresolved. There were . . . well over 100 million people, who depended on tobacco for their survival, and 120 countries were engaged in tobacco production. Tobacco was the backbone of several economies and, without the income from it many health budgets and in some cases entire government revenues would collapse.

Malawi related its concerns to the structural inequality between North and South:

It was not difficult to show that the tobacco or health programme [initiated by the WHO] would transfer to the tobacco-dependent poorer countries as many or more deaths and illnesses ascribable to the poverty caused by the loss of income from tobacco. . . . There was clearly a conflict between the economic needs of the poorer countries and the health requirements of some of the rich ones, but it always seemed to be the poor who suffered.

These forceful statements later lost some of their weight when it was discovered that the industry was behind protobacco positions of some officials from developing countries and that the International Tobacco Growers' Association, which claimed to represent the interests of tobacco farmers in the developing world and argued that the WHO tobacco campaign could destroy their livelihoods, was a "front" for the industry's lobbying activities (WHO Document, 1989, EB83/SR/10, pp. 129–130, WHO Library; WHO Document, 1980, WHA33/B/SR/15, pp. 346–347, WHO Library; Fairclough 2000).

26. WHO Document, 1986, EB77/SR/9, p. 129. WHO Library.

27. The idea of an international convention for tobacco control originated in a collaboration between Ruth Roemer, author of *Legislative Action to Combat the World Tobacco Epidemic,* and Allyn L. Taylor, who advocated that the WHO utilize its constitutional authority to advance global public health and suggested the possibility of developing a specific international regulatory mechanism for tobacco control (Roemer, Taylor, and Lariviere 2005).

of the WHO, this was a surprising goal to prioritize. A number of considerations, however, made the tobacco companies an attractive target.

First, an antismoking initiative affirmed the WHO's new commitment to noncommunicable diseases. Maybe one of the major shifts in the WHO in the late 1990s was turning noncommunicable diseases into a legitimate area of WHO involvement. The WHO staff was able to change the long-held perception that noncommunicable diseases were a concern of rich countries alone, and therefore of limited interest to the WHO, by drawing on recent data that had shown that the burden of diseases in poor countries had been shifting from infectious diseases to noncommunicable and chronic diseases. Notably, the ability to show such a shift in the burden of disease in the developing world was not simply due to increased prevalence but also to the ways the burden of diseases was then being measured. The report most widely used for asserting the global burden of various diseases, by Christopher Murray of the Harvard School of Public Health and the WHO researcher Alan Lopez (Murray and Lopez 1996), used World Bank's DALYs as the measuring unit (see chapter 5). Because DALYs incorporate information on individuals' years of partial productivity due to disease, rather than only measuring premature death, this approach led to a much greater appreciation of the cost of chronic diseases than previous measures. Using DALYs, Allyn Taylor and Douglas Bettcher, both at the Tobacco Free Initiative at the WHO, showed that cigarette smoking had become one of the largest causes of preventable death worldwide and that it would be the leading cause of premature death worldwide within thirty years (Taylor and Bettcher 2000; see also Beaglehole and Yach 2003).

Another development that permitted focus on "lifestyle" diseases such as smoking that in poor countries normally afflicted only the better-off segment of the population was the WHO's "new universalism" approach, which focused on the number of victims rather than on the socioeconomic vulnerabilities of the victims (see chapter 6). For example, in an attempt to refute a study which had concluded that noncommunicable diseases were not important to the poor by comparing causes of death in the world's poorest 20 percent of the population to the causes of death in the world's richest 20 percent (Gwatkin, Guillot, and Heuveline 1999), other researchers argued that by ignoring the middle 60 percent of the world's population, who also lived mostly in less-developed regions, the study "subvert[ed] the efforts of less-developed countries to address important policy issues related to global determinants of noncommunicable diseases," such as tobacco (Reddy 1999). Hence, Taylor and Bettcher could legitimate a WHO-led smoking campaign by showing that the majority of smokers (800 million of 1.25 billion) lived in developing countries, without having to refer to the socioeconomic status of those smokers (Taylor and Bettcher 2000).

A second incentive that led Brundtland to focus on tobacco was the fact that during the years of the WHO's relative neglect of it, the World Bank had taken the lead on the issue. In the early 1990s, a World Bank economist, Howard Barnum, published a series of articles in which he argued that the economic benefits of tobacco were more than offset by direct and indirect morbidity and mortality costs from tobacco use (Barnum 1994). A WHO antismoking campaign allowed a channel through which to reclaim the WHO's leadership in a global health matter, but one in which the WHO could complement, rather than contradict, the World Bank position.[28] What was more, smoking was not a narrowly medical issue and could therefore attract the attention of policymakers other than health ministers to the workings of the WHO, which was one of Brundtland's goals toward reviving the organization. According to Katherine Deland, of the WHO Tobacco Free Initiative:

> Brundtland saw an enormous strategic opportunity for the WHO, which had never ever been invited to talk to ministries of foreign affairs, ministries of finance, ministries of agriculture, this was not where we had entry. All of a sudden there was a tremendous opportunity to expand WHO's influence ... and to affect domestic policy.[29]

Brundtland could therefore imagine a cross-agency collaboration motivated by public health concerns:

> The Framework Convention process will activate all those areas of governance that have a direct impact on public health. Science and economics will mesh with legislation and litigation. Health ministers will work with their counterparts in finance, trade, labor, agriculture and social affairs ministries to give public health the place it deserves. (Brundtland 2000b)

While wanting the WHO to take the lead, Brundtland sought, as she had done for other projects, the collaboration and backing of the World Bank. Such collaboration provided the economic expertise that contributed to the legitimacy of the endeavor. Specifically, the WHO secretariat relied on World Bank analysis to assuage the concern that tobacco control would harm the economy in poor countries that were heavily dependent on tobacco (Jha and Chaloupka 1999, Collin 2004). The WHO also relied on the World Bank to ensure that the recommended tobacco control measures would be considered cost effective. Already in 1997, the

---

28. Interview by the author with Katherine Deland, Tobacco Free Initiative, WHO, Geneva, Switzerland, 2 June 2008.
    29. Ibid.

World Bank, in partnership with the WHO, began a global study to establish the most effective methods of curbing the prevalence and consumption of tobacco products (Ruger 2005). A report summarizing the findings of the study, *Curbing the Epidemic: Governments and the Economics of Tobacco Control,* argued that the single most effective way to reduce demand for tobacco was to raise taxes (Jha and Chaloupka 1999). Other highly cost-effective measures included improvements in the quality and extent of information, comprehensive bans on tobacco advertising and promotion, prominent warning labels, restrictions on smoking on public places, and increased access to nicotine replacement treatments (Lancaster et al. 2000).

A crusade against the powerful tobacco sector, however, could have risked the WHO's improved relations with business. The WHO secretariat was able to avoid such implications, and strategically resist the dominant probusiness logic, by presenting its attempt to regulate the tobacco industry as an exceptional case that proved the probusiness rule. Specifically, an explicit demonization of the tobacco industry was used to assure other industries that the WHO's position against tobacco companies did not reflect WHO's general position toward business: the WHO secretariat did not criticize market principles but instead emphasized all the inherent features of tobacco selling that made the tobacco sector a legitimate exception.

Hence, in defending the WHO position, Brundtland likened the role of the tobacco industry in creating health problems to that of the mosquito in causing malaria: both were blood-sucking, disease-spreading parasites (*The Economist* 2000). Unlike mosquitoes, moreover, tobacco companies were not innocent. This account provided a villain that was accountable to its deeds. According to Katherine Deland,

> It's hard to demonize a mosquito. [Mosquitoes] are not bad guys, really. They just function in the world doing what mosquitoes do. Corporate malfeasance is something that gives people a hook. Also it gets people more emotionally invested.[30]

Additionally, it was easier to demonize the tobacco industry than the producers of infant formula or sugar. There was solid scientific evidence establishing the harm caused by smoking, contrasting with the product's lack of any intrinsic benefit, and there was irrefutable legal evidence showing that tobacco companies had been long aware of the harm caused by smoking. The tobacco sector could only rely on the principles of an individual's free choice and responsibility to

---

30. Ibid.

defend itself, principles countered by the pointing to the addictiveness of nicotine and to the power of aggressive marketing.

In its criticisms of the tobacco sector, the WHO staff relied on the same rationale that it used to justify engagement with the public sector, namely, the notion that corporations could be and were socially responsible, and therefore potentially "part of the solution." According to neoliberal arguments, corporations were not only able to govern themselves more efficiently when there was less government regulation, but also to govern themselves responsibly. The WHO secretariat made use of both claims. For example, in accordance with the first claim, the organization sought to learn from Coca Cola's expertise how to deliver medicines to remote villages but, in accordance with the second claim, the secretariat also wanted Coca Cola to responsibly restrain the marketing of their sugar-inflated drinks. The WHO leadership took advantage of the new perception of business as responsible partners to lure businesses into cooperation on global health issues, but the WHO secretariat wanted to use those same claims to identify, and discipline, those businesses that were obviously not cooperating. Stella Bialous, of the WHO Tobacco Free Initiative, reported: "The unique feature of tobacco products—which kill their consumers when used as directed by the manufacturer—renders the ongoing operations of the tobacco companies incompatible with the very notion of Corporate Social Responsibility. . . . Tobacco industry and health promotion goals are mutually exclusive: no partnership is possible."[31] Through such differentiation of corporate behaviors, the WHO bureaucracy was able to strategically use the same reasoning that justified its relations with business to also mobilize against exceptional cases.

Turning the tobacco industry into a villain was used to justify the regulation of the sector; it also enabled the WHO secretariat to present its position on this particular industry as an exception to its generally positive attitude toward business, and in that way to assure other industries that the WHO's position against the tobacco industry did not reflect its position against business as a whole. Given the sinking reputation of the tobacco industry, mostly due to extensive legal cases in the United States, which demonstrated that tobacco companies had deliberately lied about their knowledge on smoking's health risks and addictiveness, it was possible to distinguish the tobacco industry from all other commercial enterprises. To set the tobacco industry apart from legitimate business, the WHO leadership and staff used particularly critical language. A cigarette, Brundtland claimed, "is the only product which when used as intended, will kill one half of its consumers" (cited in Giles and Thornhill 2000), and "a cigarette is a euphemism

31. United Nations Ad Hoc Inter-Agency Task Force on Tobacco Control, Report of the Sixth Session, Geneva, Switzerland, 30 November—1 December 2005.

for a cleverly crafted product that delivers just the right amount of nicotine to keep its user addicted for life before killing the person" (cited in Williams 1999a). Unlike other commodities, cigarettes were "*inherently* dangerous products" designed by tobacco companies to create and maintain nicotine addiction (cited in Williams 1999a). Not only the inherent danger of the product but also the marketing practices of tobacco companies were used to establish the immorality of the industry. The tobacco companies targeted young people, women, and "those less advantaged from the educational, social and economic points of view."[32] The WHO staff emphasized the unfair imbalance between the global industry and the consumers, particularly in the developing world and rejected the claims that smokers knew the risks or that they were making a deliberate choice (Giles and Thornhill 2000). Brundtland described smoking as a "communicable disease"—through advertising (Giles and Thornhill 2000)—and other WHO staff warned that many poor countries in Asia, Africa, and Latin America found it hard to fight against American, British, and Japanese multinational conglomerates (Taylor and Bettcher 2000, *The Economist* 2000).[33] Such distinctions allowed the WHO to be "unapologetic about cold-shouldering the tobacco-industry devils" (*The Economist* 2000).

In May 1999, the World Health Assembly unanimously voted to begin negotiations on a Framework Convention on Tobacco Control (Collin, Lee, and Bissell 2003: 85). The tobacco industry vigorously opposed the convention. At times, opposition was voiced by individuals who did not disclose their association with the industry, who couched their arguments as concerns that the WHO's tobacco programs diverted its attention from issues of much greater concern for poor countries (Scruton 2001). *The Economist* argued that such programs were a matter of social and economic policy far beyond the WHO's traditional medical remit and that they marked a misguided attempt at supranational regulation of a problem far better tackled by countries on their own (*The Economist* 2000), and an editorial at the *Wall Street Journal* insisted that smoking was a matter of "a free choice with health consequences" (cited in *Lancet* 2000). Imitating the tactics used by the infant formula and pharmaceutical sectors, tobacco companies also agreed on a voluntary, self-regulatory code of conduct that was presented as an alternative to the treaty (Fairclough and Branch 2001, Langley 2003). The voluntary code was announced on September 11, 2001, and as a result attracted no attention. In any event, the voluntary pact had convinced few of the supporters of

---

32. WHO Document, 1986, EB77/SR/9, p. 129. WHO Library.
33. Taylor and Bettcher (2000) also criticized international trade agreements that allowed for the liberalization of unmanufactured tobacco for enhancing the ability of multinational tobacco conglomerates to expand into other markets.

an international treaty, including at the WHO. Derek Yach from the Tobacco Free Initiative responded: "Our experience has been that a self-regulatory approach does not work" (Olson 2001).

Disclosures of past "systematic . . . effort by the tobacco industry to undermine tobacco control policy" in the UN system (Williams 1999b) and to "contain, neutralize, [and] reorient" WHO's tobacco control initiatives (Vedantam 2001) made it easy to prohibit the participation of the industry in the negotiations over the treaty (see also Godlee 2000, Zeltner et al. 2000). Still, the industry's position was represented by a number of countries with big tobacco companies or tobacco growers, including Japan, China, Germany, Argentina, Malawi, Turkey, Russia, Zimbabwe, and the United States.[34] In some cases, tobacco companies persuaded countries to send delegates who were sympathetic to the industry, typically agriculture or finance ministry officials, rather than health officials; in other cases, representatives of tobacco companies even served on member state delegations during the negotiations (Bates 2001, Gilmore and Collin 2002, Collin, Lee, and Bissell 2003: 86, Langley 2003). The companies and the governments behind them opposed many central provisions, including taxes on tobacco products, limitations on free trade, public smoking bans that failed to provide smoking areas, and "shock" images on health warnings (Roemer, Taylor, and Lariviere 2005).

Given the effective counterpressures from the tobacco sector, many of the provisions in the convention were weaker than supporters had originally hoped for. Still, in 2003 WHO member states finally agreed on an international tobacco control treaty, in which they committed to a number of steps aimed at reducing smoking in their countries. The treaty included a ban on tobacco advertising (except where a ban would violate national laws, as in the United States), encouraged nations to raise tobacco taxes, and called for specific steps to control tobacco use, such as requiring that health warnings on cigarettes packages took up 30 to 50 percent of the display area (Ruger 2005: 66, Roemer, Taylor, and Lariviere 2005). Although the U.S. government had warned the WHO that it was unlikely to sign the treaty unless governments were allowed to opt out of any provision they found objectionable, the U.S. delegation eventually voted in favor of the treaty

---

34. The United States was in an awkward position, since it had been exporting more cigarettes than any other nation in the world (more than one of every five traded), while having quite restrictive regulations at home. In the first round of negotiations, under the Clinton administration, the United States supported the treaty, but its negotiators indicated that the United States would not support a comprehensive ban on tobacco industry advertising because of constitutional protections of free speech. This attitude moved radically nearer to the tobacco industry's position under the George W. Bush administration, partly due to greater links between the industry and the Republican Party (Waxman 2002)

and the WHO's 192 members adopted the framework convention on tobacco control unanimously (Stein and Kaufman 2003). Governments had a year to decide whether to ratify the treaty, with forty ratifications needed for the treaty to come into force. The Framework Convention on Tobacco Control entered into force on February 27, 2005.

A vigorous campaign against the tobacco sector promised some institutional benefits to the WHO secretariat, but it could also be perceived as defiance of rich countries' expectations that the UN agencies improved their relations with the private sector. Given the close ties between tobacco companies and the governments of the U.S., Germany, and Japan, among others, the WHO secretariat risked punitive measures from particularly powerful governments. However, the WHO secretariat avoided such measures by justifying its opposition to the tobacco sector using reframed neoliberal probusiness sentiments. By regarding the immoral actions of the tobacco sector as an exception to the generally benevolent behavior of companies in the market, the WHO secretariat was able to present its antitobacco position as consistent with the neoliberal logic, so that even those countries objecting to the initiative did not question the WHO's commitment to probusiness principles and, while achieving significant concessions, voted in favor of the convention. In short, the WHO's campaign against the tobacco industry was made possible within a neoliberal context by justifying it in terms that reproduced, rather than rejected, the neoliberal support of a free market. A similar strategy was utilized to defend the production of generic versions of AIDS drugs.

AIDS: Access to Drugs

International organizations, including both the WHO and the World Bank, were slow to respond to the AIDS crisis as it emerged (see chapter 5). Between 1986 and 1997, the World Bank committed merely $500.5 million in credits and loans to AIDS projects, most of which were components of larger loans. During those years, the World Bank's reluctance to support AIDS projects was partly because its strategy for the health sector emphasized reform of the health systems, which was perceived as the route to improvements in all health outcomes over the longer run (see chapter 4). This focus on health systems meant a conscious lack of attention to any single disease, including HIV/AIDS. In 1992, the World Bank was still warning that "an expanded role of the Bank in AIDS should not be allowed to overtake the critical agenda for strengthening health systems" (Simms 2007).

Not long after the establishment of UNAIDS, however, the World Bank changed its course and started to consider the serious economic implications of the AIDS epidemic (World Bank 1997, World Bank 2005). In 1999, a publication by the bank, *Intensifying Action against HIV/AIDS in Africa: Responding to a Developmental Crisis,* declared that the epidemic was the main development challenge facing Africa (World Bank 1999). Following the World Bank, other international organizations also referred to AIDS as a development issue (Parker 2000). UNAIDS, too, adopted an approach to AIDS that, according to UNAIDS Executive Director Peter Piot, was "far more in the tradition of development" (cited in Hegland and Walker 2007). Advocacy, therefore, focused on the economic implications of neglect. Piot, in an interview to *National Journal,* explained:

> If we don't deal with AIDS and bring it under control, we can forget everything else, at least in Africa. It kills the teachers, it kills the doctors. . . . You can't do development with dead people. What makes AIDS so very special is that unlike any other health problem, it kills people in their most productive years of life, and it is not directly linked with poverty. Because it's transmitted through sex, you find it much more often in the more wealthy [and productive] sectors of societies: South Africa, Botswana, Swaziland, Namibia—these are by far not the poorest countries in Africa. (cited in Hegland and Walker 2007)

According to Parker (2000), the reconceptualization of AIDS as a question of economic development subjected it to cost-effective calculations "devoid of any real ethical reflection." The World Bank and others considered prevention the most cost-effective means to reduce the loss of disability-adjusted life years (World Bank 1993), enabling governments to achieve the best return for their investment in light of limited health budgets. Such cost-effective logic justified the rejection of AIDS drugs as appropriate for poor countries (World Bank 1992).

Over time, however, the World Bank, the U.S. government and others were forced to reverse their position. In 2002, UN members established the Global Fund to fight AIDS, Tuberculosis, and Malaria (see below). In 2003, President George W. Bush established the U.S. President's Emergency Plan for AIDS Relief (PEPFAR) to fight AIDS in Africa and the Caribbean. Both programs were committed to the funding and distribution of AIDS drugs. Also in 2003, the WHO and UNAIDS launched the "3 by 5" initiative, with a plan to provide antiretroviral treatment to 3 million people living with AIDS ("3") in low- and middle-income countries by the end of 2005 ("5").

A large number of factors contributed to the radical shift in the international position, including an unprecedented global mobilization of AIDS activists, an international struggle by low- and middle-income countries, and the reduction of the prices of AIDS drugs (partly due to competition coming from manufacturers of generic versions of AIDS drugs in India and elsewhere).[35] Throughout those developments, the World Health Assembly was often used as a site where low- and middle-income countries expressed their grievances, with the WHO staff playing a relatively passive role as mediator between competing interests. In earlier stages of the debate, however, the WHO staff had taken a proactive, and potentially controversial, position regarding a World Trade Organization (WTO) agreement on intellectual property rights.

In 1996, the same year that donors established UNAIDS, researchers found that new combination of therapies that included a protease inhibitor were extending the lives of HIV/AIDS patients. However, low- and middle-income countries could not afford these antiretroviral drugs (ARVs), which at the time cost more than ten thousand dollars per patient per year. One way to bypass such expense was to manufacture locally or to export generic versions of the drugs, which were much cheaper. However, an agreement signed under the auspices of the WTO in 1994—the Trade-Related Intellectual Property Rights agreement (TRIPS)—threatened the future legality of the generic manufacturing of ARVs, since the agreement required member states to grant pharmaceutical companies patent protection of any invention, including protection of both a product and the chemical production process, for a minimum of twenty years.[36]

The WHO was silent during the Uruguay Round of multilateral trade negotiations that led to TRIPS and other agreements. But starting in 1996, Executive Board members and delegates to the World Health Assemblies had contentious discussions regarding TRIPS and its effect on public health. These discussions also mobilized the WHO staff. At the World Health Assembly in May 1996, at the end of an otherwise conventional discussion on the rational use of drugs, Iran, which was not a member at the WTO, stated that it "was very much concerned about the impact of the World Trade Organization on pharmaceutical industries in developing countries," and sponsored Resolution WHA49.14 that asked the director-general to "report on the impact of the work of the . . . WTO with respect to national drug policies and essential drugs."[37] The task was given to the WHO Action Program on Essential Drugs (DAP), which a year later published a report entitled, *Globalization and Access to Drugs: Implications of the WTO/TRIPS Agreement* (WHO 1997).

35. See Bond 2003, Shadlen 2004, Sell and Prakash 2004, Friedman and Mottiar 2005, Schwartländer, Grubb, and Perriëns 2006, Klug 2008.

36. On the negotiations leading to the WTO intellectual property agreement see Sell 2003, Drahos and Braithwaite 2003.

37. The original wording of the resolution also mentioned "generic concepts," a phrase that was eventually eliminated from the resolution. WHO Document, 1996, WHA49/A/SR/5, WHO Library; interview by the author with Germán Velásquez, Drug Action Programme, World Health Organization, Geneva, Switzerland, 3 June 2008.

The DAP's position on intellectual property rights was more critical, and potentially confrontational, than the more conciliatory position the Director-General Office adopted (see below). Even the DAP, however, chose strategic rather than passive resistance, offering a strong defense for universal access to drugs without questioning the principles governing the quest for trade liberalization and intellectual property protection.

On the one hand, the WHO report did not hesitate to criticize the foundations of the TRIPS agreement and its likely uneven consequences. The report mentioned that "intellectual property rights were included in the agenda of the Uruguay Round on the initiative of industrialized countries, following pressure from a variety of economic groups," and that, "it is . . . very clear that the Uruguay Round negotiations were largely dominated by industrialized countries and that developing countries were constrained to accept commitments sometimes running counter to their economic and social development." The report also asserted that, "because the geographical distribution of know-how is concentrated in industrialized countries, this harmonization [of intellectual property laws] is likely to strengthen their existing economic superiority, in particular by prohibiting developing countries from copying a new product by reverse engineering, and thereby developing their own technology" (WHO 1997).

On the other hand, in regard to the central issue of concern to the report—the effect of TRIPS on access to drugs in developing countries—the report was able to assert its support of the principle of universal access to drugs without in any respect challenging the principle of intellectual property protection. The report first defended the concept of universal access to essential drugs in normative terms:

> Drugs . . . are an integral part of the realization of a fundamental human right—the right to health. That is why they are classified as essential goods, to emphasize that they have to be accessible for all people.
>
> The concept of accessibility . . . means that policies pursued must aim to make drugs available for all who wish to have them, and at affordable prices. (WHO 1997)

However, instead of insisting that access to drugs should overrule the liberalization of trade, the report suggested that the two principles were entirely compatible. After all, both the WHO and the WTO were concerned with improved access:

> This objective [access to drugs] *coincides* with the general objective of the GATT for the last 40 years—seeking to eliminate barriers to trade so that consumers have the greatest possible access to all the goods available in the world. (WHO 1997, emphasis added)

While arguing that "pharmaceutical products cannot be regarded as ordinary goods or products," the report did not rely on normative argumentation to justify the protection of public health. Crucially, it did not ask to exclude medicines from the realm of trade agreements. Rather, the report suggested that trade agreements, *if interpreted correctly,* already achieved an appropriate "balance between intellectual property and accessibility." To support this argument, the report provided a detailed legal interpretation of various provisions in TRIPS to show that the agreement was compatible with the health needs of developing countries.

Concretely, the report offered a legal interpretation of TRIPS that showed that the agreement "expressly provides two means of obtaining exceptions and limiting the exclusive rights conferred by the patent on its owner," and maintained that "these two provisions may be used to ensure greater accessibility to essential drugs." The first exception was compulsory licensing, which allowed the exploitation of a patent by a third person without the owner's consent. The report argued that according to Article 31 of TRIPS, "national public authorities may be allowed, within the conditions laid down in the Agreement, to issue compulsory licenses against the patent owner's will when justified by the public interest." The second exception was parallel imports. According to the WHO report, "the Agreement does not prohibit parallel imports," so governments were not prohibited from buying a patented drug from a third party without the owner's consent. In justifying their support of parallel imports, the authors again drew on general principles of free trade: "From the perspective of trade liberalization, it is considered that from the moment the product is marketed, the patent holder can no longer control its subsequent circulation" (WHO 1997).

Rather than costly defiance, then, the WHO report's resistance was consciously strategic. The report incorporated its interpretation into the dominant principles rather than trying to replace them. The report did not rely on human rights concerns to justify protection of access to drugs, it did not rely on public health expertise to challenge the legal agreement, it did not criticize the TRIPS agreement or the agenda of trade liberalization, and it did not call for the revision of TRIPS. Instead, the report used legal reasoning to make the case that TRIPS was entirely reconcilable with concerns for access to drugs. The legal interpretation of TRIPS did not attempt to negate TRIPS or the principles it stood for, but sought rather to use the same principles to defend universal access. In this way, the WHO's call for access to drugs could be presented not as reflecting opposition to neoliberalism or globalization but, to the contrary, as entirely compatible with them. Just as the WHO secretariat had utilized economic expertise to strategically comply with the World Bank's and donors' concern with economic growth (see chapter 6), here they utilized legal expertise—the WTO's own tools of expertise—to provide a more favorable interpretation of a WTO agreement.

The DAP was the first to provide a legal interpretation that allowed the use of TRIPS to defend, rather than prohibit, the manufacturing of generic drugs. This interpretation later guided the mobilization of health activists, like Oxfam, Médecins Sans Frontières (MSF), and James Love of CPTech. According to Germán Velásquez, one of the authors of the report,

> At that time, nobody was talking about the possible flexibilities of the [TRIPS] agreement. . . . There was a clear statement from WTO that there was no flexibility in the TRIPS agreement. And [the WHO report] started with a larger look into the possible flexibility, and this is the first document . . . before MSF, before Oxfam, before everybody talking about the compulsory licensing, talking about parallel importation, talking about . . . the flexibilities of the TRIPS agreement.
>
> Because we are identifying *in a very technical way* what are the flexibilities; analyzing: this is the text of the TRIPS agreement, and here there are some comments and here we are insisting what are the possibilities of all the things. If you see Article 31 of the TRIPS agreement it is not talking about compulsory licensing—this is the first time . . . "Other Use Without Authorization of the Right Holder"—this is the title of Article 31. . . . You don't have any mention of the compulsory licensing in the TRIPS agreement, and this is the first time that came. And a few months after that, probably six months after, there was Jimmy Love and some NGOs organizing a meeting here in Geneva that was called "Meeting on Article 31," and there they launched the idea of the compulsory license.[38]

The report's technical-legal interpretation of TRIPS did not completely pacify the pharmaceutical sector or the U.S. government. A letter from the vice president of the Pharmaceutical Research and Manufacturers of America (PhRMA) to the World Health Organization considered the report "a deeply flawed document that misleads the public," and the U.S. government prepared a seventeen-page paper "pointing out the inaccuracies and false implications with which the document is riddled" (cited in Velásquez, Correa, and Balasubramanlam 2004: 87). The U.S. government demanded that the WHO revise the publication and Brundtland agreed to ask independent experts to review the report. However, the new version of the report (WHO 1999b), which the United States no longer objected to, made only minor alterations to the previous one.[39]

---

38. Interview by the author with Germán Velásquez, Drug Action Programme, World Health Organization, Geneva, Switzerland, 3 June 2008. Emphasis added.
39. Velásquez, Correa, and Balasubramanlam 2004: 88; also interview by the author with Germán Velásquez, Drug Action Programme, World Health Organization, Geneva, Switzerland, 3 June 3, 2008.

Ultimately, the acceptance of the legal interpretation that allowed the use of flexibilities in TRIPS for the manufacturing and purchasing of generic versions of patented drugs was due to political struggles occurring outside the WHO, in South Africa, Brazil, Thailand, India, and the United States, as well as the WTO.[40] In November 2001, WTO members signed the *Declaration on the TRIPS Agreement and Public Health* (the Doha Declaration), which, explicitly drawing on WHO terms, stated, "We agree that the TRIPS Agreement does not and should not prevent members from taking measures to protect public health. . . . We reaffirm the right of WTO members to use, to the full, the provisions in the TRIPS Agreement, which provide flexibility for [protecting public health and promoting access to medicines for all]" (WTO 2001). After two years of further negotiations, the "30 August 2003 Decision" (WT/L/540) specified the conditions under which poor countries without pharmaceutical manufacturing capacity would be allowed to import generic versions of drugs still under patent. In subsequent WHO reports and publications, including a special issue of the *Bulletin of the World Health Organization* (Türmen and Clift 2006), WHO staff continued to critically review the effectiveness of the Doha Declaration and the 30 August Decision in increasing access to medicines in poor countries.

This successful engagement notwithstanding, the WHO under Brundtland did not seek a central role in the global fight against AIDS. It is likely that with the creation of UNAIDS in 1996 and the founding of the Global Fund to Fight AIDS, Tuberculosis, and Malaria in 2002, the WHO leadership considered any quest for leadership in this arena a lost battle (Gellman 2000a). It is also possible that, like Nakajima, Brundtland considered AIDS too controversial an issue, especially as the struggle between pharmaceutical companies and AIDS activists intensified. Brundtland therefore sought a conciliatory position, which minimized potential frictions with the pharmaceutical sector. Under Brundtland, for example, the WHO joined negotiations between UNAIDS and brand-name pharmaceutical companies for voluntary discounts, which led to the launching, in March 2000, of an Accelerated Access Initiative, in which five pharmaceutical companies agreed to cut prices for their AIDS drugs in the developing world, but under strict conditions (Gellman 2000a, 2000b, 2000c; Boseley 2002). The joint statement of intent declared, "Intellectual property rights should be protected, in compliance with international agreements, since society depends on them to stimulate innovation." On other occasions, Brundtland reiterated the principle of intellectual

---

40. It is notable, however, that the South African government, which was the first to challenge TRIPS by passing a law that gave the health ministry powers to override drug patents on public health grounds, was influenced by the WHO report. Interview by the author with Germán Velásquez, Drug Action Programme, World Health Organization, Geneva, Switzerland, 3 June 2008.

property protection as essential for innovation and therefore for improved health in poor countries. At the World Economic Forum in Davos, Switzerland, in January 2001, Brundtland announced: "We have to protect patent rights. We need them to ensure that research and development will yield badly needed new tools and technologies" (cited in Motchane 2003), and in other statements she argued that any effort to increase access to drug-company medicines should also include agreements honoring the drug makers' patents (Schoofs and Waldholz 2001). Even in Doha, in November 2001, while reiterating the WHO's principle that "access to health care is a human right," and defining health care to include, "of course, access to life-saving medicines," she was careful to assert that "the issue of patent protection for pharmaceutical products is an area where a fine balance needs to be struck between providing incentives for future inventions of new medicines and ensuring affordable access to existing medicines."[41]

Only when donor countries acceded to the idea that treatment, not only prevention and care, was a fundamental element in the response to the epidemic did the WHO become instrumental in this endeavor. In April 2002, the Twelfth Expert Committee on the Selection and Use of Essential Medicines Meeting added twelve ARVs to the WHO list of essential medicines (Zimmerman 2002). By considering AIDS drugs essential, the WHO bureaucracy expressed unqualified support in the importance of treatment and urged governments to commit their resources for the cause. Later, when donors and international organizations began to support the purchase of generic rather than brand-name AIDS drugs, the WHO Prequalification of Medicines Programme division assessed and qualified generic versions of patented AIDS drugs, mostly from India. The prequalification project had been established in 2001 to provide a reliable reference for countries procuring essential medicines by assessing product dossiers containing relevant data on safety, quality and efficacy, bio-equivalence studies (where appropriate), and manufacturing sites' compliance with WHO Good Manufacturing Practice. By qualifying generic AIDS drugs, the WHO bureaucracy used its expertise to counter opposition to the distribution of generic drugs that relied on the warning that these drugs were not safe. Finally, the WHO launched its own initiative for the provision of AIDS drugs. At the time, it was estimated that there were about 6 million people in poor countries who needed ARV therapy (Brown 2003) and at the Fourteenth International AIDS Conference in Barcelona, in July 2002, Brundtland stated, "We are aiming for 3 million people worldwide to be able to access ARVs by 2005" (Schwartländer, Grubb, and Perriëns 2006).

---

41. Statement by Dr. Gro Harlem Brundtland, Director-General of the World Health Organization, "Globalization, TRIPS, and Access to Medicines," Doha, Qatar, 9–13 November 2001. Statement WHO/17, 9 November 2001, available at http://www.who.int/inf-pr-2001/en/state2001–17.html.

Director-General Lee Jong-wook, who succeeded Brundtland in 2003, made this initiative his signature issue (Lancet 2003). In September 2003, Lee Jong-wook and Peter Piot announced before a special session of the UN General Assembly plans for the WHO and UNAIDS to work with "key partners" to meet the goal of delivering antiretroviral treatment by the end of 2005 to 3 million people living with HIV in developing countries (Lee and Piot 2003).

The argument for the WHO's involvement was that while UNAIDS was a successful advocacy body, and the Global Fund was designed to be an effective financing instrument, no international organization had assumed responsibility for controlling HIV at the country level (Lancet 2003). Hence, the WHO's role was not to provide or pay for the treatment but to give countries the advice and expertise they needed to start their own programs. According to Teguest Guerma, the associate director of the WHO HIV/AIDS Department,

> We were not the ones doing it, what we did [instead was to develop] a strategy . . . and then we told the world that this is going to happen. We prequalified generic drugs. . . . We fought for generic drugs to be used. . . . We developed standardized guidelines, and then a public health approach to be used in the less developed countries, and we really pushed countries to scale up.[42]

In short, in the initial stages of the debate over access to AIDS drugs and intellectual property protection, the WHO was able to strategically resist TRIPS. In subsequent debates over HIV/AIDS, however, the WHO more often followed rather than launched the international response, so by the time WHO initiatives took place they were usually no longer considered controversial. This relative inaction symbolizes the limits of strategic adaptation, as does, to an even greater extent, the rise of public-private partnerships independent of the WHO, as I describe in the following section.

The Limits of Strategic Adaptation: Independent Partnerships

Another explanation for the limited scope of business support for WHO programs, which I discussed above, is that some private foundations, governments, and business engaged with public health initiatives that bypassed the WHO.

---

42. Interview by the author with Teguest Guerma, HIV/AIDS Department, WHO, Geneva, Switzerland, 30 May 2008.

Public-private health partnerships (PPHPs), mostly for the development or distribution of drugs and vaccines, mushroomed in the late 1990s and early 2000s, but most functioned independently of the WHO.

The WHO and the World Bank played an important role in attracting the attention of philanthropists and business to global health issues. Bill Gates's interest in global health, for example, was first provoked by the 1993 World Bank's *World Development Report* (Specter 2005). However, the Bill and Melinda Gates Foundation, which gave more than $13 billion to global health programs between 1994 and 2010,[43] preferred creating its own initiatives to working with international organizations. This was also the case with foundations that before the 1990s had worked closely with the WHO, such as the Rockefeller Foundation.

Independent initiatives were particularly common when the goal was the development of new drugs for neglected diseases, that is, diseases common in poor countries that required drugs which the for-profit pharmaceutical sector had little or no market incentive to develop.[44] The favored solution for this "market failure" was the creation of public-private partnerships that would be financially backed by non-for-profit sources (development agencies, public research institutions, multilateral organizations, and philanthropic foundations). Drug companies were asked to contribute only in-kind or, more importantly, knowledge. Another institutional innovation, which differentiated PPHPs from existing non-for-profit research institutions, like the WHO's Special Programme for Research and Training in Tropical Diseases (TDR) or the U.S. Walter Reed Army Institute of Research, was their reliance on a "social venture capital" model. The partnerships were designed to be virtual drug makers that screened potential projects and channeled funds into selected projects conducted elsewhere (Wheeler and Berkley 2001).

The first public-private research and development partnership that followed such a structure was the International AIDS Vaccine Initiative (IAVI), with the goal of developing a preventive HIV vaccine. The initiative came out of meetings sponsored by the Rockefeller Foundation in Bellagio, Italy, where participants discussed in detail the features of the new model. In those conversations, the parties decided against the involvement of the WHO in the initiative. Seth Berkley, the CEO and founder of IAVI, recounted the considerations leading to the decision to have an independent entity.

---

43. See http://www.gatesfoundation.org/grants/Pages/overview.aspx.

44. Pharmaceutical companies, which "started to be run less by scientists and more by business people," did not invest in research into drugs where they could not see a way to recoup research costs and make a profit. The neglect was exacerbated by incredibly high costs for basic research, clinical trials and registration, and by the rise of a "blockbuster mentality" with expectations of incredibly high profits. Interview by the author with Seth Berkley, CEO and founder of IAVI, New York, 19 February 2009.

> We asked the question, "Should IAVI be part of the UN?" And the answer . . . was confidentially, no, because it won't have the flexibility to work with industry and to move with the speed and everything else. . . . The people in the UN realized that you could never do the stuff we wanted to do in IAVI within the UN. . . . [It] wouldn't have the flexibility, it would be too bureaucratic, it would be too consensus-driven, you couldn't take the risks, you couldn't stand the heat that would occur when you drop something. . . . So there was a sense this couldn't be done in the UN.[45]

As this quotation reflects, IAVI founders viewed the WHO's bureaucratic and political features as an obstacle to achieving results, and they had little trust in the capacity of an international organization to perform. These sentiments were particularly palatable in a neoliberal context that celebrated the private market and denounced political interventions and public bureaucracies (see chapter 5).

IAVI was launched in 1996. In the following years, the Rockefeller Foundation launched a number of similarly structured partnerships.[46] The Gates Foundation, which in 1999 gave $25 million to IAVI, also provided gifts to funds that sought vaccines for malaria and tuberculosis and which replicated the same model. Observers concluded that "a new model for poor-country assistance seems to have been born" (Mallaby 2000). By 2005, a study commissioned by the WHO identified twenty-four PPHPs targeting the creation of new health products for the benefit of developing countries (Ziemba 2005, CIPRIPH 2006). Private foundations contributed most of the funds, giving approximately $900 million. Bill Gates, who had a "striking faith in the transformative power of new technologies" (Timberg 2006), was the largest single contributor with more than 60 percent of the total. The Gates Foundation funded seventeen of the twenty-four partnerships, and it was the single funding source for nine organizations. Governments, in turn, contributed $244 million (of which USAID had contributed 35 percent). While the private sector contributed to partnerships more than to WHO-led initiatives, business participation in PPHPs was more limited than had been envisioned by the architects of the PPHPs, who had justified independence from the WHO as necessary to lure business. Private entities contributed $6 million to the partnerships in the study (not counting the pharmaceutical industry, which provided support in kind) (CIPRIPH 2006: 74–75).

In response to these independent initiatives, the WHO secretariat, too, sought to contribute to the development of drugs for neglected diseases by way of

---

45. Ibid.
46. Ibid.

partnerships. Discussions between the TDR (WHO's program of scientific collaboration to support global efforts to combat diseases of the poor and disadvantaged), the Rockefeller Foundation, and drug companies led to the establishment of a partnership for the development of antimalaria drugs and vaccines. Brundtland supported the initiative because it complemented her Roll Back Malaria initiative and because she was "looking to build bridges with the private sector."[47]

In this initiative the WHO was an active player and could not be easily bypassed. Nonetheless, claiming an irreconcilable tension between the institutional logic of the WHO and the desired business model, donors insisted on the need for the initiative to be organizationally independent of the WHO. The major funding agencies, including the World Bank, Wellcome Trust, and the Rockefeller Foundation emphasized the need to avoid "politically motivated decision making" and warned that locating the partnership within the WHO would subject it "to strong political influence" (Butler 1998). In the end, Brundtland had to notify WHO member states that the new initiative, named Medicines for Malaria Venture (MMV), would be outside the organization:

> In order to succeed in the long term, the Venture will need to run its affairs primarily as a not-for-profit business, with its own governing board, including an appropriate blend of expertise. This structure was felt to be essential if the Venture is to have the necessary flexibility to operate at the boundary of the public and private sectors. The Venture was therefore established as a foundation . . . and is thus independent of WHO. (Brundtland 2000a)

MMV was launched in November 1999 as a new but autonomous partner to RBM (Aginam 2002).

The aversion to a politicized decision-making process also influenced the type of governing body designed for MMV. According to Robert Ridley, who was centrally involved in the negotiations, "to be more in line with business-line practices," the founders "opposed . . . a representative-based governing body." They also opposed "a board which represented all of the donors or the founders."[48] Instead, they decided in favor of a board of experts who, according to the CEO of MMV, Chris Hentschel, "could act . . . as an enhanced management team."[49] The WHO's involvement was thereby reduced to having a representative sitting on the MMV board. In contrast, the Gates Foundation, which provided more than

47. Interview by the author with Robert Ridley, Director, TDR, Geneva, Switzerland, 3 June 2008.
48. Ibid.
49. Interview by the author with Chris Hentschel, CEO, MMV, Geneva, Switzerland, 19 May 2008.

60 percent of MMV's funds,[50] had its "own employees whose main task is to work with the management here and keep the lines of communication quite short."[51]

Institutional independence from a multilateral decision-making process was sought not only for programs seeking to develop new drugs, but also for programs for distributing drugs. In 1999, discussions among the WHO, UNICEF, the World Bank, the IFPMA, the Rockefeller Foundation, the Gates Children's Vaccine Program, and representatives of national governments resulted in the creation of the Global Alliance for Vaccines and Immunization (GAVI, later called the GAVI Alliance), in October 1999. These partners decided that GAVI would operate autonomously of the UN (Wittet 2000, Muraskin 2004, Hardon and Blume 2005: 351).

GAVI had an independent secretariat that was housed in the Program for Appropriate Technology in Health (PATH), which itself had been launched through a $100 million grant from the Gates Foundation (Muraskin 2004). As with other initiatives, the creation of an independent secretariat outside of the UN was justified as a means "to avoid delays in plan implementation associated with UN bureaucracies" (Hardon and Blume 2005: 351). In contrast to drug development partnerships, however, GAVI did not reject the concept of representation, and GAVI's board includes five permanent seats, occupied by the WHO, UNICEF, the World Bank, the Bill and Melinda Gates Foundation, and the Vaccine Fund.[52] The board also has eleven rotating seats, which represent different "constituencies," including developing countries (2 seats), developed countries (3), NGOs (1), developing country industry (1), developed country industry (1), foundations (1), technical health institutes (1) and research and academia (1).

The distribution of existing vaccines, unlike the development of new ones, had a direct and immediate effect on developing countries, and it was therefore in regard to distribution that the tensions between the WHO member states and independent partnerships were most clear. Tensions arose, for example, in regard to the GAVI's rules of eligibility: only the seventy-five countries with an annual gross domestic product below $1,000 per capita have been eligible for

---

50. The Wellcome Trust contributed 6 percent, and the Rockefeller Foundation contributed a little less than 2 percent. The United Kingdom contributed 9 percent, and the Netherlands and the United States contributed 5 percent each. The World Bank gave 1.4 percent, WHO/RBM 1.1 percent, and two companies, ExxonMobil Foundation and BHP Biliton contributed 0.9 percent and 0.2 percent respectively (MMV Annual Report 2008, available at http://www.mmv.org/newsroom/publications/mmv-annual-report-2008).

51. Interview by the author with Chris Hentschel, CEO, MMV, Geneva, Switzerland, 19 May 2008. MMV raised $330 million between 2000 and 2012 (including pledges).

52. The Vaccine Fund (originally named the Global Fund for Children's Vaccines) was established in 1999 through a grant of the Gates Foundation of $750 million over five years (Wittet 2000). Between 1999 and 2009, the Gates Foundation contributed $1.14 billion and governments contributed $1.77 billion. See http://www.gavialliance.org/support/donors/index.php.

GAVI's support, giving priority to the world's poorest countries. In some cases, eligibility has also depended on existing rates of immunization coverage. As middle-income countries that were excluded by these criteria complained, this discounted a significant criterion often used at the WHO, that of burden of disease.[53] It also prioritized interstate inequality over intrastate inequality, since it did not consider the condition of the poorest people in a country but rather the country's overall economic development.

In addition, GAVI adopted a managerial style that required countries to apply for funds, and GAVI rejected countries whose applications were deemed inadequate. Adopting Bill Gates's notion that poor nations could benefit from corporate style incentive systems, GAVI also made eligibility for additional installment of funds contingent on performance. If a country did not reach the required number of additional children immunized using GAVI aid, GAVI could withhold additional cash and could stop sending vaccines to that country (Hardon and Blume 2005: 352).

With GAVI distributing the vaccines, the WHO was left with the minimal role of serving as a stage for member states to air their frustrations. It was at an Executive Board meeting, for example, that India expressed its discontent with the eligibility criteria that disqualified "certain large countries with a heavy disease burden."[54] Others were concerned that "the eligibility criteria . . . as regards gross national product and immunization coverage rate" would disqualify countries that had had success in achieving, on their own, high immunization coverage.[55] In 2002, many countries classified as low middle-income countries, such as Swaziland and Honduras, expressed at the WHO their concern at their continued exclusion from GAVI funds and requested the GAVI board to reexamine its criteria for eligibility.[56] Given GAVI's independence of the WHO, there was little the WHO bureaucracy could do to address such concerns.

The preference for partnerships independent of the WHO was made particularly clear with donor countries' decision to establish a new international organization, the Global Fund to Fight AIDS, Tuberculosis, and Malaria, devoted to raising and distributing the requisite funds to combat these three major diseases.

There were numerous "owners" of the idea of such a fund. The possibility for a "global fund," initially intended to focus on AIDS alone, was first mentioned in 1999, by a UN commission headed by Jeffrey Sachs (Cannon 2005). In January 2001, a piece at the *Lancet* coauthored by Jeffrey Sachs and Amir Attaran again

---

53. WHO Document, 2000, EB105/SR/5. WHO Library.
54. Ibid.
55. WHO Document, 2000, WHA53/B/SR/5. WHO Library.
56. Ibid.

called for a fund for AIDS (Attaran and Sachs 2001). In the first African Summit on HIV/AIDS, tuberculosis, and other infectious diseases in Abuja, Nigeria, in April 2001, the UN secretary general, Kofi Annan, proposed the creation of a Global Fund, dedicated to the battle against HIV/AIDS and other infectious diseases (Moghalu 2006). Donor countries slowly warmed up to the idea. Already in July 2000, the possibility of an international funding mechanism was considered at a G8 summit in Okinawa (Ramsa 2002). After probing by Kofi Annan and the U.S. Secretary of State Colin Powell, among others, in May 2001, President George W. Bush pledged to support a new worldwide fund with a founding contribution of $200 million. Other wealthy nations followed suit (Cannon 2005). In June 2001, the concept of a global fund was unanimously endorsed at the UN General Assembly Special Session on HIV/AIDS (Ramsa 2002, Sell and Prakash 2004: 166).

Jeffrey Sachs had initially envisioned the Global Fund being administered under the auspices of UNAIDS and the WHO, while others thought of the World Bank as a more appropriate body.[57] Other UN agencies, including UNICEF, UNDP, and the UN Population Fund clamored for shares of the promised money (DeYoung 2001). But the Bush administration deemed multilateral organizations such as the UN agencies too top-heavy and ponderous and made it known that the U.S. government would contribute funds only to a streamlined organization that could act quickly (Cannon 2005).

In line with U.S. wishes, then, the Global Fund was to be independent of the UN. Gavin Yamey of the *British Medical Journal* noted, "By establishing the fund outside of the UN . . . donors [were] expressing a vote of no confidence in the UN's ability to deal with the AIDS epidemic" (Yamey 2002d). But others justified the decision by referring to the exceptional nature of the task. Peter Piot, executive-director of UNAIDS, argued before the WHO Executive Board that "an independent mechanism would ensure a clear focus on the . . . core business, namely to respond to countries' needs for support in planning and implementing programmes and to provide policy and technical guidance," and that "an independent mechanism [was] the best means of mobilizing additional funds, particularly from non-traditional sources."[58]

"Non-traditional sources" were also to be incorporated into the governance structure, as the U.S. government had preferred.[59] The board of the Global Fund,

---

57. Interview by the author with Cristian Baeza, Lead Health Policy Specialist in the Latin America and the Caribbean Region of the World Bank, 28 May 2009.

58. WHO Document, 2001, EB108/SR/6, p. 98. WHO Library.

59. Statement of Hon. Paula Dobriansky, Under Secretary for Global Affairs, Department of State, Washington, DC, "Halting the Spread of HIV/AIDS: Future Efforts in the U.S. Bilateral and Multilateral Response," Hearings before the Committee on Foreign Relations, U.S. Senate, One hundred and seventh Congress, Second session, February 13 and 14, 2002.

like GAVI's, attempted to incorporate all interested parties, including representatives from donor countries, beneficiary countries, NGOs, private foundations,
the private sector, and people living with AIDS, tuberculosis, and malaria. The
WHO, the World Bank, and UNAIDS were represented by nonvoting board
members (Cannon 2005).[60]

The Global Fund officially became operational in January 2002 (Ramsa 2002,
Schwartländer, Grubb, and Perriëns 2006). According to observers, the creation
of the Global Fund led to "a fundamental change in development assistance," as
it was the embodiment of a focus on "combating *priority diseases* with very clear
impact in the *short-term*."[61] Like GAVI, the Global Fund followed the principle of
performance-based financing. Although some board members maintained that
all available money should be given to as many applicants as possible no matter
the quality of the proposals, it was decided that the Global Fund would award
grants only to proposals likely to succeed, and thus funds have been released in-
crementally, based on demonstrated results against agreed targets (Zimmerman
2002, Kazatchkine 2008). Sir Richard Feachem, the first executive director of the
Global Fund explained:

> Money follows results. And if results slow, the money slows. And if re-
> sults fall below an agreed threshold, then the money stops. And it will
> go [to a place] where money is spent effectively.[62]

Helene Gayle, who represented the Gates Foundation on the Global Fund's board,
put it bluntly: "Just because you need the money, we're not giving it to you unless
you can show you can do something with it." She added, "That's very different
from the way the UN has worked [in the past], which is almost an entitlement
system" (cited in Schoofs and Phillips 2002). In a number of cases, including Tanzania, Uganda, Burma, Nigeria, and Ukraine, the Global Fund refused to provide
grants or suspended existing programs.

In discussions at the WHO before the launching of the Global Fund, some
countries expressed the need to save the WHO's centrality. The representative of
Switzerland, for example, "urged the [director-general] to endeavor to maintain
a strong position in the fund," and contended that WHO should be the lead

---

60. Developing countries, however, did not find the board sufficiently balanced. The member
states of the African region, for example, thought that the composition of the secretariat, the technical
committees, and the working groups needed to be made more equitable by ensuring that one-quarter
of the members came from their region. WHO Document, 2002, WHA55/A/SR/4. WHO Library.

61. Interview by the author with Cristian Baeza, Lead Health Policy Specialist in the Latin America and the Caribbean Region of the World Bank, 28 May 2009. Emphasis added.

62. Interview by the author with Sir Richard Feachem, former Director of the Global Fund to
fight AIDS, Tuberculosis, and Malaria, San Francisco, 27 March 2007.

agency.[63] Even after the fund had become operational, many representatives urged "strengthening WHO's role in the Global Fund."[64] By then, however, most delegates accepted the WHO's reduced role, that of helping countries file successful applications. The representative from Thailand, for example, "outlined the strong and proactive roles that WHO and UNAIDS had played . . . in the upstream processes of the Global Fund [that is, at the stage of preparing applications], and urged them to continue that participation, particularly at the country level."[65] The representative of Bhutan "urged WHO to play a strong role in providing support to Member States in the form of technical assistance, and assistance in coordination and networking."[66] Member states were especially interested in the WHO's involvement when they did not receive the funds they had applied for. The representative from Jordan, for example, "said that the Global Fund had refused applications for funding from some low-income countries with a high incidence of AIDS, tuberculosis and malaria. WHO should therefore work with the Fund to define the approval criteria and, where necessary, provide appropriate technical support through its regional offices to ensure the fulfillment of those criteria."[67] As was the case with GAVI, middle-income countries felt unfairly neglected. Argentina maintained that "without prejudicing the special attention which the poorest countries deserved, the Fund should not focus on a limited group of countries but cover all areas in need."[68] In short, given the lack of direct channels of communication between recipient countries and the Global Fund, the WHO meetings were used to complain about the Global Fund, although member states must have realized that the WHO had no ability to bring about the desired changes.

Institutionally, the most important and long-lasting impact of independent PPHPs was the loss of procedural leverage of the developing countries. Initiatives such as the Global Fund, GAVI, IAVI, and MMV greatly weakened the poor countries' influence on fundamental issues, including which health interventions to fund, which strategies to use, and which countries should receive support (Yamey 2002d). This was the result of moving authority from the World Health Assembly, where all member states had an equal voice, to boards of directors, normally dominated by northern donors (Walt and Buse 2000, Buse and Walt 2000b).[69]

---

63. WHO Document, 2001, EB108/SR/2, p. 35. WHO Library.
64. WHO Document, 2002, EB110/SR/1. WHO Library.
65. WHO Document, 2002, WHA55/A/SR/3, p. 43. WHO Library.
66. WHO Document, 2002, WHA55/A/SR/4, p. 53. WHO Library.
67. WHO Document, 2002, WHA55/A/SR/3, p. 42. WHO Library.
68. Ibid.
69. This was a continuation of the process that had already started in the 1980s, with donor countries reducing the role of interstate negotiations in the process of decision making by shifting their contributions from mandatory to voluntary funds (see chapter 5).

A study of NGO-hosted, independent, and UN-hosted partnerships found that some of the boards had no representation from southern-based institutions and none of the boards had half of their membership drawn from this group (Buse 2004, Buse and Lee 2005, see also Tucker and Makgoba 2008). Even the Global Fund board, which is equally divided between parties representing the "donors" and parties representing the "recipients," violates the one-country/one-vote principle that has allowed a majority voice for recipient countries at the UN. Justified in the name of efficiency, public-private partnerships were designed to be run by a small, functional, and apolitical team of decision makers. Craig Wheeler and Seth Berkley of IAVI, for example, promised that "by maintaining a small, effective management team that coordinates project selection and portfolio management, overhead costs are minimized, a limited number of staff are employed, and a flexible, responsive operation is maintained" (Wheeler and Berkley 2001). The head of Board and Donor Relations at the Global Fund offered a similar justification.

> [The Global Fund board] was small and the idea with it being small was to try to make it more like an NGO/private sector board, where people focus [on] what's good for the organization, what the organization's needs are—not a political forum. So not like the executive committees at one of the UN agencies or the governing bodies of some of these big [organizations] where every [member state is] on the governing body like the UN.[70]

Like its member states from the South, the WHO secretariat was also threatened by donors' support of independent health initiatives, such as the Global Fund, which came at the expense both of the organization's funds and, even more fundamentally, its scope of authority and therefore its ability to matter. An organization's capacity to act depends on member states using it as a venue for their demands, expectations, and struggles. With demands made in competing institutions and with exogenous forces no longer working through the organization, the WHO bureaucracy did not have the opportunity to respond to pressures, and it lost its ability to influence outcomes by having to respond strategically to them.

Discussion

One of the fundamental principles of neoliberal thought was faith in the capacity of organizations competing in a market, rather than public bureaucracies,

---

70. Interview by the author with Dianne Stewart, Global Fund, Geneva, Switzerland, 19 May 2008.

to develop desirable and efficient solutions to economic and social problems. Under neoliberalism, therefore, UN agencies were expected to abandon any plans to regulate the activities of multinational corporations and were encouraged to cooperate with and learn from the private sector. The WHO leadership, in spite of concerns expressed both by member states and staff, made great efforts to accommodate the interests of the private sector and reinvent the organization as a business-friendly venue. In some cases, as the confrontation with the food industry demonstrates, the WHO leadership decided to avoid antagonizing an industry even when important health issues were at stake. In two cases of great significance, however, the WHO bureaucracy was willing to risk a direct conflict with multinational companies and the member states that supported them. The WHO secretariat launched an aggressive campaign against the tobacco sector, and it sought ways to defend universal access to AIDS drugs against the position of the pharmaceutical industry. In both cases, the WHO staff was able to reduce the cost of noncompliance by means of strategic resistance. In the case of tobacco, the exceptionally unethical behavior of the industry was skillfully used by the WHO staff to establish a distinction between those industries that were part of the solution and those that were not, which also assured other companies that an antismoking campaign did not reflect broader antibusiness sentiments. In the dispute over intellectual property protection, the WHO staff avoided a conflict by suggesting there was no need for it, since intellectual property rules already incorporated the flexibilities that could be used for the manufacturing of generic versions of patented AIDS drugs. In both cases, then, the WHO bureaucracy did not directly challenge the dominant logic but, instead, was able to incorporate favorable exceptions as integral parts of that logic.

At the same time, a comparison between the WHO's strategic adaptation, including both compliance and resistance, in the 1970s and the 1990s reveals less maneuverability in the later period. Under neoliberal pressures, the WHO policies resembled quite faithfully the economic thinking of its political environment, even when it was able to employ economic reasoning to its advantage or to make legitimate exceptions to it. Two important conditions narrowed the capacity of the WHO to manipulate its environment. First, the integration of entities other than member states into WHO consultations and debates, including the private sector and nongovernmental organizations, introduced into the negotiations more bifurcated positions held by parties less willing to reach compromises. Oliver (1991) suggests that such divergence gives an organization more room for maneuver, but as we have seen also in the WHO's leadership response to debates over codes of conduct in the 1970s, the opposite is normally the case. Even more so in the 1990s, the explicit debates and negotiations among interested parties, including, for example, the pharmaceutical sector and AIDS activists, allowed little room for the WHO staff to exercise influence. Nonetheless, as long as the World Health Assembly was used as a site for those debates, the organization could still attempt to influence the outcome. The second condition that narrowed the capacity of the WHO to manipulate its environment was donors' bypassing of the WHO altogether, by the creation of PPHPs independent of the WHO. The rise of partnerships did not lead to an authority crisis, as the involvement of the World Bank and the creation of UNAIDS had in the early 1990s, partly because the creation of partnerships was justified without directly questioning the legitimacy of the WHO. Nonetheless, the partnerships had a direct effect on the WHO's capacity to act. In the next, and final, chapter, I offer a summary of the central insights drawn from the history of the World Health Organization, and I consider recent transformations in the battle of the WHO to become central again.

STRUCTURAL TRANSFORMATIONS OF THE GLOBAL HEALTH REGIME

In the previous chapters I offered an account of the response of the WHO bureaucracy to external pressures. I showed how both in the 1970s–1980s and the 1990s–2000s, the WHO secretariat adapted to changes in the political environment by advocating policies and programs that could be reconciled with the new dominant logic. In the 1970s–1980s, the WHO secretariat, which was attentive to the majority of votes of the developing countries, sought to follow the call for a New International Economic Order. In the 1990s–2000s, the WHO secretariat, which relied heavily on developed countries' financial contributions, made sure to adhere to the neoliberal logic. However, the adherence to the external demands was often selective. The changes introduced by the WHO bureaucracy as gestures of compliance were based on an interpretation of the original demands that allowed the new policies and programs to also protect or even advance the WHO material needs or ideational preferences. The WHO bureaucracy often presented its actions as if they were congruous with the original demands even when resisting them.

Because of its dependence on external actors, the WHO secretariat was compelled to shift its position and programs in a way compatible with the dominant logic—to function, the WHO relied on member states' funds, votes, and recognition of the WHO's legitimacy. The successful introduction of health policies and programs that deviated from exogenous prescriptions, however, reveals the capacity of international bureaucracies to respond strategically in the face of such pressures. I identified two types of strategies that the WHO secretariat employed, which by avoiding the common dichotomy of compliance/resistance, reveal new dimensions of organizational behavior: strategic compliance, when the international bureaucracy is able to alter the meaning of the demands before it adheres to them in a way that reduces the incongruity of the required changes with the organization's interests; and strategic resistance, when the international bureaucracy is able to reframe the demands so that it is no longer expected to conform to them and in a way that minimizes the risk of sanctions. The WHO secretariat's need to rely on *strategic* responses acknowledges the difficulty of international bureaucracies to act against the will of their member states and other external actors. In turn, the success of such strategies indicates that international bureaucracies are not only actors with independent positions but also that they are important protagonists with capacity to shape outcomes in accordance with those independent preferences.

In the 1970s–1980s, developing countries expected the WHO to contribute to the making of a New International Economic Order. The NIEO emphasized principles important to the social and economic development of poor countries, including equity, economic sovereignty, universal international organizations, and collective self-reliance. To fit these new international sensibilities, the WHO secretariat developed new priorities and programs. However, the new WHO programs shifted the original NIEO focus on economic development to a focus on social development, which, by defining individuals' quality of life independently of economic capabilities, was more suitable to the WHO's ideational goals. In addition, the WHO secretariat altered the focus of concern from equity among states to equity within states, which allowed the WHO to prioritize initiatives concerned with those "most in need." The WHO secretariat also broadened the principle of collective self-reliance so as to encourage the full participation of developing countries in the decision-making process of the WHO, to encourage the participation of communities at the local level, and to justify countries' reliance on their own economic resources for health programs. Finally, the WHO secretariat utilized the demand from developing countries for transfers of technology to call for the transfer only of appropriate technology. It was due to these alterations of the original demands that the WHO leadership could successfully present its call for Health for All by the Year 2000, its support of the primary health care approach, and the launching of a model list of essential drugs, as complying with the New International Economic Order. Resistance to the external demands of developing countries was similarly strategic. Realizing that international codes of conduct undermined the organization's legitimacy, the WHO leadership exploited the principle of political sovereignty to convince developing countries against turning the WHO into a supranational organization and drop their call for an international code of marketing of pharmaceutical products.

During the 1990s–2000s, the U.S. government and other rich countries pressed the WHO to follow neoliberal principles, which emphasized economic growth, to be achieved through private enterprise, individual initiative, and free competitive markets. Following a neoliberal logic, also at the international level, goals were to be defined, priorities listed, and success measured in purely economic terms. In response to the new pressures, the WHO secretariat abandoned the social logic that had dominated the organization's programs during the previous era and turned to economic logic as the foundation for its decisions and policies. However, by providing economic evidence that improved health contributed to economic development, the WHO leadership was able to exploit the neoliberal focus on economic growth to call for enhanced investment in health. In addition, the WHO leadership used donor countries' concern with economic growth and cost effectiveness to promote the concept of "new universalism"— the delivery of high-quality essential care to all—as a viable alternative not only to the primary health care approach of the past but also to the neoliberal-informed market-oriented approach favored by the World Bank and others. Resistance to exogenous expectations was again strategic: by emphasizing the unethical characteristics of the tobacco industry, the WHO bureaucracy was able to present its campaign against smoking as a legitimate exception to the general probusiness principle it followed. Likewise, by providing a legal interpretation of TRIPS that reconciled patent protection with access to drugs, the WHO staff was able to defend access to AIDS drugs without questioning the principle of intellectual property rights claimed by the pharmaceutical industry.

The ability of the WHO bureaucracy to strategically respond to the demands of developing countries for a New International Economic Order and, some decades later, to the demands of developed countries for neoliberal reforms, clarifies numerous arguments made by the constructivist and principal-actor theories of international organizations. The WHO secretariat's embrace of new policies and programs following transformations in the exogenous political environment illustrates the vulnerability of international bureaucracies to pressures, due to their dependence on countries' material resources, votes, and normative support. However, the response of the WHO secretariat shows that international bureaucracies have the capacity to act on their independent goals and perceptions. In this book, I emphasize that this capacity stems not from formal authority but from practices, particularly the ability to act strategically. I argue that international bureaucracies are able to exercise their partial autonomy and pursue their own agendas—even when those clash with the preferences of member states—by employing strategic, rather than passive, responses. Strategic responses that alter the meaning of external demands enable international bureaucracies to protect their goals and principles without alienating member states and other supporters.

I suggested that the choice of response—whether to respond passively or strategically, whether to comply or resist—depends on a number of institutional conditions, including the capacity of the international bureaucracy to develop preferences and interests independent from the external environment, the hierarchical position of member state representatives at the national level, the degree of conflict among member states over the issue in question, the precision of demands, and whether the head of the international organization is a strong leader, well positioned in the environment, and recently appointed. International bureaucracies will not always choose strategic over passive responses, and not all strategic responses will bring the desired results. Nonetheless, the potential capacity of international bureaucracies to manipulate their political environment suggests their influence on international policies and programs, which depends on, but cannot be reduced to, the will of member states. International outcomes should not be regarded as a reflection of member states' demands but of a strategic interplay between member states and the international bureaucracies that selectively adhere to those demands.

As a way of conclusion, in the next section, I consider the implications of this study on the capacity of international bureaucracies to influence policies by strategically responding to external demands for our understanding of the emergence and transformation of international regimes. Drawing on a systematic comparison of global health policies and programs in the 1970s–1980s and in the 1990s–2000s, which I present below, I evaluate the structural transformations of the global health regime over time and what they reveal about the institutional and political differences between the "international organizations" of the 1970s–1980s and the "global governance" of the 1990s–2000s. In the final section of the chapter, I draw on the analytical conclusions of this study and on recent attempts of the WHO bureaucracy to respond to the still-evolving post-neoliberal global order to speculate on the likely future of the WHO.

The Global Health Regime in Comparative-Historical Perspective

As suggested in chapter 2, even successful strategic responses entail organizational changes. Also in the case of the WHO, policies and institutional arrangements have changed quite radically in response to the call for a New International Economic Order and then again in response to neoliberal demands. Each era is therefore characterized by distinct qualities in regard to a number of institutional aspects (see table C.1).

Rationale for intervention: from social development to economic growth. In the 1970s–1980s, the WHO bureaucracy advanced the concept of social development, which is concerned with improvements in living conditions and quality of life, as distinct from economic development. Having social development as the rationale for intervention enabled the WHO secretariat to defend the position

TABLE C.1   Comparing global health regimes in the 1970s–1980s and in the 1990s–2000s

	1970s–1980s	1990s–2000s
Rationale for intervention	Social development	Economic growth
Principle of intervention	Equity	Cost effectiveness
Flagship initiatives	Horizontal interventions Appropriate technology Basic health needs	Vertical/disease specific Technological solutions Noncommunicable diseases
Sources of funds	Obligation Mandatory (rich countries)	Charity Voluntary (rich countries, private foundations, business)
Relations with the private sector	Part of the problem (with strategic exceptions)	Part of the solution (with strategic exceptions)
Institutional focus	Member-driven UN agency	In-house and independent public- private partnerships
Forms of expertise	Public health	Economics, law, and business
Type of management	Public sector mentality	Private sector mentality

that health was a fundamental goal in its own right. Moreover, the notion that social development could be secured in conditions of economic scarcity and independently of economic growth made Health for All by the Year 2000 and the primary health care approach compatible with the call for a New International Economic Order. Under neoliberalism, however, social development as a goal independent of economic considerations was no longer defendable. In strategic response to the neoliberal focus on economic growth, the WHO justified investment in health by accepting the primacy of economic growth while offering evidence, provided by the Commission on Macroeconomics and Health, that improved health would advance the desired economic development.

Principle of intervention: from equity to cost-effectiveness. In the 1970s–1980s, the overarching principle guiding WHO programs was that of intranational equity. The question of affordability was crucial, but not the question of effectiveness: the population that merited the most attention was identified by its need rather than by the cost-effectiveness of the interventions that could help it. In the 1990s–2000s, the new governing principle gave precedence to the most cost-effective interventions. Even when "need" was taken into consideration, it was defined in national terms, so priority was given to the poorest countries, not necessarily the poorest populations (Motchane 2003, Kickbusch and Buse 2001,

Poku and Whiteside 2002). Nonetheless, the WHO bureaucracy was able to use cost-effectiveness to promote a "new universalism"—the delivery of high-quality essential care to all.

Flagship initiatives: from primary health care to technological solutions for specific diseases. To achieve the goal of Health for All by the Year 2000, the flagship initiatives in the 1970s–1980s focused on primary health care: WHO programs advocated the provision of basic services for those most in need, and the use only of appropriate and affordable technology. In the 1990s–2000s, a number of factors—including cost-effective calculations, the desire to lure private sector funding, and the influence of the Gates Foundation and of disease-specific health activists—led to a renewed embrace of disease-specific programs, with corresponding focuses on medical treatment, particularly the distribution of drugs and vaccines, and on the allocation of resources to the development of technological solutions. In addition to communicable diseases, in the 1990s–2000s the WHO developed an unprecedented interest in noncommunicable diseases as well.

Sources of funds: from mandatory to voluntary contributions. In the 1970s–1980s, poor countries and most wealthy countries viewed the transfer of funds as an obligation, partly linked to the colonial past, and partly linked to the contemporary uneven distribution of economic benefits. While during the NIEO period WHO funds did not radically increase, more of the mandatory funds were devoted to operational assistance and the Geneva Group failed in its attempt to significantly reduce the annual growth in the WHO budget. By the mid-1980s, however, rich countries refused to accept their contributions as a nonnegotiable obligation and, now seeing themselves as "donors," considered contributions a voluntary act of charity. Mandatory assessments were frozen, and the WHO budget drew mostly from voluntary contributions. In response to the drying up of mandatory funds, the WHO welcomed voluntary contributions not only from rich member states but also from private philanthropists and business. In 2008, the Gates Foundation's giving to global health programs was more than $10 billion; by comparison, the WHO's budget for the biennium 2008–2009 was around $5 billion.[1]

The shift from mandatory contributions, which were decided by the World Health Assembly, to voluntary contributions meant that the director-general and developing countries lost their influence over the amount of funds and over how these funds were to be spent. The WHO's loss of control over the amount and use of funds was further extended with the creation of partnerships independent of the WHO, such as GAVI and the Global Fund. Also, since donors no longer

---

1. For the financial reports of the Gates Foundation, see Foundation Center, at http://dynamo data.fdncenter.org/990s/990search/ffindershow.cgi?id=GATE023); on the WHO budget see WHO, Programme Budget 2008–2009, at apps.who.int/gb/ebwha/pdf_files/AMTSP-PPB/a-mtsp_4en.pdf.

considered funds for health programs an entitlement of poor countries, funds could be distributed based on the quality of countries' proposals and conditioned on performance and other criteria. This was the case in GAVI and the Global Fund, as well as the WHO's Tobacco Free Initiative.

Relations with the private sector: from "part of the problem" to "part of the solution." In the 1970s–1980s, the relations between the WHO bureaucracy and multinational corporations were formally hostile. In defiance of multinational companies' expressed interest, the WHO opposed "inappropriate" technology, promoted the notion of essential drugs, and sponsored a code of conduct for infant formula. However, to protect the legitimacy of the organization, the WHO leadership lobbied against a binding code for the marketing of infant formula and also objected to a code of conduct for the marketing of pharmaceutical products. In the 1990s–2000s, in comparison, the WHO bureaucracy developed a much closer relationship with the private sector, invited companies to become partners in WHO initiatives, and welcomed monetary, in-kind, and other contributions from industry. This led to concerns that WHO decisions would cater to the interests of business (Walt and Buse 2000), and NGOs warned of "a slippery slope toward the partial privatization and commercialization of the UN system itself" (Utting 2000). In other cases, the WHO secretariat strategically resisted business influence. The WHO secretariat took a leading position in an international antismoking crusade against the tobacco industry, and WHO officials offered an early and important critique of the international agreement for intellectual property protection because of the effect it had on access to drugs, particularly AIDS drugs.

Institutional focus: from a member-driven UN agency to public-private partnerships (PPHPs). In the 1970s–1980s, the WHO was the sole authority over health issues at the international level, and the secretariat was mostly accountable to member states, with most other actors, particularly the private sector, having to work through member states to influence the organization. Some parties, however, such as the Rockefeller Foundation, did have a disproportionate impact on the intellectual development and policy initiatives of the organization. The 1990s–2000s saw the rise of a very different global health architecture, wherein the WHO integrated into the internal process of decision-making entities other than member states, including nongovernmental organizations, private foundations, and businesses and their associations. Even more important, the WHO became just one of many entities with an interest in global health, including the World Bank, UNAIDS, and the Global Fund, as well as GAVI, IAVI, and MMV, among others. Many of the new entities were designed as partnerships, incorporating both the private and the public sectors.

Forms of expertise: from public health knowledge to economics, law, and business. While in the 1970s–1980s, leadership in global health initiatives was given to medical and public health experts, in the 1990s–2000s such initiatives were designed and managed also by economists, lawyers, and those with "private sector experience."[2] Brundtland, who was a medical doctor but not a public health expert, explicitly deferred to economic expertise in creating the Commission on Macroeconomics and Health and establishing the Evidence and Information for Policy Unit, for which she hired many economists. As part of the Tobacco Free Initiative, in turn, the WHO welcomed many lawyers, who brought with them legal expertise. Public-private partnerships were often managed by experts from the public sector with experience in international organizations, but many partnerships hired individuals who had experience primarily in the private sector. For example, the founder and CEO of IAVI, Seth Berkley, previously at the Rockefeller Foundation, had served on a number of company boards in the vaccine world, which, he argued, gave him "a fair amount [of experience] in the vaccine industry";[3] and the CEO of MMV, Chris Hentschel, started off his career as an academic but moved to the biotech world, including being the chief scientific advisor for a U.S. biotech company. As Hentschel describes it: "I was completely in the private sector, not only the private sector, but probably the most aggressive and commercial private sector on earth, which was the U.S. biotech industry."[4] However, it was not only CEOs hired for their experience in the private sector. In a conscious attempt to resemble for-profit companies, many PPHPs sought to recruit people from the business world.[5]

Type of management: from a public sector to a private sector mentality. In the 1970s–1980s, the WHO bureaucracy was an explicitly political organization, motivated by the demands of its member states, but it was also an unapologetically public bureaucracy. In the 1990s, this public sector mentality was replaced with a private sector mentality. This new type of management was often instituted through the philanthropic activities of former businessmen, particularly Bill Gates. The Gates Foundation used the enormous funds it contributed to global health projects not only to shape the research priorities in health issues, but also to impose a strictly private-sector managerial logic for the undertakings of its funds.[6] As observers described it, Bill Gates has brought to the global health arena an "entrepreneurial . . . culture" (Kehaulani Goo 2006)—and in particular, has applied "a relentlessly competitive business model" to his philanthropic initiatives (Masters and Noguchi 2006) and a "business-like focus on results and effectiveness" (Kehaulani Goo

---

2. Interview by the author with Seth Berkley, CEO and founder of IAVI, New York, 19 February 2009.
3. Ibid.
4. Interview by the author with Chris Hentschel, CEO, MMV, Geneva, Switzerland, 19 May 2008.
5. Ibid.
6. According to one interviewer, "all the projects supported by Gates today are the priority, and all the others that are not supported . . . are not at all the priority for public health." Interview by the author, Drugs for Neglected Diseases initiative (DNDi), Geneva, Switzerland, June 2008.

2006). In pursuing such a managerial logic, Gates was from early on helped by an emergent global health elite, those who had the task of heading the growing numbers of PPHPs and, also coming from the private sector, were themselves invested in making their partnerships "more private sector in the management style and management ethos of running [them],"[7] and in basing their procedures "on operational paradigms of industry, not the public sector" (Buse and Walt 2000a). This managerial logic meant that public health initiatives were now expected to behave as if they were companies functioning in conditions of market competition and were encouraged to use the sorts of strategies and solutions used by business.

This comparison of the global health regime in the 1970s–1980s to the regime in the 1990s–2000s reveals some of the core differences between the institutional arrangements of international organizations in the postwar, state-centered era and in the more recent era of economic globalization and alleged political fragmentation. Much has been said about the drastic economic transformations since the 1970s (Block 1996, Dicken 1998) and the equally dramatic political changes at the national and the international levels. At the national level, scholars first warned of the "eclipse" or "retreat" of the nation-state (Evans 1997, Strange 1996), and later carefully analyzed the structural transformation of the still-standing state (Sassen 2006, Morgan and Campbell 2011). At the international level, on the contrary, initial analyses suggested that international organizations have been gaining authority and taking over some of the functions of sovereign states (Jessop 1997, Abbott et al. 2000). Other scholars, however, have also identified important structural transformations, in particular, the introduction of new actors into the process of decision making. While some have focused on the emergence of a transnational capitalist class with a growing political influence (van der Pijl 1998, Robinson and Harris 2000, Sklair 2000), others, on the contrary, referred to the emergence of pluralistic "global governance," in which state and nonstate actors alike are involved in processes of decision making in a manifestly decentralized way (Rosenau and Czempiel 1992, Cerny 2001).

Indeed, in contrast to the shift that followed the call for a New International Economic Order, the neoliberal transformation affected not only the nature of global health programs but also the field's organizational features, in particular the decentralization of global health authority. This decentralization, as the literature on global governance suggests, is partly institutional. Rather than one World Health Organization with a de facto monopoly over global health issues, today there are many organizations that take responsibility over various aspects of the field: the World Health Organization, UNAIDS, and the Global Fund, but importantly, also the World Bank on the one hand and PPHPs on the other.

---

7. Interview by the author with Chris Hentschel, CEO, MMV, Geneva, Switzerland, 19 May 2008.

This decentralization is also expressed in the rise of new types of participants (Hewson and Sinclair 1999, Avant, Finnemore, and Sell 2010). The global health regime has seen the growing importance of philanthropic foundations, business, and NGOs. No doubt many global health policies and programs today owe more to the support and influence of the Bill and Melinda Gates Foundation, multinational pharmaceutical companies, or Médecins Sans Frontières, among others, than they do to the WHO bureaucracy and at least some of its member states. While philanthropists, businesses, and NGOs already had great influence in the 1970s–1980s, their involvement has been greatly enhanced with their "institutional defection" from the WHO and their establishment of global health initiatives elsewhere. Of course, the introduction of additional actors does not guarantee a pluralistic process of decision making. As we have seen, the current institutional arrangements have increased the bargaining leverage of private foundations, civil society actors, and business, but at the expense of the WHO bureaucracy and, most importantly, of developing countries themselves.

In addition to philanthropists, corporations, and representatives of global civil society, another important actor in the global health field that is less commonly analyzed in the literature is the professional manager who comes from the private sector into a top position in the field. As we have seen, PPHPs, in particular, are often run by former businesspeople who manage the partnerships as if they were entities functioning in a competitive market. These professional managers have introduced a completely new logic of governance, based on private-sector management rather than public-sector mentality. Arguably, it is the new logic of governance, more than the greater influence of interested actors such as business and NGOs, that defines the essence of today's global governance.

However, just as the WHO programs of the 1970s–1980s did not survive the dismantling of the NIEO, we should not expect the global health programs and institutions of the 1990s–2000s to survive the dismantling of neoliberalism. At the time of this writing, neoliberal logic had been fundamentally undermined by the financial crisis of 2008, but there are still no clear signs of what logic will replace it. The WHO secretariat has responded to this liminal stage by taking some important steps in rejecting past perceptions, but without yet having a clear alternative, as I describe below.[8]

What Future for the WHO?

In the last few years, global health initiatives have seen important shifts, linked to the financial insecurity of relying on voluntary contributions from private

---

8. I thank Ted Brown for alerting my attention to the significance of these new developments.

foundations and for-profit companies. The future of PPHPs, in particular, has been intimately linked to the financial well-being of the Bill and Melinda Gates Foundation, which, in the course of the financial crisis, lost one-fifth of its assets in 2008. Even before the financial crisis, there had been a clear decline in the number of new partnerships created: while sixteen new development partnerships were established in 2000, only three were established in 2003. No new partnerships were created between 2004 and 2007 (Meredith and Ziemba 2008). Public-private partnerships have also learned that R&D pharmaceutical companies are difficult to attract as partners and have looked for alternatives: for example, IAVI has been working with biotech companies, and MMV has been working with generic manufacturers from developing countries.[9]

Also, the focus on technological solutions for specific diseases, which had been celebrated both by philanthropists and health activists, has been under increasing attack. A central concern, which echoes the response to the vertical programs of the 1950s, is that diseases cannot be eradicated without the strengthening of the entire health system and that partnerships that focus only on product development or distribution underestimate the difficulties of delivering drugs and vaccines when health systems are weak. Drugs, some have concluded, offer "technology in a vacuum" that has not been able to overcome the political, logistical, and managerial difficulties in getting them to the people in the poorer regions of the world who most need them (Jack 2006; see also Walt and Buse 2000, Utting and Zammit 2006). Indeed, the WHO, UNAIDS, and the Global Fund have all discovered that paying for drugs was no assurance they would get where they were needed. The WHO, for example, missed its initial target to supply AIDS drugs to half a million patients in the first six months of 2004. Some of the reasons for this failure include lack of capacities in place to store medicines, track inventory, and truck drugs to remote outposts, and a shortage of people trained to deliver AIDS care (Naik 2004, 2005). Cristian Baeza of the World Bank, describes the issue as follows:

> So the single disease programs and donors are rediscovering that to be able to actually reach people with malaria treatments, well, you need to have . . . a primary health center. You need to have incentives to actually work in the rural areas. You need to have a logistical system in place. You need to have a way to pay them. You need all these things that a [health] system is.[10]

---

9. Interview by the author with Seth Berkley, CEO and founder of IAVI, New York, 19 February 2009; interview by the author with Chris Hentschel, CEO, MMV, Geneva, Switzerland, 19 May 2008.
10. Interview by the author with Cristian Baeza, Lead Health Policy Specialist in the Latin America and the Caribbean Region of the World Bank, 28 May 2009.

A related criticism has been that the focus on three "private" diseases—AIDS, malaria and tuberculosis—came at the significant expense of other priorities.[11] In particularly harsh terms, an article in the *British Medical Journal* criticized the "AIDS industry" for being too vertical, at the expense in particular of health care systems:

> It is no longer heresy to point out that far too much is spent on HIV relative to other needs and that this is damaging health systems. Although HIV causes 3.7% of mortality, it receives 25% of international healthcare aid and a big chunk of domestic expenditure. HIV aid often exceeds total domestic health budgets themselves, including their HIV spending. It has created parallel financing, employment, and organizational structures, weakening national health systems at a crucial time and sidelining needed structural reform. (England 2008)

While such recent calls for new health priorities have often been justified by pointing out inherent faults stemming from existing programs, they are also made in a new political context that once again tolerates support for strengthening health systems. The emergence of a new global order is still tentative but Joseph Stiglitz—who has served as World Bank senior vice president and chief economist and has been an adamant critic of the neoliberal development program—has termed it "post-neoliberalism" or the "post–Washington consensus." According to Stiglitz, Washington Consensus policies had produced only limited growth, and even when growth did occur, it was not equitably shared. Rather than seeking policies intended to increase economic growth, therefore, the post–Washington Consensus calls for policies that seek sustainable and equitable democratic development.[12] The website of the World Health Organization has its own take on the rise of a new logic:

> For many supporters, the post-Washington consensus differs fundamentally from the original. While the Washington consensus made economic growth the main goal of development, the new consensus moves away from the neo-liberal, market-friendly approach and places sustainable, egalitarian and democratic development at the heart of the agenda. It includes a more poverty-focused approach that protects and supports the poor and prioritizes social spending on education and health. Others argue that the original neo-liberal agenda still underpins the post-Washington consensus, saying that the social safety net aspects

---

11. Interview by the author with Badara Samb, Health Systems Strengthening, Department of HIV/AIDS, WHO, Geneva, Switzerland, 3 June 2008; Shiffman 2007.

12. See http://www.policyinnovations.org/ideas/policy_library/data/01232.

of the new policies are put in place as an add-on to deal with market failure.[13]

It is too early to identify the specific principles of the alleged consensus, and the WHO's lack of clear response to the new sentiments reflects the general uncertainty at the global level regarding what is now expected of international organizations. Nonetheless, a WHO report by the Commission on Social Determinants of Health (CSDH), *Closing the Gap in a Generation: Health Equity through Action on the Social Determinants of Health* (CSDH 2008), explicitly rejected neoliberal principles and the WHO's adaptation to them and offered a possible new direction that the WHO may take.

The Commission on Social Determinants of Health was called for in 2004 by Director-General Lee Jong-wook and was charged with recommending policies to narrow health inequalities specifically through action on social, rather than economic, determinants (Banerji 2006). The focus on inequalities rather than growth and the study of social conditions rather than economic ones implied a search for a new direction for the WHO.

The report was published in August 2008. In a provocative disregard to the more recent perceptions dominating the WHO logic, the authors described the report as emerging from the "inspiring declarations" of both the WHO Constitution and the Alma-Ata Conference (CSDH 2008). Echoing the emerging sentiments of a post-neoliberal order, the report emphasized the problem of inequity both between *and* within countries. The report lamented: "Our children have dramatically different life chances depending on where they were born. In Japan or Sweden they can expect to live more than 80 years; in Brazil, 72 years; India, 63 years; and in one of several African countries, fewer than 50 years" (CSDH 2008). But the report did not ignore inequities within countries. "In Glasgow, an unskilled, working-class person will have a lifespan 28 years shorter than a businessman in the top income bracket in Scotland" (Navarro 2009). Nonetheless, the integration of inter- and intracountry comparison brought the authors to a conclusion more in line with the "new universalism" of the 2000s than the "most in need" principle of the 1970s, as the report recommended "interventions that affect the whole of society not only those at the bottom" (Marmot and Friel 2008). In addition, the report recommended the prioritization of the poorest countries, which was in line with GAVI's eligibility criteria more than with the WHO's traditional concern with "burden of disease."

Still, the report's response to inequality challenged neoliberal thinking in a number of important ways. First, it criticized inequality from a normative, rather than a

---

13. See http://www.who.int/trade/glossary/story074/en/index.html.

utilitarian perspective. Explicitly reversing the logic developed by the Commission on Macroeconomics and Health, the new commission advocated an approach to health and human development in which equity mattered in its own right and was the fundamental objective of reform (Lancet 2008). The report used explicit references to "social justice" and "fairness" to express its dismay with inequality:

> Where systematic differences in health are judged to be avoidable by reasonable action they are, quite simply, unfair. . . . Putting right these inequities—the huge and remediable differences in health between and within countries—is a matter of social justice. Reducing health inequities is . . . an ethical imperative. (CSDH 2008)

The report challenged neoliberal thinking also by rejecting the notion that economic growth was sufficient to resolve inequality: "Growth by itself, without appropriate social policies to ensure reasonable fairness in the way its benefits are distributed, brings little benefit to health equity" (CSDH 2008). Rather than smoothing potential differences between the approach developed in the report and previous WHO perceptions, the authors of the report provocatively emphasize them. Michael Marmot and Sharon Friel (2008) wrote,

> At various points in the Commission's life, the point was put to us strongly that, for the Commission's recommendations to be taken seriously, we had to show that taking action on health equity would be good for the economy. A previous WHO Commission, on Macroeconomics and Health, had argued for massive investment in disease control in order to promote economic development. . . . But the Commission did not revisit this territory. Our starting position was the social determinants of health—social included economic—not the health determinants of economics.

More radically, the report suggested that economic growth, if achieved through the marketplace, could lead to negative health results: "The marketplace can . . . generate negative conditions for health in the form of economic inequalities, resource depletion, environmental pollution, unhealthy working conditions, and the circulation of dangerous and unhealthy goods" (CSDH 2008). Finally, the report criticized a number of macroeconomic policy reforms, some of which had been opposed by the WHO before, including "encouragement of user fees, performance-related pay, [and] separation of the provider and purchaser functions," but others had been earlier strongly endorsed by the WHO, including "determination of a package that privileges cost-effective medical interventions at the expense of priority interventions to address social determinants" and "a stronger role for private sector agents" (CSDH 2008).

In its recommendations, the report urged three principles of action. First, improving the conditions of daily life; second, tackling the inequitable distribution of power and resources that shaped these daily conditions and in that way explicitly bringing social justice and broad political and economic determinants to the forefront of the world's health agenda; third, showing that the authors have not abandoned concerns with efficiency, measuring the problems, and assessing the impact of actions (Muntaner et al. 2009). From these principles the report drew a number of more specific recommendations: improving living and learning conditions in early childhood; strengthening social programs to provide fairer employment conditions and access to labor markets, particularly for vulnerable social groups; policies and interventions to protect people in informal employment; policies to improve living conditions in urban slums; and programs to address key determinants of women's health, such as access to education and economic opportunities (CSDH 2008). In line with the policy focus in these recommendations, the commission called for the creation of strong public sectors—"committed, capable, and adequately financed" (Lancet 2008). Although inspired by the Alma-Ata Declaration, therefore, the concrete recommendations were significantly different from the primary health care approach: both targeted the most vulnerable populations (now more often residing in urban slums than in rural areas), but the recommendations of the 2008 report focused less on environmental issues, such as clean water, and more on social welfare issues, particularly education and employment.

The Commission on the Social Determinants of Health Report, a piece about the CSDH report published in the *Lancet* by Director-General Margaret Chan that celebrated the "Return to Alma Ata" (Chan 2008), and the 2008 World Health Report entitled, *Primary Health Care (Now More Than Ever)* all signify a potential U-turn in the WHO orientation. The election of Margaret Chan as director-general, following the untimely death of Lee Jong-wook in 2006, is another indication of the same transformation. Another strong candidate, Julio Frenk, had been the minister of health in Mexico and had solid neoliberal credentials in the field of health, having been the WHO executive director of Evidence and Information for Policy, and the chair of the steering committee that directed the World Health Report 2000. Margaret Chan, in contrast, had no known neoliberal inclinations (Lancet 2006).

The recent rejection of some neoliberal principles and the revival of the Alma-Ata Declaration imply that the WHO secretariat has been responding to the likely emergence of a new dominant logic in the same way that it responded in the past: the WHO bureaucracy is adapting strategically, embracing the new expectations, but in ways that allow the organization to protect its material and ideational goals while minimizing the risk of direct confrontations. Future global health policies, like the ones they replace, will largely depend on geopolitical and global financial developments. But, as in the past, the response of the WHO secretariat to the new exogenous logic will have a major effect on whether, and how, that new logic will be translated into specific health policies. International organizations function under strenuous exogenous constraints, but they are still part of history.

References

Abbasi, Kamran. 1999. "The World Bank and World Health: Changing Sides." *British Medical Journal* 318(7187): 865–869.

Abbott, Kenneth W., Robert O. Keohane, Andrew Moravcsik, Anne-Marie Slaughter, and Duncan Snidal. 2000. "The Concept of Legalization." *International Organization* 54(3): 385–400.

Abdelal, Rawi. 2007. *Capital Rules: The Construction of Global Finance.* Cambridge, MA: Harvard University Press.

Abrams, Elliott. 1981. "Infant Formula Code: Why the U.S. May Stand Alone." *Washington Post,* May 21.

Adams, Nassau A. 1993. *Worlds Apart: The North-South Divide and the International System.* London: Zed Books.

Adelman, Kenneth L. 1982. "Biting the Hand That Cures Them." *Regulation* 6: 16–18.

Aginam, Obijiofor. 2002. "Public Health and International Law: From the Core to the Peripheries: Multilateral Governance of Malaria in a Multi-Cultural World." *Chicago Journal of International Law* 3: 87.

Akin, John, Nancy Birdsall, and David de Ferranti. 1987. "Financing Health Services in Developing Countries: An Agenda for Reform." Washington, DC: World Bank.

Albert, Stuart, and David A. Whetton. 1985. "Organizational Identity." *Research in Organizational Behavior* 7: 263–295.

Al-Mazrou, Yagob, and Barry Bloom. 1997. "A Vital Opportunity for Global Health." *Lancet* 350(9080): 750.

Amrith, Sunil. 2002. "Plague of Poverty? The World Health Organization, Tuberculosis, and International Development, c. 1945–1980." Thesis. Christ's College, Cambridge, UK.

Amsden, Alice H. 2001. *The Rise of "The Rest": Challenges to the West from Late-Industrializing Economies.* New York: Oxford University Press.

———. 2003. "Comment: Good-bye Dependency Theory, Hello Dependency Theory." *Studies in Comparative International Development* 38(1): 32–38.

Anderson, Jack. 1981. "Formula Flap: Story Behind the Lone 'No.'" *Washington Post,* June 2.

Armada, Francisco, Carlos Muntaner, and Vicente Navarro. 2001. "Health and Social Security Reforms in Latin America: The Convergence of the World Health Organization, the World Bank, and Transnational Corporations." *International Journal of Health Services* 31: 729–768.

Arrow, Kenneth J., Claire Panosian, and Hellen Gelband, eds. 2004. *Saving Lives, Buying Time: Economics of Malaria Drugs in an Age of Resistance.* Washington, DC: Institute of Medicine of the National Academies.

Ascher, Robert. 1983. "New Development Approaches and the Adaptability of International Agencies: The Case of the World Bank." *International Organization* 37(3): 1–21.

Ashraf, Haroon. 2000. "WHO Assembles Leading Economists to Study Poverty Reduction and Health." *Lancet* 355(9201): 387.

——. 2001. "WHO Commission Announces Bold Plan for World's Poor." *Lancet* 358(9299): 2133.

Attaran, Amir, Karen I. Barnes, Christopher Curtis, Umberto d'Alessandro, Caterina I. Fanello, Mary R. Galinski, Gilbert Kokwaro, Sornchai Looareesuwan, Michael Makanga, Theonest K. Mutabingwa, Ambrose Talisuna, Jean François Trape, and William M. Watkins. 2004. "WHO, The Global Fund, and Medical Malpractice in Malaria Treatment." *Lancet* 363(9415): 237–240.

Attaran, Amir, and Jeffrey Sachs. 2001. "Defining and Refining International Donor Support for Combating the AIDS Epidemic." *Lancet* 357(9249): 57–61.

Avant, Deborah D., Martha Finnemore, and Susan K. Sell, eds. 2010. *Who Governs the Globe?* Cambridge, UK: Cambridge University Press.

Awuonda, Moussa. 1995. "Swedes Support UNAIDS." *Lancet* 345(8964): 1563.

Babb, Sarah. 2007. "Embeddedness, Inflation, and International Regimes: The IMF in the Early Postwar Period." *American Journal of Sociology* 113: 128–164.

——. 2009. *Behind the Development Banks.* Chicago, IL: University of Chicago Press.

Balter, Michael. 1998. "Healer Needed for World Health Body." *Science* 279(5348): 166–169.

Bandow, Doug. 1985. "Totalitarian Global Management: The UN's War on the Liberal International Economic Order." Cato Policy Analysis No. 61. Washington, DC: Cato Institute.

Banerji, Debabar. 1999. "A Fundamental Shift in the Approach to International Health by WHO, UNICEF, and the World Bank: Instances in the Practice of 'Intellectual Fascism' and Totalitarianism in Some Asian Countries." *International Journal of Health Services* 29(2): 227–259.

——. 2002. "Report of the WHO Commission on Macroeconomics and Health: A Critique." *International Journal of Health Services* 32(4): 733–754.

——. 2006. "Serious Crisis in the Practice of International Health by the World Health Organization: The Commission on Social Determinants of Health." *International Journal of Health Services* 36(4): 637–650.

Banta, David. 2002. "Economic Development Key to Healthier World." *Journal of the American Medical Association* 287(24): 3195–3197.

Barber, Tony, and Demetri Sevastopulos. 2003. "UN Backs Off from Battle with Sugar Industry over Health Tips." *Financial Times,* April 24.

Barnett, Michael N. 1997. "Bringing in the New World Order: Liberalism, Legitimacy, and the United Nations." *World Politics* 49(4): 526–551.

Barnett, Michael, and Liv Coleman. 2005. "Designing Police: Interpol and the Study of Change in International Organizations." *International Studies Quarterly* 49: 593–619.

Barnett, Michael, and Martha Finnemore. 1999. "The Politics, Power, and Pathologies of International Organizations." *International Organization* 53(4): 699–732.

——. 2004. *Rules for the World: International Organizations in Global Politics.* Ithaca, NY: Cornell University Press.

——. 2005. "The Power of Liberal International Organizations." In *Power in Global Governance,* edited by Michael Barnett and Raymond Duvall. Cambridge, UK: Cambridge University Press.

Barnum, Howard. 1994. "The Economic Burden of the Global Trade in Tobacco." *Tobacco Control* 3: 358–361.

Bates, Clive. 2001. "Developing Countries Take the Lead on WHO Convention." *Tobacco Control* 10(3): 209.

Battilana, Julie, Bernard Leca, and Eva Boxenbaum. 2009. "How Actors Change Institutions: Towards a Theory of Institutional Entrepreneurship." *Academy of Management Annals* 3(1): 377–419.

Beaglehole, Robert, and Derek Yach. 2003. "Globalization and the Prevention and Control of Non-Communicable Disease: The Neglected Chronic Diseases of Adults." *Lancet* 362(9387): 903–908.

Beer, Linda, and Terry Boswell. 2002. "The Resilience of Dependency Effects in Explaining Income Inequality in the Global Economy: A Cross-National Analysis, 1975–1995." *Journal of World-Systems Research* 8(1): 30–59.

Beigbeder, Yves, Mahyar Nashat, Marie-Antoinette Orsini, and Jean-François Tiercy. 1998. *The World Health Organization.* Leiden: Martinus Nijhoff.

Berlin, Michael. 1975. "Rich and Poor Nations Reach Accord on World Economy." *New York Post,* September 16.

Birdsall, Nancy, and Estelle James. 1993. "Health, Government, and the Poor: The Case for the Private Sector." In *Policy and Planning Implications of the Epidemiological Transition,* edited by James Gribble and Samuel Preston. Washington, DC: National Academy of Sciences.

Birmingham, Karen. 1999. "Bruntdland Makes Waves in Her First Six Months at the WHO." *Nature Medicine* 5(3): 249.

Blau, Peter M. 1964. *Exchange and Power in Social Life.* New York: Wiley.

Block, Fred. 1977. "The Ruling Class Does Not Rule: Notes toward a Marxist Theory of the State." *Socialist Revolution* 7: 6–28.

———. 1996. *The Vampire State and Other Myths and Fallacies about the U.S. Economy.* New York: New Press.

Bond, Patrick. 2003. *Against Global Apartheid: South Africa Meets the World Bank, IMF, and International Finance.* London: Zed Books.

Booth, Karen M. 1995. "Technical Difficulties: Experts, Women, and the State in Kenya's AIDS Crisis." Ph.D. diss., University of Wisconsin.

Boseley, Sarah. 1999. "Malaria Fears at Planned DDT Ban." *Guardian,* August 30.

———. 2000. "Poor Stung by Malaria's Hidden Cost." *Guardian,* April 25.

———. 2001. "WHO Says Breastfeed for Six Months" *Guardian,* April 3.

———. 2002. "Unhealthy Influence: There Is a Danger That WHO's New Partnership with Drug Companies Will Skew its Health Policies." *Guardian,* February 6.

———. 2003a. "Obesity Attack on Soft Drink Firms." *Guardian,* March 3.

———. 2003b. "Sugar Industry Threatens to Scupper WHO." *Guardian,* April 21.

Bradshaw, York W., and Jie Huang. 1991. "Intensifying Global Dependency: Foreign Debt, Structural Adjustment, and Third World Underdevelopment." *Sociological Quarterly* 32(3): 321–342.

Braveman, Paula, Barbara Starfield, and H. Jack Geiger. 2001. "World Health Report 2000: How It Removes Equity from the Agenda for Public Health Monitoring and Policy." *British Medical Journal* 323(7314): 678–680.

Broad, Robin, and Zahara Heckscher. 2003. "Before Seattle: The Historical Roots of the Current Movement against Corporate-Led Globalization." *Third World Quarterly* 24(4): 713–728.

Brody, Jane E. 2005. "As America Gets Bigger, The World Does, Too." *New York Times,* April 19.

———. 2003. "WHO Set to Announce Details of Global Effort To Fight HIV and AIDS." *Washington Post,* December 1.

Brown, Theodore M., and Marcos Cueto. 2011. "The World Health Organization and the World of Global Health." In *Handbook on Global Public Health,* edited by Richard Parker and Marni Sommer. London: Routledge.

Brown, Theodore M., Marcos Cueto, and Elizabeth Fee. 2006. "The World Health Organization and the Transition from 'International' to 'Global' Public Health." *American Journal of Public Health* 96(1): 62–72.

Brundtland, Gro Harlem. 1998. "Editorial: Reaching Out for World Health." *Science* 280(5372): 2027.

——. 1999a. "WHO—The Way Ahead. Statement by the Director-General to the Executive Board at its 103rd Session. Geneva. 25 January 1999." EB103/2. Geneva: WHO.

——. 1999b. "Looking Ahead for WHO after a Year of Change. Summary of *The World Health Report 1999*." Dr. Gro Harlem Brundtland, Director-General. 30 March 1999. Fifty-Second World Health Assembly. Provision agenda item 3. A52/4. Geneva: WHO.

——. 1999c. "Environment and Health: Europe's Partnerships Can Be a Model." *British Medical Journal* 318(7199): 1635.

——. 2000a. "Public-Private Partnership for Health. Medicines for Malaria Venture. Report by the Director-General." 6 January 2000. EB105/8 Add. 1. Geneva: WHO.

——. 2000b. "WHO's International Conference on Global Tobacco Control Law: Towards a WHO Framework Convention on Tobacco Control." New Delhi, available at http://www.who.int/director-general/speeches/2000/english/20000107_new_delhi.html.

——. 2000c. "Speech at the Opening of the Third Meeting of the Commission for Macroeconomics and Health." Third Meeting of the Commission on Macroeconomics and Health, Paris, November 8, 2000, available at http://www.who.int/director-general/speeches/2000/english/20001108_paris.html.

——. 2002. "Reducing Risks to Health, Promoting Healthy Life." *Journal of the American Medical Association* 288(16): 1974.

Bruno, Kenny. 2000. "Perilous Partnerships: The UN's Corporate Outreach Program." *Journal of Public Health Policy* 21(4): 388–393.

Bryant, John H. 1969. *Health and the Developing World*. Ithaca, NY: Cornell University Press.

——. 1980. "WHO's Program of Health for All by the Year 2000: A Macrosystem For Health Policy Making—A Challenge to Social Science Research." *Social Science and Medicine* 14A: 381–386.

Buehrig, Edward H. 1976. "The Tribulations of UNESCO." *International Organization* 30(4): 679–685.

Bundy, Harvey H. 1947. "An Introductory Note." *International Organization* 1(1): 1.

Buse, Kent. 1994. "Spotlight on International Organizations: The World Bank." *Health Policy and Planning* 9(1): 95–99.

——. 2004. "Governing Public-Private Infectious Disease Partnerships." *Brown Journal of World Affairs* 10(2): 225–242.

Buse, Kent, and Catherine Gwin. 1998. "World Health: The World Bank and Global Cooperation in Health: The Case of Bangladesh." *Lancet* 351(9103): 665–669.

Buse, Kent, and Kelley Lee. 2005. "Business and Global Health Governance." Discussion Paper No. 5. Centre on Global Change and Health: London School of Hygiene and Tropical Medicine.

Buse, Kent, and Gill Walt. 2000a. "Global Public-Private Partnerships: Part I—A New Development in Health?" *Bulletin of the WHO* 78(4): 549–561.

——. 2000b. "Global Public-Private Partnerships: Part II—What Are the Health Issues for Global Governance?" *Bulletin of the WHO* 78(5): 699–709.

Butler, Declan. 1998. "Malaria Research Deal Seeks to Make Up for Industry's Retreat." *Nature* 395: 417–418.

Cannon, Carl M. 2005. "Bush and AIDS." *National Journal* 37(26): 2063–2065.

Castells, Manuel, and Roberto Laserna. 1989. "The New Dependency: Technological Change and Socioeconomic Restructuring in Latin America." *Sociological Forum* 4(4): 535–560.

Central Intelligence Agency (CIA). August 1975. "Politicization of International Technical Organizations." Directorate of Intelligence Office of Political Research.

Cerny, Phil. 2001. "From 'Iron Triangles' to 'Golden Pantangles'? Globalizing the Policy Process." *Global Governance* 7(4): 397.

Chan, Margaret. 2008. "Return to Alma-Ata." *Lancet* 372(9642): 865–866.

Chetley, Andrew. 1988. "New Challenges for the World Health Organization." *Lancet* 331(8596): 1216.

Chorev, Nitsan. 2007. *Remaking U.S. Trade Policy: From Protectionism to Globalization.* Ithaca, NY: Cornell University Press.

Chorev, Nitsan, and Sarah Babb. 2009. "The Crisis of Neoliberalism and the Future of International Institutions: The IMF and the WTO in Comparative Perspective." *Theory and Society* 38: 459–484.

Chwieroth, Jeffrey. 2008a. "Normative Change from Within: The International Monetary Fund's Approach To Capital Account Liberalization." *International Studies Quarterly* 52: 129–158.

——. 2008b. "Organizational Change 'From Within': Exploring the World Bank's Early Lending Policies." *Review of International Political Economy* 15(4): 481–505.

Cleaver, Harry. 1977. "Malaria and the Political Economy of Public Health." *International Journal of Health Services* 7(4): 557–579.

Cline, William R. 1995. *International Debt Reexamined.* Washington, DC: Institute for International Economics.

Collin, Jeff. 2004. "Tobacco Politics." *Development* 47(2): 91–96.

Collin, Jeff, Kelley Lee, and Karen Bissell. 2003. "The Framework Convention on Tobacco Control: The Politics of Global Health Governance." In *Global Health and Governance,* edited by Nana Poku and Alan Whiteside. New York: Palgrave.

Commission on Intellectual Property Rights, Innovation, and Public Health (CIPRIPH). 2006. *Public Health, Innovation and Intellectual Property Rights.* Geneva: WHO.

Commission on Macroeconomics and Health (CMH). 2001. *Macroeconomics and Health: Investing in Health for Economic Development.* Geneva: WHO.

Commission on Social Determinant of Health (CSDH). 2008. "Closing the Gap in a Generation: Health Equity through Action on the Social Determinants of Health." Final Report of the Commission on Social Determinants of Health. Geneva: WHO.

Conti, Joseph. 2010. *Between Law and Diplomacy: Disputing at the World Trade Organization in its Social Contexts.* Palo Alto, CA: Stanford University Press.

Cox, Robert. 1969. "The Executive Head: An Essay on Leadership in the ILO." *International Organization* 23(2): 205–229.

——. 1986. *Production, Power, and World Order.* New York: Columbia University Press.

Cox, Robert, and Harold Jacobson, eds. 1973. *Anatomy of Influence: Decision Making in International Organization.* New Haven, CT: Yale University Press.

Crane, Barbara, and Jason L. Finkle. 1981. "Organizational Impediments to Development Assistance: The World Bank's Population Program." *World Politics* 33(4): 516–553.

Crossette, Barbara. 1998. "U.N. and World Bank Unite To Wage War on Malaria." *New York Times,* October 31.

Cueto, Marcos. 2004. "The Origins of Primary Health Care and Selective Primary Health Care." *American Journal of Public Health* 94: 1864–1874.

——. 2007. *Cold War, Deadly Fevers: Malaria Eradication in Mexico 1955–1975.* Baltimore, MD: Johns Hopkins University Press.

Das, Pam, and Udani Samarasekera. 2008. "What Next for UNAIDS?" *Lancet* 372(9656): 2099–2102.

de Ferranti, David. 1985. "Paying for Health Services in Developing Countries: An Overview." World Bank Staff Working Papers. Number 721.

de Kadt, Emanuel. 1985. "Of Markets, Might, and Mullahs: A Case for Equity, Pluralism, and Tolerance in Development." *World Development* 13(4): 549–556.

de Montbrial, Thierry. 1975. "For a New World Economic Order." *Foreign Affairs* 54(1): 61–78.

DeYoung, Karen. 2001. "Global AIDS Strategy May Prove Elusive." *Washington Post,* April 23.

Dicken, Peter. 1998. *Global Shift: Transforming the World Economy.* 3rd ed. New York: Guilford Press.

DiMaggio, Paul J. 1983. "State Expansion and Organizational Fields." In *Organizational Theory and Public Policy,* edited by Richard H. Hall and Robert E. Ouinn. Beverly Hills, CA: Sage.

——. 1988. "Interest and Agency in Institutional Theory." In *Institutional Patterns and Organizations: Culture and Environment,* edited by Lynne Zucker. Cambridge, UK: Ballinger.

——. 1991. "Constructing an Organizational Field as a Professional Project: U.S. Art Museums, 1920–1940." In *The New Institutionalism in Organizational Analysis,* edited by Walter W. Powell and Paul J. DiMaggio. Chicago, IL: University of Chicago Press.

DiMaggio, Paul J., and Walter W. Powell. 1983. "The Iron Cage Revisited: Institutional Isomorphism and Collective Rationality in Organizational Fields." *American Sociological Review* 48(2): 147–160.

——, eds. 1991. *The New Institutionalism in Organizational Analysis.* Chicago, IL: University of Chicago Press.

Djukanovic, V., and E. P. Mach, eds. 1975. *Alternative Approaches to Meeting Basic Health Needs of Populations in Developing Countries.* A Joint UNICEF/WHO Study. Geneva: WHO.

Doyle, Michael W. 1983. "Review: Stalemate in the North-South Debate: Strategies and the New International Economic Order." *World Politics* 35(3): 426–464.

Drahos, Peter, and John Braithwaite. 2003. *Information Feudalism.* New York: Free Press.

Drezner, Daniel. 2001. "Globalization and Policy Convergence." *International Studies Review* 3(1): 53–78.

Dutton, Jane E., and Janet M. Dukerich. 1991. "Keeping an Eye on the Mirror: Image and Identity in Organizational Adaptation." *Academy of Management Journal* 34(3): 517–554.

Economist, The. 2000. "The tobacco war goes global." 357(8192): 97–98.

Edelman, Lauren B. 1992. "Legal Ambiguity and Symbolic Structures: Organizational Mediation of Civil Rights." *American Journal of Sociology* 97(6): 1531–1576.

Einhorn, Jessica. 2001. "The World Bank's Mission Creep." *Foreign Affairs* 80(5): 22–35.

England, Roger. 2008. "The Writing Is on the Wall for UNAIDS." *British Medical Journal* 336(7652): 1072.

Enserink, Martin. 2008. "Malaria Drugs, the Coca-Cola Way." *Science* 322(5905): 1174.

Evans, Peter. 1997. "The Eclipse of the State? Reflections on Stateness in an Era of Globalization." *World Politics* 50: 62–87.

Evans, Peter, Dietrich Rueschemeyer, and Theda Skocpol, eds. 1985. *Bringing the State Back In.* New York: Cambridge University Press.

Evans, Peter, and William H. Sewell, Jr. Forthcoming. "The Neoliberal Era: Ideology, Policy, and Social Effects." In *Social Resilience in the neoliberal Era,* edited by Peter Hall and Michèle Lamout.

Evans, Tony, and Peter Wilson. 1992. "Regime Theory and the English School of International Relations: A Comparison." *Millennium: Journal of International Studies* 21(3): 329–351.

Fabricant, Stephen J., and Norbert Hirschhorn. 1987. "Deranged Distribution, Perverse Prescription, Unprotected Use: The Irrationality of Pharmaceuticals in the Developing World." *Health Policy and Planning* 2(3): 204–213.

Fairclough, Gordon. 2000. "Philip Morris and Other Cigarette Firms Tried to Foil WHO." *Wall Street Journal,* August 2.

Fairclough, Gordon, and Shelly Branch. 2001. "Tobacco Giants Prepare New Marketing Curbs Ahead of U.N. Treaty." *Wall Street Journal,* September 11.

Fazal, Anwar. 1983. "The Right Pharmaceuticals at the Right Prices: Consumer Perspectives." *World Development* 11(3): 265–269.

Ferriman, Annabel. 2000. "WHO Accused of Stifling Debate about Infant Feeding." *British Medical Journal* 320(7246): 1362.

Finnemore, Martha. 1993. "International Organizations as Teachers of Norms." *International Organization* 47(4): 565–597.

———. 1996. *National Interests in International Society.* Ithaca, NY: Cornell University Press.

Fourcade, Marion, and Sarah Babb. 2002. "The Rebirth of the Liberal Creed: Paths to Neoliberalism in Four Countries." *American Journal of Sociology* 108: 533–579.

Frenk, Julio, Jaime Sepúlveda, Octavio Gómez-Dantés, Michael J. McGuinness, and Felicia Knaul. 1997. "The Future of World Health: The New World Order and International Health." *British Medical Journal* 314(7091): 1404–1407.

Frieden, Jeffry. 2006. *Global Capitalism: Its Fall and Rise in the Twentieth Century.* New York: Norton.

Friedman, Steven, and Shauna Mottiar. 2005. "A Rewarding Engagement? The Treatment Action Campaign and the Politics of HIV/AIDS." *Politics and Society* 33(4): 511–565.

Fröbel, Folker, Jürgen Heinrichs, and Otto Kreye. 1980. *The New International Division of Labor.* Cambridge, UK: Cambridge University Press.

Gellman, Barton. 2000a. "Death Watch: The Global Response to AIDS in Africa." *Washington Post,* July 5.

———. 2000b. "An Unequal Calculus of Life and Death." *Washington Post,* December 27.

———. 2000c. "A Turning Point That Left Millions Behind." *Washington Post,* December 28.

Gereffi, Gary. 1989. "Rethinking Development Theory: Insights from East Asia and Latin America." *Sociological Forum* 4(4): 505–533.

Ghebali, Victor-Yves. 1991. "The Politicization of UN Specialized Agencies: A Preliminary Analysis." In *Peace by Pieces—United Nations Agencies and Their Roles: A Reader and Selective Bibliography,* edited by Robert N. Wells. New Jersey: Scarecrow Press.

Gibbons, Ann. 1990. "New Head for the WHO Global Program on AIDS." *Science* 248(4961): 1306–1307.

Giles, Warren, and John Thornhill. 2000. "Gloves Off In WHO Tobacco Campaign." *Financial Times,* September 22.

Gillies, Rowan, Tido von Schoen-Angerer, and Ellen 't Hoen. 2006. "Historic Opportunity for WHO to Reassert Leadership." *Lancet* 368(9545): 1405–1406.

Gilmore, Anna B., and Jeff Collin. 2002. "The World's First International Tobacco Control Treaty." *British Medical Journal* 325(7369): 846–847.

Gilson, Lucy, Denny Kalyalya, Felix Kuchler, Sally Lake, Hezron Oranga, and Marius Ouendo. 2001. "Strategies for Promoting Equity: Experience with Community Financing in Three African Countries." *Health Policy* 58(1): 37–67.

Gilson, Lucy, Steven Russell, and Kent Buse. 1995. "The Political Economy of User Fees with Targeting: Developing Equitable Health Financing Policy." *Journal of International Development* 7(3): 369–401.

Gish, Oscar. 1983. "The Relation of the New International Economic Order to Health."
    Journal of Public Health Policy 4(2): 207–221.

Glynn, Mary Ann. 2000. "When Cymbals Become Symbols: Conflict Over Organizational
    Identity within a Symphony Orchestra." *Organization Science* 11(3): 285–298.

Godlee, Fiona. 1994a. "WHO in Crisis." *British Medical Journal* 309(6966): 1424–1428.

——. 1994b. "WHO in Retreat: Is It Losing Its Influence?" *British Medical Journal*
    309(6967): 1491–1495.

——. 1995. "WHO's Special Programmes: Undermining from Above." *British Medical
    Journal* 310(6973): 178–182.

——. 1997. "WHO Reform and Global Health." *British Medical Journal* 314(7091):
    1359–1360.

——. 2000. "WHO Faces Up to Its Tobacco Links." *British Medical Journal* 321(7257):
    314–315.

Golden-Biddle, Karen, and Hayagreeva Rao. 1997. "Breaches in the Boardroom: Orga-
    nizational Identity and Conflicts of Commitment in a Nonprofit Organization."
    Organization Science 8(6): 593–611.

Goodrick, Elizabeth, and Gerald R. Salancik. 1996. "Organizational Discretion in Re-
    sponding to Institutional Practices: Hospitals and Cesarean Births." *Administra-
    tive Science Quarterly* 41(1): 1–28.

Goodstein, Jerry D. 1994. "Institutional Pressures and Strategic Responsiveness: Em-
    ployer Involvement in Work-Family Issues." *Academy of Management Journal*
    37(2): 350–382.

Goshko, John M. 1998. "UN Agencies Launch Anti-Malaria Campaign." *Washington Post*,
    October 31.

Gosovic, Branislav, and John G. Ruggie. 1976. "On the Creation of a New International
    Economic Order: Issue Linkage and the Seventh Special Session of the UN Gen-
    eral Assembly." *International Organization* 30(2): 309–345.

General Accounting Office (GAO). 1977. "US participation in the World Health Organi-
    zation Still Needs Improvement." ID-77–15. Report to the Senate Committee on
    Government Affairs. Washington, DC: GAO.

——. 1986. "United Nations. Implications of Reductions in U.S. Funding. Briefing Re-
    port to Congressional Requesters." Washington, DC: GAO.

——. 1998. "HIV/AIDS: USAID and U.N. Response to the Epidemic in the Developing
    World." Washington, DC: GAO.

Griffin, Charles C. 1989. *Strengthening Health Services in Developing Countries through
    the Private Sector*. Washington, DC: World Bank.

Gruber, Lloyd. 2000. *Ruling the World: Power Politics and the Rise of Supranational Insti-
    tutions*. Princeton, NJ: Princeton University Press.

Guardian. 1994. "Swedes Cut WHO Aid," December 24.

Gwatkin, Davidson R., Michel Guillot, and Patrick Heuveline. 1999. "The Burden of Dis-
    ease among the Global Poor." *Lancet* 354(9178): 586–589.

Haas, Ernst B. 1964. *Beyond the Nation-State: Functionalism and International Organiza-
    tion*. Palo Alto, CA: Stanford University Press.

——. 1992. "Introduction: Epistemic Communities and International Policy Coordina-
    tion." *International Organization* 46(1): 1–35.

Hafner-Burton, Emilie N., and Kiyoteru Tsutsui. 2005. "Human Rights in a Globalizing
    World: The Paradox of Empty Promises." *American Journal of Sociology* 110(5):
    1373–1411.

Hallett, Timothy. 2010. "The Myth Incarnate: Recoupling Processes, Turmoil, and Inhab-
    ited Institutions in an Urban Elementary School." *American Sociological Review*
    75(1): 52–74.

Halliday, Terence C., Susan Block-Lieb, and Bruce G. Carruthers. 2009. "Attainting the Global Standard." In *Bankrupt: Global Lawmaking and Systemic Financial Crisis.* Palo Alto, CA: Stanford University Press.

Halliday, Terence C., and Bruce G. Carruthers. 2009. *Bankrupt: Global Lawmaking and Systemic Financial Crisis.* Palo Alto, CA: Stanford University Press.

Hardon, Anita. 1992. "Consumers versus Producers: Power Play behind the Scenes." In *Drugs Policy in Developing Countries,* edited by Najmi Kanji, Anita Hardon, Jan Willen Harnmeijer, Masuma Mamdani, and Gill Walt. London: Zed Books.

———. 2005. "Confronting the HIV/AIDS Epidemic in Sub-Saharan Africa: Policy versus Practice." Paris: UNESCO.

Hardon, Anita, and Stuart Blume. 2005. "Shifts in Global Immunization Goals (1984–2004): Unfinished Agendas and Mixed Results." *Social Science and Medicine* 60: 345–356.

Harris, Lloyd C., and Emmanuel Ogbonna. 1999. "The Strategic Legacy of Company Founders." *Long Range Planning* 32(3): 333–343.

Hart, Jeffrey A. 1983. *The New International Economic Order: Conflict and Cooperation in North-South Economic Relations, 1974–77.* New York: St. Martin's Press.

Harvey, David. 2005. *A Brief History of Neoliberalism.* New York: Oxford University Press.

Hawkins, Darren G., and Wade Jacoby. 2006. "How Agents Matter." In *Delegation and Agency in International Organizations,* edited by Darren G. Hawkins, David A. Lake, Daniel L. Nielson, and Michael J. Tierney. New York: Cambridge University Press.

Hawkins, Darren G., David A. Lake, Daniel L. Nielson, and Michael J. Tierney, eds. 2006. *Delegation and Agency in International Organizations.* New York: Cambridge University Press.

Hegland, Corine, and Courtney O. Walker. 2007. "UNAIDS Chief: 'There Is Progress.'" *National Journal* 39(15): 44–46.

Helleiner, Gerald K. 1976. *A World Divided: The Less Developed Countries in the International Economy.* Cambridge, UK: Cambridge University Press.

Helms, Robert. 2000. "Sick List: Health Care a la Karl Marx." *Wall Street Journal,* June 29.

Hewson, Martin, and Timothy J. Sinclair, eds. 1999. *Approaches to Global Governance Theory.* New York: State University of New York Press.

Hirschman, Albert O. 1970. *Exit, Voice, and Loyalty: Responses to Decline in Firms, Organizations, and States.* Cambridge, MA: Harvard University Press.

Holm, Petter. 1995. "The Dynamics of Institutionalization: Transformation Processes in Norwegian Fisheries." *Administrative Science Quarterly* 40(3): 398–422.

Hornblower, Margot, and Philip J. Hilts. 1981. "House Condemns Administration Opposition to Baby Formula Code." *Washington Post,* June 17.

Horton, Richard. 2002. "WHO: The Casualties and Compromises of Renewal." *Lancet* 359(9317): 1605–1611.

Hurd, Ian. 2007. *After Anarchy: Legitimacy and Power in the United Nations Security Council.* Princeton, NJ: Princeton University Press.

Imber, Mark F. 1989. *The USA, ILO, UNESCO AND IAEA: Politicization and Withdrawal in the Specialized Agencies.* London: Macmillan.

Italian Global Health Watch. 2008. "From Alma Ata to the Global Fund: The History of International Health Policy." *Social Medicine* 3(1): 36–48.

Jack, Andrew. 2006. "Gates Learns That Even in Charity There Can Be Controversy." *Financial Times,* June 13.

Jacobson, Harold K. 1984. "U.S. Withdrawal from UNESCO: Incident, Warning, or Prelude?" *PS* 17(3): 581–585.

Jankowitsch, Odette, and Karl P. Sauvant. 1981. "The Initiating Role of the Non-Aligned Countries." In *Changing Priorities on the International Agenda: The New International Economic Order,* edited by Karl. P. Sauvant. Oxford: Pergamon.

Jayasuriya, Dayanath, Adrian Griffiths, and Raymond Rigoni. 1984. *Judgement Reserved: Breast-Feeding, Bottle-Feeding, and the International Code.* Sri Lanka: Asian Pathfinder Publishers.

Jepperson, Ron. 1991. "Institutions, Institutional Effects, and Institutionalism." In *The New Institutionalism in Organizational Analysis,* edited by W. W. Powell and Paul DiMaggio. Chicago, IL: University of Chicago Press.

Jessop, Bob. 1997. "Capitalism and Its Future: Remarks on Regulation, Government, and Governance." *Review of International Political Economy* 4(3): 561–581.

Jha, Prabhat, and Frank J. Chaloupka. 1999. *Curbing the Epidemic: Governments and the Economics of Tobacco Control.* Washington, DC: World Bank.

Johnson, Victoria. 2008. *Backstage at the Revolution: How the Royal Paris Opera Survived the End of the Old Regime.* Chicago, IL: University of Chicago Press.

Jolly, Richard. 1991. "Adjustment with a Human Face: A UNICEF Record and Perspective on the 1980s." *World Development* 19(12): 1807–1821.

Jonsson, Christer. 1986. "Interorganizational Theory and International Organizations." *International Studies Quarterly* 30(1): 39–57.

Kapp, Clare. 2003. "Brundtland Meets Food and Drink Leaders but Declines Coke Cocktail." *Lancet* 361(9370): 1707.

Katz, Alison. 2004. "The Sachs Report: *Investing in Health for Economic Development*—Or Increasing the Size of the Crumbs from the Rich Man's Table? Part I." *International Journal of Health Services* 34(4): 751–773.

———. 2005. "The Sachs Report: *Investing in Health for Economic Development*—or Increasing the Size of the Crumbs from the Rich Man's Table? Part II." *International Journal of Health Services* 35(1): 171–188.

Kazatchkine, Michel. 2008. Blog-interview at The Herald Tribune, March 12, available at http://blogs.iht.com/tribtalk/business/globalization/?p = 672.

Kehaulani Goo, Sara. 2006. "Bill Gates, Version 2.0: Full-Time Philanthropist." *Washington Post,* June 16.

Kentor, Jeffrey, and Terry Boswell. 2003. "Foreign Capital Dependence and Development: A New Direction." *American Sociological Review* 68: 301–313.

Keohane, Robert. 1984. *After Hegemony: Cooperation and Discord in the World Political Economy.* Princeton, NJ: Princeton University Press.

Keohane, Robert, and Lisa L. Martin. 1995. "The Promise of Institutionalist Theory." *International Security* 20(1): 39–51.

Keohane, Robert O., and Joseph S. Nye, Jr. 1985. "Two Cheers for Multilateralism." *Foreign Policy* 60: 148–167.

Kickbusch, Ilona. 2000. "The Development of International Health Policies—Accountability Intact?" *Social Sciences and Medicine* 51: 979–989.

———. 2002. "Influence and Opportunity: Reflections on the US Role In Global Public Health." *Health Affairs* 21(6): 131–141.

Kickbusch, Ilona, and Kent Buse. 2001. "Global Influences and Global Responses: International Health at the Turn of the Twenty-First Century." In *International Public Health: Diseases, Programs, Systems, and Policies,* edited by M. H. Merson, R. E. Black, and A. J. Mills. Gathersburg, MD: Aspen.

Kiewiet, D. Roderick, and Mathew D. McCubbins. 1991. *The Logic of Delegation.* Chicago, IL: University of Chicago Press.

Kim, Soo Yeon, and Bruce Russett. 1996. "The New Politics of Voting Alignments in the United Nations General Assembly." *International Organization* 50(4): 629–652.

Kirkpatrick, Jeane J. 1993. "Defining a Conservative Foreign Policy." The Heritage Lectures. Washington, DC: The Heritage Foundation.

Klug, Heinz. 2008. "Law, Politics, and Access to Essential Medicines in Developing Countries." *Politics and Society* 36(2): 207–245.

Koremenos, Barbara, Charles Lipson, and Duncan Snidal, eds. 2001. *The Rational Design of International Institutions.* New York: Cambridge University Press.

Krasner, Stephen D. 1985. *Structural Conflict: The Third World Against Global Liberalism.* Berkeley, CA: University of California Press.

——. 1987. "The United States and the Third World: Institutional Conflicts and Particular Agreements." In *America's Changing Role in the World-System,* edited by Terry Boswell and Albert Bergesen. Westport, CT: Praeger.

Kratochwil, Friedrich, and John G. Ruggie. 1986. "International Organization: A State of the Art on the Art of the State." *International Organization* 40(4): 753–775.

Krücken, Georg, and Gili S. Drori, eds. 2009. *World Society: The Writings of John W. Meyer.* New York: Oxford University Press.

Laing, Richard, Brenda Waning, Andy Gray, Nathan Ford, and Ellen 't Hoen. 2003. "25 Years of the WHO Essential Medicines Lists: Progress and Challenges." *Lancet* 361(9370): 1723–1729.

Lall, Sanjaya. 1978. *The Growth of the Pharmaceutical Industry in Developing Countries: Problems and Prospects.* Study prepared by Lall in cooperation with the UNIDO Secretariat. ID/204. Vienna: UNIDO.

Lancaster, Tim, Lindsay Stead, Chris Silagy, and Amanda Sowden. 2000. "Effectiveness of Interventions to Help People Stop Smoking: Findings from the *Cochrane Library.*" *British Medical Journal* 321(7257): 355–358.

Lancet. 1993. "Editorial: World Bank's Cure for Donor Fatigue." *Lancet* 342(8863): 63–64.

——. 1997. "Editorial: WHO: Where There Is No Vision, The People Perish." *Lancet* 350(9080): 749.

——. 2000. "Editorial: A Manipulated Dichotomy in Global Health Policy." *Lancet* 355(9219): 1923.

——. 2002a. "Editorial: The Globalization of the NHS." *Lancet* 359(9316): 1447–1448.

——. 2002b. "Editorial: The Future of the World Health Organization." *Lancet* 360(9348): 1798.

——. 2003. "Editorial: WHO 2003–08: A Programme of Quiet Thunder Takes Shape." *Lancet* 362(9379): 179.

——. 2006. "13 candidates compete to be next WHO Director-General." *Lancet* 368(9540): 977–980.

——. 2008. "Editorial: Addressing the inequities in health: a new and vital mandate." *Lancet* 372(9640): 689.

Langley, Alison. 2003. "Anti-Tobacco Pact Gains despite Firms' Lobbying." *New York Times,* May 20.

Lavelle, Kathryn C. 2011. "Multilateral Cooperation and Congress: The Legislative Process of Securing Funding for the World Bank." *International Studies Quarterly* 55(1): 199–222.

Lee, Jong-wook, and Peter Piot. 2003. "Turning the Tide." *Washington Post,* September 22.

Lee, Kelley. 2009. *The World Health Organization (WHO).* London: Routledge.

Lee, Kelly, Sue Collinson, Gill Walt, and Lucy Gilson. 1996. "Who Should be Doing What in International Health: A Confusion of Mandates in the United Nations?" *British Medical Journal* 312(7026): 302–307.

Lee, Kelley, and Richard Dodgson. 2000. "Globalization and Cholera: Implications for Global Governance." *Global Governance* 6(2): 213–236.

Lee, Kelley, and Gill Walt. 1992. "What Role for WHO in the 1990s?" *Health Policy and Planning* 7: 387–390.

Lerer, Leonard, and Richard Matzopoulos. 2001. "'The Worst of Both Worlds': The Management Reform of the World Health Organization." *International Journal of Health Services* 31(2): 415–438.

Litsios, Socrates. 1997. "Malaria Control, the Cold War, and the Postwar Reorganization of International Assistance." *Medical Anthropology* 17(3): 255–278.

——. 2002. "The Long and Difficult Road to Alma-Ata: A Personal Reflection." *International Journal of Health Services* 32(4): 709–732.

——. 2004. "The Christian Medical Commission and the Development of the World Health Organization's Primary Health Care Approach." *American Journal of Public Health* 94(11): 1884–1893.

Livingston, Steven G. 1992. "The Politics of International Agenda-Setting: Reagan and North-South Relations." *International Studies Quarterly* 36(3): 313–329.

Magarinos, Carlos A., George Asaf, Sanjaya Lall, John D.-Martinussen, Rubens Ricupero, and Francosco Sercovich. 2001. *Reforming the UN System: UNIDO's Need-Driven Model.* The Hague: Kluwer Law International.

Magnussen, Lesly, John Ehiri, and Pauline Jolly. 2004. "Comprehensive versus Selective Primary Health Care: Lessons For Global Health Policy." *Health Affairs* 23(3): 167–176.

Mallaby, Sebastian. 2000. "The Fight for an AIDS Vaccine." *Washington Post,* January 18.

Mamdani, Masuma. 1992. "Early Initiatives in Essential Drugs Policy." In *Drugs Policy in Developing Countries,* edited by Najmi Kanji, Anita Hardon, Jan Willen Harnmeijer, Masuma Mamdani, and Gill Walt. London: Zed Books.

Mamdani, Masuma, and Godrey Walker. 1986. "Essential Drugs in the Developing World." *Health Policy and Planning* 1(3): 187–201.

Manela, Erez. 2010. "A Pox on Your Narrative: Writing Disease Control into Cold War History." *Diplomatic History* 34(2): 299–323.

Mann, Jonathan, and Kathleen Kay. 1991. "Confronting the Pandemic: the WHO's GPA 1986–9," *AIDS* 5 (Supp. 2): S221–S229.

Marmot, Michael, and Sharon Friel. 2008. "Global Health Equity: Evidence for Action on the Social Determinants of Health." *Journal of Epidemiology and Community Health* 62(12): 1095–1097.

Marton, Katherin. 1986. *Multinationals, Technology, and Industrialization: Implications and Impact in Third World Countries.* Lexington, MA: Lexington Books.

Masters, Brooke A., and Yuki Noguchi. 2006. "Corporate Titans Create a Colossal Charity." *Washington Post,* June 27.

McCarthy, Michael. 2002. "Special Report: What's Going On at the World Health Organization?" *Lancet* 360(9340): 1108–1110.

McMichael, Philip. 2000. *Development and Social Change: A Global Perspective.* 2d ed. California: Pine Forge Press.

McNeil, Donald G. Jr. 2000. "Study Says Combating Malaria Would Cost Little." *New York Times,* April 25.

——. 2008. "Revisions Sharply Cut Estimates on Malaria." *New York Times,* September 23.

Mearsheimer, John. 1994. "The False Promise of International Institutions." *International security* 19(3): 5–49.

Melanson, Richard A. 1979. "Human Rights and the American Withdrawal from the ILO." *Universal Human Rights* 1(1): 43–61.

Melrose, Dianna. 1983. "Double Deprivation: Public and Private Drug Distribution from the Perspective of the Third World Poor." *World Development* 11(3): 181–186.

Meredith, Stefanie, and Elizabeth Ziemba. 2008. "The New Landscape of Product Development Partnerships (PDPs)." *Global Forum for Health Research:* 11–15.

Meyer, John W., John Boli, George M. Thomas, and Francisco O. Ramirez. 1997. "World Society and the Nation-State." *American Journal of Sociology* 103(1): 144–181.

Meyer, John, and Brian Rowan. 1977. "Institutional Organizations: Formal Structure as Myth and Ceremony." *American Journal of Sociology* 83(2): 340–363.

Mintz, Morton. 1981a. "Infant-Formula Maker Battles Boycotters by Painting Them Red." *Washington Post,* January 4.

———. 1981b. "Baby Formula Producers Challenge UN Agencies." *Washington Post,* March 18.

Moghalu, Kingsley C. 2006. "Kofi Annan and the HIV/AIDS Pandemic: The Global Fund as a Metaphor of War." The International Conference on the Legacy of Kofi Annan. Georgetown University, Washington, DC, October 30–31.

Morgan, Kimberly, and Andrea L. Campbell. 2011. *The Delegated Welfare State: Medicare, Markets, and the Governance of American Social Policy.* New York: Oxford University Press.

Mortimer, Robert A. 1984. *The Third World Coalition in International Politics.* Boulder, CO: Westview Press.

Motchane, Jean-Loup. 2003. "Health For All or Riches for Some: WHO's Responsible?" *International Journal of Health Services* 33(2): 395–400.

Muntaner, Carles, Sanjeev Sridharan, Orielle Solar, and Joan Benach. 2009. "Commentary: Against Unjust Global Distribution of Power and Money: The Report of the WHO Commission on the Social Determinants of Health: Global Inequality and the Future of Public Health Policy." *Journal of Public Health Policy* 30: 163–175.

Muraskin, William. 1998. *The Politics of International Health: The Children's Vaccine Initiative and the Struggle to Develop Vaccines for the Third World.* New York: State University of New York Press.

———. 2004. "The Global Alliance for Vaccines and Immunization: Is It a New Model for Effective Public-Private Cooperation in International Public Health?" *American Journal of Public Health* 94(11): 1922–1926.

Murphy, Craig. 1983. "What the Third World Wants: An Interpretation of the Development and Meaning of the New International Economic Order Ideology." *International Studies Quarterly* 27(1): 55–76.

———. 1984. *Emergence of the NIEO Ideology.* Boulder, CO: Westview Press.

Murray, Christopher J. L., and Alan D. Lopez. 1996. *The Global Burden of Disease.* Cambridge, MA: Harvard University Press.

Nabarro, David, and Elizabeth Tayler. 1998. "The 'Roll Back Malaria' Campaign." *Science* 280(5372): 2067.

Naik, Gautam. 2003. "Unhealthy Habits Span the Globe." *Wall Street Journal,* March 4.

———. 2004. "WHO Misses Half-Year Target For Distributing AIDS Drugs." *Wall Street Journal,* July 12.

———. 2005. "WHO Is Likely to Miss Its AIDS-Program Goal." *Wall Street Journal,* June 30.

Nájera, José A. 1989. "Malaria and the Work of WHO." *Bulletin of WHO* 67(3): 229–243.

National Intelligence Council (NIC). 2000. "The Global Infectious Disease Threat and Its Implications for the United States." NIE 99–17D, available at http://www.fas.org/irp/threat/nie99–17d.htm.

Navarro, Vicente. 2000. "Assessment of the World Health Report 2000." *Lancet* 356(9241): 1598–1601.

——. 2001. "The New Conventional Wisdom: An Evaluation of the WHO Report *Health Systems: Improving Performance.*" *International Journal of Health Services* 31(1): 23–33.

——. 2002. "The World Health Report 2000: Can Health Care Systems Be Compared Using a Single Measure of Performance?" *American Journal of Public Health* 92(1): 31–34.

——. 2009. "What We Mean by Social Determinants of Health." *International Journal of Health Services* 39(3): 423–441.

Ness, Gayl D., and Steven R. Brechin. 1988. "Bridging the Gap: International Organizations as Organizations." *International Organization* 42(2): 245–273.

Newell, Kenneth. 1988. "Selective Primary Health Care: The Counter Revolution." *Social Science and Medicine* 26(9): 903–906.

Newton, Lisa H. 1999. "Truth Is the Daughter of Time: The Real Story of the Nestle Case." *Business and Society Review* 104(4): 367–395.

Nielson, Don, and Michael Tierney. 2003. "Delegation to International Organizations: Agency Theory and World Bank Environmental Reform." *International Organization* 57(2): 241–276.

Noor, Abdisalan M., Abdinasir A. Amin, Willis S. Akhwale, and Robert W. Snow. 2007. "Increasing Coverage and Decreasing Inequity in Insecticide-Treated Bed Net Use among Rural Kenyan Children." *PLoS Med* 4(8): e255, 1341–1348.

Okie, Susan. 1999. "TB Fights Back." *Washington Post,* August 17.

——2008. "A New Attack on Malaria." *New England Journal of Medicine* 358(23): 2425–2428.

Oliver, Christine. 1991. "Strategic Responses to Institutional Pressures." *Academy of Management Review* 16(1): 145–179.

Ollila, Eeva. 2003. "Health-Related Public-Private Partnerships and the United Nations." In *Global Social Governance: Themes and Prospects,* edited by Bob Deacon, Eeva Ollila, Meri Koivusalo, and Paul Stubbs. Helsinki: Ministry for Foreign Affairs of Finland, Department for International Development Cooperation.

Ollila, Eeva, and Meri Koivusalo. 2002. "The World Health Report 2000: World Health Organization Health Policy Steering Off Course—Changed Values, Poor Evidence, and Lack of Accountability." *International Journal of Health Services* 32(3): 503–514.

Olson, Elizabeth. 2001. "Talks, and Accusations, Resume Over a World Tobacco Treaty." *New York Times,* November 25.

Packard, Randall. 1989. *White Plague, Black Labor: Tuberculosis and the Political Economy of Health and Disease in South Africa.* Pietermaritzburg: University of Natal Press.

——. 1997. "Malaria Dreams: Postwar Visions of Health and Development in the Third World." *Medical Anthropology* 17: 279–296.

——. 2009. "'Roll Back Malaria, Roll in Development'? Reassessing the Economic Burden of Malaria." *Population and Development Review* 35(1): 53–87.

Parker, Richard. 2000. "Administrating the Epidemic: HIV/AIDS Policy, Models of Development, and International Health." In *Global Health Policy, Local Realities: The Fallacy of the Level Playing Field,* edited by Linda M. Whiteford and Lenore Manderson. Boulder, CO: Lynn Reinner Publishers.

——. 2002. "The Global HIV/AIDS Pandemic, Structural Inequalities, and the Politics of International Health." *American Journal of Public Health* 92(3): 343–346.

Patel, Surendra J. 1983. "Editor's Introduction." *World Development* 11(3): 165–167.

People's Health Movement, Medact, and Global Equity Gauge Alliance. 2008. *Global Health Watch 2: An Alternative World Health Report.* London: Zed Books.

Peretz, S. Michael. 1983. "An Industry View of Restricted Drugs Formularies." *Journal of Social and Administrative Pharmacy* 1(3): 130–133.

Pfeffer, Jeffrey, and Gerald R. Salancik. 1978. *The External Control of Organizations: A Resource Dependence Perspective.* New York: Harper and Row.

Phelps, James R. 1982. "The New International Economic Order and the Pharmaceutical Industry." *Food Drug Cosmetic Law Journal* 37: 200–211.

Pilkington, Edward. 1995. "A Samaritan Extends A Battered Hand." *Guardian,* May 19.

Piot, Peter. 2000. "Global AIDS Epidemic: Time to Turn the Tide." *Science* 288(5474): 2176–2178.

Poku, Nana K. 2002. "The Global AIDS Fund: Context and Opportunity." *Third World Quarterly* 23(2): 283–298.

Poku, Nana K., and Alan Whiteside. 2002. "Global Health and the Politics of Governance: An Introduction." *Third World Quarterly* 23(3): 191–195.

Powell, Walter W. 1988. "Institutional Effects on Organizational Structure and Performance." In *Institutional patterns and organizations: Culture and environment,* edited by Lynne G. Zucker. Cambridge, UK: Ballinger.

Prasad, Monica. 2006. *The Politics of Free Markets: The Rise of Neoliberal Economic Policies in Britain, France, Germany, and the United States.* Chicago, IL: University of Chicago Press.

Ramsa, Sarah. 2002. "Global Fund Makes Historic First Round of Payments." *Lancet* 359(9317): 1581–1582.

Raviglione, Mario C., and Antonio Pio. 2002. "Evolution of WHO Policies for Tuberculosis Control, 1948–2001." *Lancet* 359(9308): 775–780.

Reddy, K. Srinath. 1999. "Correspondence: The Burden of Disease Among The Global Poor." *Lancet* 354(9188): 1477.

Reich, Michael R. 1987. "Essential Drugs: Economics and Politics in International Health." *Health Policy* 8: 39–57.

Revzin, Philip. 1988. "Money Squeeze." *Wall Street Journal,* April 7.

Rich, Bruce. 1994. *Mortgaging the Earth: The World Bank, Environmental Impoverishment, and the Crisis of Development.* Boston: Beacon Press.

Rich, Spencer. 1981. "Rules on Infant Formula Called Unconstitutional." *Washington Post,* May 13.

Richter, Judith. 2004. "Public-Private Partnerships for Health: A Trend with No Alternatives?" *Development* 47(2): 43–48.

Robinson, William, and Jerry Harris. 2000. "Towards a Global Ruling Class? Globalization and the Transnational Capitalist Class." *Science and Society* 64(1): 11–54.

Rochester, J. Martin. 1986. "The Rise and Fall of International Organization as a Field of Study." *International Organization* 40(4): 777–813.

Roemer, Milton. 1986. "Priority for Primary Health Care: Its Development and Problems." *Health Policy and Planning* 1(1): 58–66.

Roemer, Ruth, Allyn Taylor, and Jean Lariviere. 2005. "Origins of the WHO Framework Convention on Tobacco Control." *American Journal of Public Health* 95(6): 936–938.

Rosenau, James N., and Ernet-Otto Czempiel, eds. 1992. *Governance without Government: Order and Change in World Politics.* Cambridge, UK: Cambridge University Press.

Rothstein, Robert L. 1979. *Global Bargaining: UNCTAD and the Quest for a New International Economic Order.* Princeton, NJ: Princeton University Press.

Ruger, Jennifer Prah. 2005. "Global Tobacco Control: An Integrate Approach to Global Health Policy." *Development* 48(2): 65–69.

Ruggie, John G. 1985. "The United States and the United Nations: Toward a New Realism." *International Organization* 39(2): 343–356.

Sanders, Ron. 1991. "An Assessment of UNCTAD's Effectiveness as an Instrument to Promote the Interests of the Third World." In *Peace by Pieces—United Nations Agencies and Their Roles: A Reader and Selective Bibliography,* edited by Robert N. Wells. New Jersey: Scarecrow Press.

Sassen, Saskia. 2006. *Territory, Authority, Rights: From Medieval to Global Assemblages.* Princeton, NJ: Princeton University Press.

Sauvant, Karl P. 1981. "The Origins of the NIEO Discussions." In *Changing Priorities on the International Agenda: The New International Economic Order,* edited by Karl. P. Sauvant. Oxford: Pergamon.

Schickler, Eric. 2001: *Disjointed Pluralism: Institutional Innovation and the Development of the U.S. Congress.* Princeton, NJ: Princeton University Press.

Schofer, Evan, and John W. Meyer. 2005. "The Worldwide Expansion of Higher Education in the Twentieth Century." *American Sociological Review* 70: 898–920.

Schoofs, Mark, and Michael M. Phillips. 2002. "Global Disease Fund to Be Strict For Better Chance to Get Results." *Wall Street Journal,* February 13.

Schoofs, Mark, and Michael Waldholz. 2001. "New Regimen." *Wall Street Journal,* March 7.

Schwartländer, Bernhard, Ian Grubb, and Jos Perriëns. 2006. "The 10-Year Struggle to Provide Antiretroviral Treatment to People With HIV in the Developing World." *Lancet* 368(9534): 541–546.

Schwartz, Harry. 1981. "A Drug-Code Warm Up." *Pharmaceutical Executive.*

———. 1985. "Will WHO Give Drug Firms a Fair Diagnosis?" *Wall Street Journal,* November 25.

Scott, W. Richard. 1981. *Organizations: Rational, Natural and Open Systems.* New Jersey: Prentice-Hall.

———. 2008. "Approaching Adulthood: The Maturing of Institutional Theory." *Theory and Society* 37: 427–442.

Scott, W. Richard, and John W. Meyer. 1983. "The Organization of Societal Sectors." In *Organizational Environments: Ritual and Rationality,* edited by John W. Meyer and W. Richard Scott. Beverly Hills, CA: Sage.

Scruton, Roger. 2001. *Who, What, and Why? Transnational Government, Legitimacy, and the World Health Organization.* London: Institute of Economic Affairs.

Seers, Dudley. 1977. "The New Meaning of Development." *International Development Review* 19(3): 2–7.

Segall, Malcolm. 2003. "District Health Systems in a Neoliberal World: A Review of Five Key Policy Areas." *International Journal of Health Planning and Management* 18: S5–S26.

Sell, Susan K. 2003. *Private Power, Public Law: The Globalization of Intellectual Property Rights.* Cambridge, UK: Cambridge University Press.

Sell, Susan K., and Aseem Prakash. 2004. "Using Ideas Strategically: The Contest between Business and NGO Networks in Intellectual Property Rights." *International Studies Quarterly* 48: 143–175.

Selznick, Philip. 1949. *TVA and the Grass Roots: A Study of Politics and Organization.* Berkeley, CA: University of California Press.

———. 1957. *Leadership in Administration: A Sociological Interpretation.* New York: Harper and Row.

Sethi, S. Prakash. 1994. *Multinational Corporations and the Impact of Public Advocacy on Corporate Strategy: Nestle and the Infant Formula Controversy.* Boston: Kluwer Academic.

Seytre, Bernard, and Mary Shaffer. 2005. *The Death of a Disease: A History of the Eradication of Poliomyelitis.* New Brunswick, NJ: Rutgers University Press.

Shadlen, Kenneth C. 2004. "Patents and Pills, Power and Procedure: The North-South Politics of Public Health in the WTO." *Studies in Comparative International Development* 39(3): 76–108.

Shiffman, Jeremy. 2008. "Has Donor Prioritization of HIV/AIDS Displaced Aid for Other Health Issues?" *Health Policy and Planning* 23: 95–100.

Shubber, Sami. 1998. *The International Code of Marketing of Breast-milk Substitutes: An International Measure to Protect and Promote Breast-feeding.* The Hague: Kluwer Law International.

Siddiqi, Javed. 1995. *World Health and World Politics: The World Health Organization and the UN System.* Columbus, SC: University of South Carolina Press.

Sikkink, Kathryn. 1986. "Codes of Conduct for Transnational Corporations: The Case of the WHO/UNICEF Code." *International Organization* 40(4): 815–840.

Silverman, Milton. 1976. *The Drugging of the Americas.* Berkeley, CA: University of California Press.

Simmons, Beth A., Frank Dobbin, and Geoffrey Garrett. 2006. "The Diffusion of Liberalism." *International Organization* 60: 781–810.

Simms, Chris. 2007. "The World Bank and Sub-Saharan Africa's HIV/AIDS crisis." *Canadian Medical Association Journal* 176(12): 1728–1730.

Sklair, Leslie. 2000. *The Transnational Capitalist Class.* Oxford: Wiley-Blackwell.

Skocpol, Theda. 1992. *Protecting Soldiers and Mothers: The Political Origins of Social Policy in the United States.* Cambridge, MA: Harvard University Press.

Slutkin, Gary. 2000. "Global AIDS 1981–1999: The Response." *International Journal of Tuberculosis and Lung Disease* 4(2 Supp. 1): S24–S33.

Smith, Duane, and John H. Bryant. 1988. "Building the Infrastructure for Primary Health Care: An Overview of Vertical and Integrated Approaches." *Social Science Medicine* 26(9): 909–917.

Somers, Margaret R. 2008. *Genealogies of Citizenship: Markets, Statelessness, and the Right to Have Rights.* Cambridge, UK: Cambridge University Press.

Specter, Michael. 2005. "What Money Can Buy: Million of Africans Die Needlessly of Disease Each Year. Can Bill Gates Change That?" *New Yorker,* October 24, 56–71.

Standing, Guy. 2008. "The ILO: An Agency for Globalization?" *Development and Change* 39(3): 355–384.

Starrels, John M. 1985. *The World Health Organization: Resisting Third World Ideological Pressures.* Washington, DC: Heritage Foundation.

Stein, Rob, and Marc Kaufman. 2003. "U.S. Backs Pact Curbing Tobacco Use Worldwide." *Washington Post,* May 19.

Steinmo, Sven, Kathleen Thelen, and Frank Longstreth, eds. 1992. *Structuring Politics: Historical Institutionalism in Comparative Analysis.* Cambridge, UK: Cambridge University Press.

Stenson, Bo, and Goran Sterky. 1994. "What Future WHO?" *Health Policy* 28: 235–256.

Strange, Susan. 1996. *The Retreat of the State: The Diffusion of Power in the World Economy.* Cambridge, UK: Cambridge University Press.

Streeck, Wolfgang, and Kathleen A. Thelen. 2005. "Introduction: Institutional Change in Advanced Political Economies." In *Beyond Continuity: Institutional Change in Advanced Political Economies,* edited by Wolfgang Streeck and Kathleen A. Thelen. New York: Oxford University Press.

Suchman, Mark. 1995. "Managing Legitimacy: Strategic and Institutional Approaches." *Academy of Management Review* 20(3): 571–610.

Tarantola, Daniel, Sofia Gruskin, Theodore Brown, and Elizabeth Fee. 2006. "Jonathan Mann Founder of the Health and Human Rights Movement." *American Journal of Public Health* 96(11): 1942–1943.

Taylor, Allyn L., and Douglas W. Bettcher. 2000. "WHO Framework Convention on To-
    bacco Control: A Global 'Good' For Public Health." *Bulletin of WHO* 78(7): 920–929.
Taylor, Carl E., ed. 1976. *Doctors for the Villages: Study of Rural Internships in Seven In-
    dian Medical Colleges.* New York: Asia Publishing House.
Tejada de Rivero, David A. 2003. "Alma-Ata Revisited." *Perspective in Health Magazine:
    The Magazine of the Pan American Health Organization* 8: 1–6.
Thomas, Caroline, and Martin Weber. 2004. "The Politics of Global Health Governance:
    Whatever Happened to 'Health for All by the year 2000'?" *Global Governance* 10:
    187–205.
Thompson, James D. 1967. *Organizations in Action.* New York: McGraw-Hill.
Thornton, Patricia H., and William Ocasio. 1999. "Institutional Logics and the Histori-
    cal Contingency of Power in Organizations: Executive Succession in the Higher
    Education Publishing Industry, 1958–1990." *American Journal of Sociology* 105(3):
    801–843.
Tickner, J. Ann. 1990. "Reaganomics and the Third World: Lessons from the Founding
    Fathers." *Polity* 23(1): 53–76.
Timberg, Craig. 2006. "In Africa, The Gateses Define Limit Of Giving." *Washington Post,*
    July 23.
Torfason, Magnus, and Paul Ingram. 2010. "The Rise of Global Democracy: A Network
    Account." *American Sociological Review* 75(3): 355–377.
Tucker, Tim J., and Malogapuru W. Makgoba. 2008. "Public Health: Public-Private Part-
    nerships and Scientific Imperialism." *Science* 320(5879): 1016–1017.
Türmen, Tomris, and Charles Clift. 2006. "Public Health, Innovation and Intellectual
    Property Rights: Unfinished Business." *Bulletin of the World Health Organization*
    84(5): 338.
Ugalde, Antonio, and Jeffrey T. Jackson. 1995. "The World Bank and International
    Health Policy: A Critical Review." *Journal of International Development* 7(3):
    525–542.
ul Haq, Mahbub. 1976. *The Poverty Curtain: Choices for the Third World.* New York: Co-
    lumbia University Press.
United Nations Chronicle. 1994. "Acting Now to Make a Difference." Interview with Mi-
    chael Merson.
United Nations Conference on Trade and Development (UNCTAD). 1979 "Transna-
    tional Corporations and the Pharmaceutical Industry." ST/CTC/9. New York:
    UNCTAD.
United Nations Development Programme (UNDP). 1990. *Human Development Report.*
    New York: Oxford University Press.
United Nations Programme on HIV/AIDS (UNAIDS). 2008. *UNAIDS: The First Ten
    Years, 1996–2006.* Geneva: UNAIDS.
———. 2010. Report on the Global AIDS Epidemic. Geneva: UNAIDS.
Unger, J. P., and J. Killingsworth. 1986. "Selective Primary Health Care: A Critical View of
    Methods and Results." *Social Science and Medicine* 20: 1001–1013.
Utting, Peter. 2000. "UN-Business Partnerships: Whose Agenda Counts?" Paper pre-
    sented at seminar on Partnerships for Development or Privatization of the Multi-
    lateral System? organized by the North-South Coalition. Oslo, Norway.
Utting, Peter, and Ann Zammit. 2006. "Beyond Pragmatism: Appraising UN-Business
    Partnerships." Markets, Business, and Regulation Programme. Paper
    No. 1. United Nations Research Institute for Social Development.
van der Pijl, Kees 1998. *Transnational Classes and International Relations.* London: Rout-
    ledge.

Vaughan, Patrick J., Sigrun Mogedal, Stein-Erik Kruse, Kelley Lee, Gill Walt, and Koen de Wilde. 1996. "Financing the World Health Organization: Global Importance of Extrabudgetary Funds." *Health Policy* 35: 229–245.

Vedantam, Shankar. 2001. "Big Tobacco Accused of Destroying Evidence." *Washington Post*, December 7.

Velásquez, German, Carlos M. Correa, and Thurkumaran Balaubramanlam. 2004. "WHO in the Frontlines of the Access to Medicines Battle: The Debate on Intellectual Property Rights and Public Health." In *Intellectual Property in the Context of the WTO TRIPS Agreement: Challenges for Public Health*, edited by Jorge A. Z. Bermudez and Maria A. Oliveira. Rio de Janeiro: Escola Nacional de Saúde Pública, Fundação Oswaldo Cruz.

Voeten, Erik. 2000. "Clashes in the Assembly." *International Organization* 54(2): 185–215.

Waitzkin, Howard. 2003. "Report of the WHO Commission on Macroeconomics and Health: A Summary and Critique." *Lancet* 361(9356): 523–526.

Walgate, Robert. 1997. "WHO Leader to Step Down." *British Medical Journal* 314(7091): 1365.

Walsh, Julia A., and Kenneth S. Warren. 1979. "Selective Primary Health are: An Interim Strategy for Disease Control in Developing Countries." *New England Journal of Medicine* 301: 967–974.

Walt, Gill, and Kent Buse. 2000. "Editorial: Partnership and Fragmentation in International Health: Threat or Opportunity?" *Tropical Medicine and International Health* 5(7): 467–471.

Walt, Gill, and Jan Willem Harnmeijer. 1992. "Formulating an Essential Drugs Policy: WHO's Role." In *Drugs Policy in Developing Countries*, edited by Najmi Kanji, Anita Hardon, Jan Willen Harnmeijer, Masuma Mamdani, and Gill Walt. London: Zed Books.

Warren, Kenneth S. 1988. "The Evolution of Selective Primary Health Care." *Social Science and Medicine* 26(9): 891–898.

Waxman, Henry A. 2002. "The Future of the Global Tobacco Treaty Negotiations." *New England Journal of Medicine* 346(12): 936–939.

Weaver, Catherine. 2008. *Hypocrisy Trap: The World Bank and the Poverty of Reform*. Princeton, NJ: Princeton University Press.

Weaver, Catherine, and Ralf J. Leiteritz. 2005. "'Our Poverty Is a World Full of Dreams': Reforming the World Bank." *Global Governance* 11(3): 369–388.

Wells, Robert N. 1991. "Introduction: the UN's Specialized Agencies: Adaptation and Role Changes in an Altered International Environment." In *Peace by Pieces— United Nations Agencies and Their Roles: A Reader and Selective Bibliography*, edited by Robert N. Wells. New Jersey: Scarecrow Press.

Wheeler, Craig, and Seth Berkley. 2001. "Initial Lessons from Public-Private Partnerships in Drug and Vaccine Development." *Bulletin of WHO* 79(8): 728–734.

Williams, Alan. 2001. "Science or Marketing at WHO? A Commentary on 'World Health 2000.' *Health Economics* 10: 93–100.

Williams, Douglas. 1987. *The Specialized Agencies for the United Nations: The System in Crisis*. London: Hurst.

Williams, Frances. 1999a. "WHO Wants Tobacco to Be Regulated Like Other Drugs." *Financial Times*, April 28.

——. 1999b. "US Called to Act Over Tobacco." *Financial Times*, October 30.

——. 2003. "Food Executives Meet WHO Chief." *Financial Times*, May 10.

——. 2004. "Global Anti-Obesity Agreement Near." *Financial Times*, May 22.

Williamson, John. 1990. "What Washington Means by Policy Reform." In *Latin American Adjustment: How Much Has Happened?* edited by John Williamson. Washington, DC: Institute for International Economics.

Wittet, Scott. 2000. "Introducing GAVI and the Global Fund for Children's Vaccines." *Vaccine* 19(4–5): 385–386.

World Bank. 1992. "AIDS Assessment and Planning Study. Tanzania. A World Bank Country Study." Report No. 11540. Washington, DC: IBRD.

——. 1993. *World Development Report: Investing in Health.* 1993. Washington, DC: IBRD.

——. 1997. *Confronting AIDS: Public Priorities in a Global Epidemic.* New York: Oxford University Press.

——. 1999. "Intensifying Action against HIV/AIDS in Africa: Responding to a Development Crisis." Washington, DC: World Bank.

——. 2005. *Committing to Results: Improving the Effectiveness of HIV/AIDS Assistance: An OED Evaluation of the World Bank's Assistance for HIV/AIDS Control.* Washington, DC: World Bank.

World Health Organization (WHO). 1958. *The First Ten Years of the World Health Organization.* Geneva: WHO.

——. 1968. *The Second Ten Years of the World Health Organization: 1958–1967.* Geneva: WHO.

——. 1973. *Organizational Study on Methods of Promoting the Development of Basic Health Services. Official Records of the World Health Organization,* No. 206, Annex 11. Geneva: WHO.

——. 1975. *Health by the People.* Geneva: WHO.

——. 1978. "Declaration of Alma-Ata: International Conference on Primary Health Care, Alma-Ata, USSR, 6–12 September 1978." Geneva: WHO.

——. 1980a. "Technical Discussions on the Contribution of Health to The New International Economic Order." A33/Technical Discussions/1. Geneva: WHO.

——. 1980b. "Report of the Technical Discussions at the Thirty-Third World Health Assembly. The Contribution of Health to the New International Economic Order." A33/Technical Discussions/5. Geneva: WHO.

——. 1993a. "Report of the Executive Board Working Group on the WHO Response to Global Change." EB92/4. Geneva: WHO.

——. 1993b. "Evaluation of Recent Changes in the Financing of Health Services." WHO Technical Report Series 829. Geneva: WHO.

——. 1997. *Globalization and Access to Drugs: Implications of the WTO/TRIPS Agreement.* Geneva: WHO.

——. 1999a. "Public-private partnerships for health. Report by the Director-General." Provisional agenda item 2. 105th Session 14 December 1999. Executive Board EB105/8. Geneva: WHO.

——. 1999b. *Globalization and Access to Drugs: Implications of the WTO/TRIPS Agreement.* 2d ed. Geneva: WHO.

——. 2000a. *World Health Report 2000. Health Systems: Improving Performance.* Geneva: WHO.

——. 2000b. "The African Summit on Roll Back Malaria." Abuja, April 25, 2000. WHO/CDS/RBM/2000.17, available at whqlibdoc.who.int/hq/2000/WHO_CDS_RBM_2000.17.pdf.

——. 2001. "Public-Private Interactions for Health: WHO's Involvement. Note by the Director-General." Provisional agenda item 3.2. 109th Session. 5 December 2001. Executive Board EB109/4. Geneva: WHO.

——. 2002. *World Health Report 2002. Reducing Risk, Promoting Healthy Life.* Geneva: WHO.

——. 2003. "Giving Tuberculosis a Human Face; Global Advocacy Report 2003." WHO/CDS/TB/2003.321 Geneva: WHO.

——. 2005a. *World Health Report 2005. Make Every Mother and Child Count.* Geneva: WHO.

——. 2005b. "The Practice of Charging User Fees at The Point of Service Delivery for HIV/AIDS Treatment and Care." WHO Discussion Paper. WHO/HIV/2005.11. Geneva: WHO.

——. 2006. *World Health Report 2006. Working Together for Health.* Geneva: WHO.

——. 2008. *The Third Ten Years of the World Health Organization: 1968–1977.* Geneva: WHO.

——. 2009. "Financial Report and Audited Financial Statements for the Period 1 January 2008–31 December 2009." Document A63/32. Geneva: WHO.

World Health Organization / Food and Agriculture Organization (WHO/FAO). 2003. "Diet, Nutrition, and the Prevention of Chronic Diseases: Report of a joint WHO/FAO Expert Consultation." Geneva: WHO.

World Trade Organization (WTO). 2001. *Declaration on the TRIPS Agreement and Public Health.* Ministerial Conference. Fourth Session. Doha. WT/MIN(01)/DEC/W/2.

Yamey, Gavin. 2002a. "Global Vaccine Initiative Creates Inequity, Analysis Concludes." *British Medical Journal* 322(7289): 754.

——. 2002b. "WHO in 2002: Have the Latest Reforms Reversed WHO's Decline?" *British Medical Journal* 325(7372): 1007–1112.

——. 2002c. "WHO in 2002: Faltering Steps towards Partnership." *British Medical Journal* 325(7374): 1236–1240.

——. 2002d. "WHO in 2002: Why Does the World Still Need WHO?" *British Medical Journal* 325(7375): 1294.

——. 2002e. "WHO in 2002: Interview with Gro Brundtland." *British Medical Journal* 325(7376): 1355–1358.

Zeltner, Thomas, David Kessler, Anke Martiny, and Fazel Randera. 2000. "Tobacco Company Strategies to Undermine Tobacco Control Activities at the World Health Organization." Committee of Experts on Tobacco Industry Documents. World Health Organization. Geneva: WHO.

Ziemba, Elizabeth. 2005. "Public-Private Partnerships for Product Development: Financial, Scientific and Managerial Issues as Challenges to Future Success." Research Report for the WHO Commission on Intellectual Property Rights, Innovation and Public Health, available at http://www.who.int/intellectualproperty/studies/Ziemba.pdf.

Zimmerman, Rachel. 2002. "WHO Characterizes AIDS Drugs as Essential." *Wall Street Journal,* April 23.

Index

Note: Page numbers followed by *f* or *t* indicate figures or tables.